CURRENT CONCEPTS IN KIDNEY TRANSPLANTATION

Edited by **Sandip Kapur**

Current Concepts in Kidney Transplantation
http://dx.doi.org/10.5772/3048
Edited by Sandip Kapur

Contributors

Cheguevara Afaneh, Choli Hartono, Leila Kamal, David Serur, Dhaval Patel, Jun Lee, Meredith J. Aull, Anthony Watkins, Sandip Kapur, Jim Kim, John R. Lee, Thangamani Muthukumar, Dinesh Kannabhiran, Michelle L. Lubetzky, Darshana Dadhania, Sarah A. Hosgood, James P. Hunter, Michael L. Nicholson, Mithat Tabaković, Nermin N. Salkić, Fahir Baraković, Senaid Trnačević, Taqi Toufeeq Khan, Mirza Anzar Baig, Joseph J. Del Pizzo, Wui-Chiang Lee, Shu-Yun Tsao, Che-Chuan Loong

Published by InTech

Janeza Trdine 9, 51000 Rijeka, Croatia

Copyright © 2012 InTech

Notice

Publishing Process Manager Romina Skomersic
Technical Editor InTech Prepress, Novi Sad
Cover InTech Design team

Additional hard copies can be obtained from orders@intechopen.com

Current Concepts in Kidney Transplantation, Edited by Sandip Kapur
p. cm.
ISBN 978-953-51-0900-6

For EU product safety concerns:
IN TECH d.o.o., Prolaz Marije Krucifikse Kozulić 3, 51000 Rijeka, Croatia,
info@intechopen.com or visit our website at intechopen.com.

Meet the editor

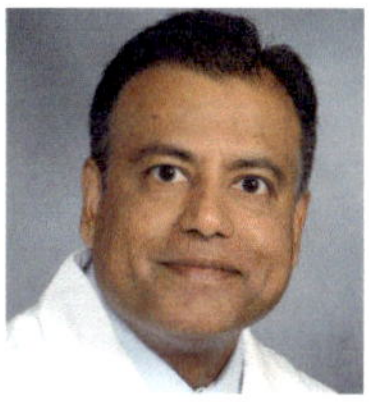

Dr. Sandip Kapur is Chief of Transplantation and Director of the Kidney and Pancreas Transplant Programs at NewYork-Presbyterian Hospital/Weill Cornell Medical Center. Dr. Kapur is an internationally recognized pioneer in advancing innovative strategies that allow more recipients to receive successful transplants, including high risk kidney transplantation and expanding opportunities for living donor kidney transplantation. Dr. Kapur led Cornell in performing one of the first living donor kidney transplant chains, a novel concept that is revolutionizing transplantation and dramatically improves the opportunity for kidney transplant candidates to find a compatible living donor. Dr. Kapur's areas of research include translating molecular monitoring techniques from bench to bedside and clinical trials on immunosuppression, ischemia-reperfusion injury, and immunosuppression minimization strategies.

Dr. Afaneh earned his medical degree from The Chicago Medical School in 2007. He is a resident in General Surgery at New York-Presbyterian Hospital/Weill Cornell Medical College. In 2009, he pursued a two-year research fellowship in the Department of Transplantation Medicine, where his worked focused on renal allograft recipients and urinary cell gene expression patterns, predicting and prognosticating outcomes. He has won several awards including the Genzyme's Clinical Science Award, TTS/Astellas Young Investigator Award, and the ERA-EDTA: Best Abstract by a Young Investigator Award. He is finishing his General Surgery residency in 2014.

Dr. Aull received her bachelor's degree in pharmacy and Doctor of Pharmacy degree from Saint John's University College of Pharmacy and Allied Health Professions and completed a Specialty Residency in Transplantation and Clinical Research at the University of Cincinnati. At Weill Cornell Medical College, Dr. Aull serves as the Director of Clinical Research and Quality for the Kidney & Pancreas Transplant Program, coordinating all aspects of transplant-related investigator-initiated and industry-sponsored research for the Division of Transplant Surgery. Her research interests include steroid-sparing immunosuppression regimens and hepatitis C virus infection in kidney transplant recipients. Dr. Aull is an author on numerous transplant publications, and has presented her research at local, national, and international transplant conferences.

Contents

Preface XI

Section 1 Evaluation and Management of the Kidney Transplant Patient 1

Chapter 1 **Evaluation of Kidney Transplant Candidates: An Update in 2012 3**
Cheguevara Afaneh and Choli Hartono

Chapter 2 **Evaluation of Potential Living Kidney Donors 29**
Leila Kamal and David Serur

Chapter 3 **Medical Management of the Kidney Transplant Recipient 55**
Dhaval Patel and Jun Lee

Chapter 4 **Surgical Management of the Kidney Transplant Recipient 79**
Cheguevara Afaneh, Meredith J. Aull, Anthony Watkins, Sandip Kapur and Jim Kim

Section 2 Immunologic Considerations in Kidney Transplantation 97

Chapter 5 **Immunologic Concepts in Kidney Transplantation 99**
John R. Lee and Thangamani Muthukumar

Chapter 6 **Transplanting Against Histocompatibility Barriers 117**
Dinesh Kannabhiran, Michelle L. Lubetzky and Darshana Dadhania

Chapter 7 **Modern Immunosuppression Regimens in Kidney Transplantation 145**
Cheguevara Afaneh, Meredith J. Aull and Sandip Kapur

Chapter 8 **Complications of Kidney Transplantation: Effects of Over-Immunosuppression 169**
Meredith J. Aull, Cheguevara Afaneh and Sandip Kapur

Chapter 9 **BK Virus Infection in Renal Allograft Recipients 199**
Darshana Dadhania

Section 3 Selected Topics in Kidney Transplantation 215

Chapter 10 **Cold Ischaemic Injury in Kidney Transplantation 217**
Sarah A. Hosgood, James P. Hunter and Michael L. Nicholson

Chapter 11 **Hypertension After Renal Transplantation 243**
Mithat Tabaković, Nermin N. Salkić,
Fahir Baraković and Senaid Trnačević

Chapter 12 **Transplant Renal Artery Stenosis 259**
Taqi Toufeeq Khan and Mirza Anzar Baig

Chapter 13 **Surgical Advances in Laparoscopic Donor Nephrectomy 273**
Cheguevara Afaneh, Meredith J. Aull,
Joseph J. Del Pizzo and Sandip Kapur

Chapter 14 **Higher Volume and Better Outcomes Relationship in Kidney Transplant 285**
Wui-Chiang Lee, Shu-Yun Tsao and Che-Chuan Loong

Chapter 15 **Expanding Opportunities for Kidney Transplantation 301**
Cheguevara Afaneh, Meredith J. Aull, Anthony Watkins,
Jim Kim and Sandip Kapur

Preface

Although renal transplantation is a relatively young field in medicine, with the first successful kidney transplant occurring in 1954, the past 15 years have shown rapid advances in many areas within transplantation, and the next 15 hold great promise for further advancement. The armamentarium of immunosuppressive agents has grown significantly since the mid-to-late 1990's, and currently, the immunosuppressive therapies available are potent enough to prevent rejection in the vast majority of low risk patients. Utilization of non-traditional immunosuppressive agents such as IVIG and rituximab has enabled successful transplantation of incompatible pairs (due to blood type or crossmatch incompatibility) in recent years as well. Rapid advances in kidney paired donation registries has reduced the need for incompatible transplantation in more recent years, although desensitization in the setting of kidney paired donation remains an important option for highly sensitized patients. However, with the use of potent immunosuppressive therapies, we must be cognizant of the balance needed to protect patients from the complications of over-immunosuppression. The need for tools to monitor transplant recipients and therapies to treat these patients for the complications of over-immunosuppression is an important target for research and development.

The deceased donor organ shortage continues to be the major limiting factor in transplantation, particularly as the waiting list grows in the setting of an aging population. Successful transplant programs must work diligently to maximize opportunities for transplantation for their patients, which includes utilization of marginal donor organs, pediatric organs, and hepatitis C positive organs. By considering the use of such organs in carefully selected recipients, the organs that are available can be utilized to the greatest extent possible, with acceptable if not excellent outcomes.

Medical management of kidney transplant recipients is also of utmost importance since the population is aging and often present with multiple co-morbidities that may complicate their care. Death with allograft function is the leading cause of kidney allograft loss, and the leading cause of death is cardiovascular death. Therefore, management of co-morbidities such as diabetes, hypertension, and hyperlipidemia are essential to success in maximizing both patient and graft survival.

We hope that the reader finds this textbook to be a comprehensive resource on the topics mentioned above as well as others that can help you to offer transplantation to as many candidates as possible, and improve post-transplant outcomes in order to maximize the grafts that are donated.

I would like to thank my assistant editors Cheguevara Afaneh, M.D. and Meredith J. Aull, Pharm.D. for their instrumental roles in the completion of this textbook.

Dr. Sandip Kapur
Department of Surgery, Division of Transplant Surgery New York - Presbyterian Hospital/Weill Cornell Medical College New York, NY, USA

Section 1

Evaluation and Management of the Kidney Transplant Patient

Chapter 1

Evaluation of Kidney Transplant Candidates: An Update in 2012

Cheguevara Afaneh and Choli Hartono

Additional information is available at the end of the chapter

http://dx.doi.org/10.5772/53540

1. Introduction

The first successful kidney transplant between identical twins at the Peter Bent Brigham Hospital took place in Boston on December 23, 1954. This momentous event ushered in the modern era of organ transplantation. Kidney transplantation is now considered a routine procedure and is the treatment of choice for suitable patients with end-stage renal disease (ESRD). In 2001, approximately 100000 patients were predicted to be on the kidney transplant waiting list by 2010 [1]. In 2012, the waiting list is fast approaching that predicted number. A successful transplant affords independence from and provides a survival advantage over dialysis treatment [2]. However, patients with ESRD reap the benefit of renal transplant invariably at the expense of potential morbidity and mortality. The requirement to fully assess the benefit and risk of transplant ultimately is in the best interest of the candidate. By thoroughly evaluating a transplant candidate, the transplant program anticipates potential complications that may arise during the perioperative period. Moreover, appropriate kidney organs are in short supply relative to patients on the wait-list supporting the need to screen and identify candidates who are not eligible.

In the United States of America (US), kidney transplant candidates may receive either a live-donor (LD) or deceased-donor (DD) kidney. Live-donor kidneys may come from biologically related relatives or completely unrelated altruistic individuals. Increased potency of immunosuppressive agents has decreased the risk of acute rejection enabling transplantation from unrelated LD and DD kidneys. Harvesting marginal kidneys from deceased donors is gaining acceptance in response to organ shortages due to an expanding recipient pool. Organ Procurement Transplantation Network/United Network for Organ Sharing (OPTN/UNOS) implemented a new allocation system (UNOS Policy 3.5) in October 2002 to reclassify DD and better define the marginal kidney donor [3]. In the new classification schema, expanded criteria donor (ECD) is defined by any DD over the age of 60 or if aged between 50 to 59 with the addition of at least two of the following three criteria: cerebrovascular accident as a cause of death, history of hypertension, and terminal serum creatinine above 1.5 mg/dL. Standard criteria donors (SCD) are DDs who do not meet the criteria for ECD. SCD or ECD kidneys may be procured from donation after brain death (DBD) or donation after cardiac death (DCD) donors. Potential candidates should be made aware that transplantation of marginal kidneys from deceased donors may result in delayed graft function (DGF), defined as the need for dialysis during the first week after kidney transplant.

Kasiske et al. provided for the American Society of Transplantation (AST) an in-depth discussion and reviewed guidelines for evaluation of renal transplant candidates in 2001 [4]. The British and Canadian guidelines for kidney transplant evaluation as well as recent reviews by Bunnapradist et al. and Scandling are referenced in [5-8]. The transplant candidate should be aware of various short- and long-term considerations, as listed in Table 1. In this chapter, updates will be presented on key issues such as age for candidacy, cardiovascular risk, recurrent disease, malignancies, viral infections, endocrine issues, hematology considerations, dual organ transplants, and high-risk candidates. Table 2 lists the standard initial kidney transplant candidate evaluation at New York-Presbyterian/Weill Cornell Medical Center.

Topics of Discussion for the Kidney Transplant Candidate
Perioperative risk factors: - Cardiopulmonary reserve - Extent of vascular disease - Obesity - Patient specific comorbid conditions, i.e. type 1 diabetes mellitus, end-stage liver disease, human immunodeficiency virus, [see references 4-8]
Extent of histocompatibility and type of organ donor regarding short- and long-term outcomes
Availability and suitability of a living donor
Discuss the willingness to accept marginal donor kidneys, pediatric donors, and high-risk kidney donors
Reasonable expectations of deceased donor waitlist times
Financial considerations of life-long immunosuppression as well as adverse event costs
Lifelong Immunosuppression Risks - Infections - Malignancies, with a predominance of skin cancers
Need for lifelong follow-up with frequent regular blood testing
Risks of graft failure and death following transplantation at various time points

Table 1. Kidney Transplant Candidate Considerations

2. Age as a factor for transplant candidates

The ESRD population is graying and in comparison to a decade ago, transplant programs are wait listing more individuals who are greater than 65 years old [9-12]. What are some of the concerns for transplanting an older ESRD patient? A senior recipient in his or her seventh and eighth decades of life has a natural lifespan that is shorter than a younger patient hence reducing the predicted life years gained after transplant. Trepidation for the senior recipient is also the issue of further shortening patient survival after transplant due to the increased risk of transplant-associated morbidity. Indeed, Veroux et al. [13] observed that in a single center study in Italy, elderly recipients older than 65 years of age had a worsened survival rate after renal transplants from older donors when compared to wait-listed candidates. However, the functional status of elderly patients deteriorated if they have ESRD and require dialysis treatment [14]. Data from the United States Renal Data System (USRDS) demonstrated that the life expectancy of a 75-year-old patient on dialysis is only a third of a similar aged individual not receiving dialysis [15]. The 1-year survival rate of an 80- to 84-year-old patient on dialysis is 63% based on data from the USRDS [16]. Because the waiting time may be an obstacle for older transplant candidates, they may elect to receive ECD kidneys with a shorter waiting time [17]. Realistically, to fully address whether dialysis or transplant is a better option for this age group, a randomized study will have to be performed. Short of that, we are able to gleaned new insights into transplantation of seniors from the Scientific Registry of Transplant Recipients (SRTR) database.

In a study by Rao et al. [18], using data from the SRTR, the mortality risk of 5667 patients with age greater than or equal to 70 years old and listed between January 1, 1990 to December 31, 2004 were analyzed. There were 4475 (79%) patients with age between 70 to 74 years old and 1192 (21%) patients with age above 75 years old. Of the 5667 wait-listed candidates, 2078 (36.7%) had received a DD transplant, 360 (6.4%) had received a LD transplant, 1849 (32.6%) were deceased before transplant, and 1380 (24.4%) had not received a transplant prior to the cut-off period for analysis in December 2005. A third of the DD transplants were from ECD kidneys. The authors observed that kidney transplantation in patients greater or equal to 70 years of age was associated with a 41% reduction in mortality risk when compared to similar patients on the wait list [18]. The survival benefit was statistically significant in patients carrying a primary diagnosis of hypertension or diabetes mellitus but not significant for patients with glomerulonephritis [18]. Compared to wait-listed individuals, recipients of ECD kidneys enjoyed a 25% reduction in the risk of death whereas recipients of LD kidneys had a 57% reduction in mortality risk [18]. Analysis of relative mortality risk demonstrated that the risk of death at 45 days after transplant was 2.26 fold the risk of wait-listed candidates with the mortality risk equalizing at day 125 after transplant [18].

Huang et al. using data from OPTN/UNOS, compared the outcomes of recipients older than 80 years of age with recipients in the 60 to 69 and 70 to 79 age groups [19]. The 80 years and older cohort had 199 recipients (median age of 81 years) and represented 0.6% of the entire elderly cohort (age greater or equal to 60 years) that was transplanted between 2000 and 2008 in the US. The 60 to 69 years group had 24877 recipients whereas the 70 to 79 years group had 6103 recipients. The use of induction agents such as IL-2 receptor antagonist, antithymocyte globulin, and alemtuzumab were similar in the 3 groups. The rate of DGF

Consultations
Nephrology consultation Transplant Surgery consultation Social Work evaluation Nutritional assessment Pharmacy screening
Laboratory Data
Laboratory evaluation: 1. Serum chemistry 2. Serum hematology 3. ABO blood group verification on two separate dates 4. Viral serologies 5. Histocompatibility testing 6. Tubuerculosis screening (Quantiferon Gold) if PPD unavailable 7. Additional testing may be indicated based on co-morbidities
Other Baseline Data
Radiographic evaluation: 1. Chest x-ray 2. Complete abdominal ultrasound 3. MRI or CT Brain in patients with Polycystic Kidney Disease 4. Further testing may be indicated based on co-morbidities Electrocardiogram (EKG)
Routine Screening
Routine health maintenance screening: 1. Colonoscopy after the age of 50 years, and repeated as deemed appropriate 2. Mammogram in female candidates after the age of 40 years, and repeated as deemed appropriate 3. Pap smear in female candidates after the age of 21 years, and repeated as deemed appropriate 4. Prostate specific antigen (PSA) in male candidates over the age of 50 years, and repeated as deemed appropriate
Referrals
Referral to specialists as indicated based on candidate co-morbidities including: 1. Cardiologist 2. Gastroenterologist 3. Hematologist 4. Urologist 5. Psychiatrist

Table 2. New York-Presbyterian/Weill Cornell Medical Center Evaluation

defined as the need for dialysis therapy during the first week after transplant was similar in the 3 groups. The authors observed no difference in the rate of acute rejection during the initial hospitalization or at 1 year [19]. In the analysis, 73% of transplant recipients in the 80 years and older group were alive at 2 years [19] exceeding the expectation of the 2-year survival rate of 44% for a dialysis patient aged 80 to 84 years according to the USRDS database [15]. The overall perioperative mortality risk at 30 days was low at 1.5% for the overall cohort of elderly patients with a trend towards a higher perioperative mortality rate at 2.5% for the aged 80 years and older cohort [19]. Among the 80 years and older cohort, death-censored graft failure did not occur more frequently and the mortality rates were similar for SCD or ECD transplant recipients [19]. When comparing the 3 cohorts of elderly recipients, no differences were observed in the proportion of cardiovascular (P=0.64), infectious (P=0.47), malignant (P=0.27) and cerebrovascular (P=0.89) causes of death [19].

The recommendation from the AST is to avoid setting a cut-off age limit for eligible senior renal transplant candidates without medical contraindications [4]. When evaluating elderly patients for renal transplant, attention should be focused on the early perioperative mortality risk from cardiovascular comorbidity. ECD kidneys should be considered and offered to this age group to potentially shorten the waiting period [17].

3. Cardiovascular risk factors

Patients with ESRD are at risk for cardiovascular disease with 50% of all mortality in this population attributable to cardiac complications [20]. A retrospective analysis of 1460 renal transplant recipients at a major transplant center from 2000 to 2009 was performed to assess preoperative cardiovascular risk [20]. Among 962 patients with complete records, 357 patients (37.1%) underwent coronary angiogram demonstrating coronary artery disease (CAD) in 212 patients (59.4%) [20].

Death with graft function (DWGF) was the most common reason for graft loss observed in 10.4% of 1317 kidney transplants performed at a single major transplant center from 1996 to 2006 [21]. Of the 318 graft failures identified over the study period, DWGF occurred in 138 recipients (43.4%) [21]. The causes of DWGF include cardiovascular at 28.2%, infections at 15.2%, malignancies at 13.8%, and others or unknown represented 42.8% respectively [21]. In recent years, the rising imbalance between wait-listed candidates and available organs for procurement has necessitated the use of once discarded organs such as ECD and DCD kidneys. The expanded use of ECD and DCD kidneys has increased the incidence of DGF when compared to SCD transplants. According to the SRTR, the incidence of DGF was 31.2% for ECD, 37.1% for DCD, and 21.6% for SCD kidney transplants [22]. Tapiawala et al. investigated the relationship between DGF and risk of DWGF using data from the USRDS [23]. An increased risk of DWGF was observed among kidney transplant recipients with DGF (relative hazard of 1.53; 95% confidence interval 1.45 to 1.63 for fully adjusted models). Cardiovascular causes of death were slightly more prevalent in patients with DGF [23].

Diabetes mellitus is the most common etiology cited for ESRD in the US and a large proportion of renal transplants are done in patients with diabetes mellitus [24]. Diabetes mellitus confers a poor prognosis for survival after renal transplant in association with cardiovascular disease that is often present before transplantation [24]. Ramanathan et al. investigated the prevalence of silent CAD in 97 asymptomatic type 1 and 2 diabetic kidney and kidney-pancreas transplant candidates by analyzing their cardiac angiogram records [25]. The authors observed that 33% of type 1 and 48% of type 2 asymptomatic diabetic patients had significant lesions (greater than or equal to 70%) in one or more coronary vessels [25]. A Norwegian study by Witczak et al. [26] also showed a high incidence of significant CAD in 155 diabetic renal transplant candidates who underwent compulsory coronary angiogram testing. Among the 155 patients, 69 patients (45%) were found to have significant stenosis (greater than 50%) resulting in 39 patients (57%) who required revascularization [26].

Pulmonary hypertension is highly prevalent in patients with ESRD resulting in increased mortality [27]. Identification of pulmonary hypertension may impact early graft function in renal transplant recipients [28]. Zlotnick et al. analyzed the impact of pulmonary hypertension defined as pulmonary artery systolic pressure (PASP) of greater than or equal to 35 mmHg by echocardiographic measurements on DGF and slow graft function (serum creatinine of greater than 3 mg/dL on post-transplant day 5) [27]. The authors demonstrated that pulmonary hypertension was an independent risk factor for early graft function in DD kidney transplants. An increased incidence of early graft dysfunction from 11.7% to 56% (P=0.01) was seen in DD transplant recipients with pulmonary hypertension [27].

In summary, cardiovascular risk should be addressed when assessing renal transplant candidates. A wait-list conference convened in 2002 recommended annual cardiovascular surveillance for diabetic ESRD patients [29]. Asymptomatic patients with diabetes mellitus should undergo rigorous cardiac testing for CAD including coronary angiogram if noninvasive studies are suspicious for pathology. Efforts to optimize cardiovascular care should be afforded to candidates at risk for DGF if they are potential recipients of ECD and DCD kidneys. Pulmonary hypertension should also be identified and addressed for wait-listed individuals at risk for DGF.

4. Malignancies

Malignancy is the third most common cause of mortality after renal transplant [21]. The risk of cancer is increased in solid organ transplant recipients [30]. A recent report suggests that renal transplant tourism in older individuals may be associated with a higher risk of post-transplant malignancy [31]. Because immunosuppressive agents could negatively impact existing and contribute to the emergence of malignancy after transplant, examining transplant candidates for the presence of malignancy is an important aspect of pre-transplant evaluation. Common malignancies encountered in the dialysis population include cancer in the kidney, bladder, and thyroid [32]. The AST guideline for most cancer encountered in patients on the wait-list is to delay transplant for 2 years to ensure no recurrence and up to 5 years for some cancer with a high incidence of recurrence [see reference 4]. However, certain malignancies may not warrant a long wait time [4] and should be evaluated on a case-by-case basis at the transplant center. Herein, updates to challenging malignancies during evaluation and after transplant will be presented.

Post-transplant lymphoproliferative disorder (PTLD) has an incidence of 1-2% in renal transplant recipients and occurs at a rate 20-fold higher than in the general population [33]. Sampaio et al. investigated the risk of PTLD using the OPTN/UNOS database [34]. Between 2000 and 2009 and among 137939 kidney transplant recipients, 913 developed PTLD. The authors found that Epstein-Barr virus (EBV) donor (D) and recipient (R) status impacted on the risk of PTLD. Specifically, EBV D+/R- when compared to D-/R- was associated with an increase in PTLD incidence of 35% and 42% in adult DD and LD renal transplants respectively [34]. A relationship between monoclonal gammopathy of undetermined significance (MGUS) and PTLD was observed in a recent single center retrospective study [35]. In the study, MGUS was defined as a serum M protein of less than 3.0 g/dL, bone marrow biopsy with less than 10% plasma cells, and the absence of end-organ involvement. Of 42 patients with MGUS, 23 were identified prior to kidney transplant. After a median follow-up of 8.5 years, 4 (17.4%) patients with pretransplant MGUS went on to develop 2 cases each of smoldering multiple myeloma and PTLD [35]. Of the 19 posttransplant MGUS cases, none developed multiple myeloma but 2 patients were found to have EBV-negative T cell lymphoproliferative disorders at 16 and 26 years after transplant [35]. The authors concluded that patients with MGUS, a common disease that occurs in 2% of the population under the age of 50 could safely receive a kidney transplant [35].

Transplant recipients have an increased risk of various skin malignancies such as squamous cell carcinoma, melanoma, and basal cell carcinoma [36]. Pretransplant melanoma is often a malignancy cited as needing a long recurrence-free waiting time [4]. A recent report from a melanoma collaborative working group provided guidance when evaluating a potential candidate with a history of melanoma for organ transplant [37]. The recommendation is for no wait time in candidates with a prior history of melanoma *in situ* [37]. The working group suggests that the risk of recurrence is lower in thin melanoma (Breslow depth < 1mm) without any clinical evidence of metastasis and warrants a waiting time of a minimum of 2 years [37]. A shorter wait time may be reasonable for melanoma depth of < 1 mm and a negative sentinel lymph node (SLN) biopsy. Candidates with melanoma depth of > 2 mm should delay transplant until after a 5-year recurrence-free waiting period [37]. Transplant may be contraindicated in potential renal transplant recipients with lymph node involvement or frank metastatic disease from melanoma [37]. The data is lacking for transplant patients with melanoma depth of > 1 mm and < 2mm with a negative SLN biopsy. However, since the prognosis of immunocompetent patients with melanoma depth of < 2mm is favorable, renal transplant candidates with similar melanoma thickness may be eligible for a 2-year waiting period prior to transplant [37].

5. Recurrent disease

In a recent large retrospective single center study, recurrent glomerulonephritis (GN) was the cause in approximately 15% of kidney allograft failure after censoring for death [21].

Recurrence of prominent GN in the allograft namely focal segmental glomerulosclerosis (FSGS) and membranoproliferative GN (MPGN) will be discussed in this section.

Idiopathic FSGS has a high rate of recurrence after renal transplant. The rate of recurrence is estimated at 30% to 50% for the first kidney transplant and as high as 100% in subsequent kidney transplants [38]. Recurrence of disease may emerge within hours to days after kidney transplant or months to years later. Known risk factors for recurrence are Caucasian or Hispanic recipients, history of bilateral native kidney nephrectomy, mesangial hypercellularity, young recipients, progression to ESRD within 3 years after the diagnosis of FSGS is made, retransplant after failed allograft from FSGS recurrence [38-39]. Genetic and acquired mutations have been reported in 15% of idiopathic FSGS affecting slit diaphragm proteins such as podocin (NPHS2), nephrin (NPHS1), α-actinin 4, CD2AP, and TRPC6 [40-41]. Recurrence of FSGS may occur in less than 10% of patients with mutations in NPHS2 and commercial testing for this mutation could help to define the risk for donors [42]. The USRDS data reported that living donor transplants do not increase the risk of graft loss in FSGS [43]. Krishnan N et al. also reported successful renal transplant between monozygotic twins [44]. Cibrik et al. estimated the risk for death-censored graft loss to be 1% per year in adult FSGS recipients of zero HLA mismatch live-donor kidney in comparison to 4.4% per year for FSGS recipients of zero HLA mismatch deceased-donor kidney [45]. Because FSGS recurrence may in some recipients be unavoidable, efforts should be made to educate both donors and recipients of the risk with frank discussions about early graft loss. The previous finding of a circulating factor (30 to 50 kDa glycoprotein) being responsible for FSGS recurrence supports the use of plasmapheresis to manage at risk patients with idiopathic FSGS before and after kidney transplants [46]. Recent studies by Wei et al. implicated circulating urokinase receptor (suPAR) as a causative factor for FSGS recurrence [47]. In their report, the presence of suPAR in the serum was predictive of FSGS recurrence after transplant and lowering serum suPAR by plasmapheresis was associated with clinical remission [47]. Nozu et al. and Pescovitz et al. described the first two successful cases utilizing rituximab in children with recurrent FSGS and subsequent PTLD [48-49]. Followup reports by other investigators demonstrated complete, partial, and no response to rituximab [reviewed in reference 50]. Rituximab appears to play a direct role by targeting podocytes in recurrent FSGS and inducing remission [51]. More studies are needed to clarify recurrent FSGS cases that will respond to rituximab.

MPGN is the most common cause of recurrent GN in renal transplant allografts [38]. Among the 3 subtypes of MPGN, MPGN type II is now known as dense deposit disease with recurrence occurring in as high as 100% of transplant candidates [38]. On examination via electron microscopy, Dense deposit disease (DDD) is manifested by a ribbon-like electron-dense deposition in the glomerular basement membrane. Patients with DDD tend to have a low serum C3 level and up to 80% has a circulating autoantibody to C3Bb known as C3 nephritic factor (C3Nef) [38]. Evaluation of potential transplant candidates with DDD should include a search for the type of complement dysregulation. This is accomplished by assessing factor H, I, and membrane cofactor protein levels [38]. Consideration should be given to providing fresh frozen plasma prior to and after kidney engraftment in DDD patients with complement dysregulation [38]. Vivarelli et al. recently reported the use of eculizumab, an anti-C5 antibody on a young 17-year-old patient with DDD and positive C3Nef but normal levels of factor H and factor B. [52]. Eculizumab was administered approximately seven years after the disease onset with a baseline focal sclerosis documented prior to therapy at 40% of glomeruli. The authors reported a reduction in proteinuria and microhematuria following administration of eculizumab. Repeat biopsies at 18 months after therapy showed a decrease in dense deposits in the glomerular basement membrane albeit with progression of glomerular sclerosis and tubular atrophy [52]. The authors observed an increased in the proteinuria when eculizumab was stopped after 18 months [52]. Following resumption of eculizumab therapy, the patient again responded with a reduction in proteinuria and had a normal renal function and blood pressure despite a persistently low serum C3 levels [52]. Daina et al. similarly reported a favorable clinical response to eculizumab in a young patient who had previously received rituximab for DDD [53]. Radhakrishnan et al. reported on the successful treatment of refractory MPGN type I in a 16-year-old girl using eculizumab [54]. In the kidney transplant arena, a recent report by McCaughan et al. described the successful use of eculizumab in a recipient with recurrent DDD [55]. The patient was a 29-year-old female with ESRD from DDD and she received a kidney transplant from her brother after requiring renal replacement therapy for 6 years. She received triple immunosuppression with tacrolimus, mycophenolate mofetil, and prednisone without any induction and her best serum creatinine was 0.9 mg/dL. A recurrence, which was confirmed by biopsy that showed cellular crescents and polymorphs in the glomeruli with endocapillary proliferation was noted at 4 weeks after transplant. The patient was given a course of methylprednisolone, plasmapheresis, and rituximab with progressive deterioration of renal function with a rise in serum creatinine to 4.93 mg/dL. After a second biopsy to confirm the diagnosis of DDD at 10 weeks after transplant, eculizumab was provided with a loading dose of 900mg for 2 doses given a week apart followed by a maintenance dose of 600mg given every 2 weeks. The authors observed an immediate response with a dramatic decline in serum creatinine and reduction in proteinuria during the first 2 weeks of eculizumab therapy [55].

In summary, MPGN and FSGS may recur at a high rate following kidney transplant. Although allograft outcome is typically poor following recurrence, new approaches to therapy described herein may improve allograft survival.

6. Infections

Encountering chronic viral infections in the prospective renal transplant candidate is not uncommon. Viral hepatitides may be a known comorbidity or newly diagnosed during the transplant evaluation process. Patients with failed kidney transplant due to polyomavirus type BK induced nephropathy may present for retransplant evaluation. Increasingly, HIV patients with ESRD are also being referred for renal transplant. A list of the most common infections of kidney transplant recipients in a chronological order following transplant are listed in Table 3. Guidelines on the medical evaluation of hepatitis B or C infections in potential transplant candidates were reviewed in reference [4]. Herein, updates on the evaluation of BK virus or HIV infected transplant candidates will be discussed.

Perioperative Infections in the Recipient
Nosocomial Infections -Methicillin-resistant *Staphylococcus aureus* (MRSA) -Vancomycin-resistant *Enterococcus* (VRE) -Hospital acquired pneumonia (HAP) *-Clostridium difficile* -Central venous catheter-associated infections -Urinary catheter-associated infections
Candida
Aspergillus
Infections Post-Transplant (1 to 6 months)
Viral infections -CMV -HSV -Shingles (VZV) -HBV or HCV recurrence or new infection -BKV -Community acquired viral infections (adenovirus, parainfluenza, respiratory syncytial virus, metapneumovirus)
Opportunistic infections *-Pneumocystis carinii (jiroveci)* *-Listeria monocytogenes* *-Toxoplasma gondii* *-Mycoplasma tuberculosis* *-Nocardia* *-Strongyloides* *-Leishmania* *-Aspergillus*
Infections Post-Transplant (>6 months)
Community-acquired pneumonia (CAP) CMV BKV Urinary tract infections Colitis *Aspergillus* EBV (associated with PTLD)

BKV: BK (polyoma) virus, CMV: cytomegalovirus, EBV: Epstein-Barr virus, HBV: hepatitis B virus, HCV: hepatitis C virus, herpes virus, HSV: herpes simplex virus, PTLD: post-transplant lymphoproliferative disorder

Table 3. Infections in Kidney Transplant Donors and Recipients

A prospective nonrandomized multicenter trial was conducted on HIV-infected ESRD patients who underwent live- or deceased-donor renal transplantation at 19 US transplant centers [56]. Eligible participants had a $CD4^+$ T-cell count of greater or equal to 200 per cubic millimeter and undetectable plasma HIV-1 RNA levels. Participants were on a stable regimen of HAART for 16 weeks prior to kidney transplant. A history of treated opportunistic infections with the exception of progressive multifocal leukoencephalopathy, chronic intestinal cryptosporidiosis, primary central nervous system lymphoma, and visceral Kaposi's sarcoma were permitted for participants in the trial. Patients with hepatitis B coinfection must demonstrate undetectable hepatitis B virus surface antigen whereas patients coinfected with hepatitis C were offered pretransplant interferon therapy if eligible. Patients with hepatitis B and C coinfection had to demonstrate an absence of liver cirrhosis by biopsy. Induction with interleukin-2 receptor blocker and/or antithymocyte globulin was provided at the discretion of the transplant center. Participants received calcineurin inhibitor (CNI) cyclosporine or tacrolimus, mycophenolate mofetil, and glucocorticoid for maintenance therapy. CNI was replaced by sirolimus in patients with CNI-related toxicity. Among the 150 participants who were enrolled between November 2003 and June 2009, 1 subject withdrew consent at 6 months whereas 53 subjects had completed at least 3 years of follow-up at the time of analysis. The authors observed that the 1 year and 3 years patient survival rates (±SD) (94.6±2.0% and 88.2±3.8%) as well as graft survival rates (90.4% and 73.7%) were similar to the SRTR database for all kidney transplant recipients during the study period [56]. Both univariate and multivariate proportional-hazards models showed an increased risk of graft loss that was associated with treatment of rejection and the use of antithymocyte globulin induction whereas transplant using living donor graft was protective [56]. Of concern, the allograft rejection rate was unexpectedly 2 to 3 fold higher in participants of the trial when compared to the SRTR rejection rate at 1-year. Furthermore, approximately half of the rejection episodes were steroid-resistant indicative of severe rejection. Also unexpected, the authors did not observe any progression of HIV disease in the trial in spite of the initial decrease in $CD4^+$ T-cell count and that maintenance immunosuppression did not promote HIV viremia. Among the 150 participants, 57 required hospitalization for 140 reported infections during the trial with 60% of serious infections occurring during the first 6 months after transplant. Of note, 5 cases of BK nephropathy and no cases of PTLD were observed during the study. The authors concluded that kidney transplant is a safe alternative to dialysis therapy for a select group of HIV-infected ESRD patients [56].

With the current reliance on immunosuppression, BK virus nephropathy (BKVN) may affect up to 8% of kidney allografts [57]. The negative impact of persistent BK viremia following BKVN-induced allograft failure on retransplant is a concern during re-evaluation. Womer et al. reported successful preemptive retransplant in 2 patients with active BK viremia [58]. The first patient was a 20-year-old Asian female deceased-donor renal transplant recipient with ESRD due to FSGS. Within approximately 3 years after transplant, BKVN was diagnosed along with transplant rejection. Severe allograft dysfunction ensued with glomerular filtration rate (GFR) falling to 14 mL/min despite therapy using intravenous immunoglobulin (IVIG), intravenous cidofovir, and reduction in overall immunosuppression.

Preemptive live-donor renal transplant from a 6 antigen-mismatched biological sister was performed with simultaneous allograft nephrectomy. No induction therapy was provided and maintenance immunosuppression consisted of prednisone, mycophenolate mofetil, and rapamycin. The authors observed a decline in plasma BK virus levels by PCR from 26000 copies/mL prior to retransplantation to undetectable at 14 days after retransplant. Plasma BK viral level of 9300 copies/mL was detected at 5 months after retransplant but had disappeared at 8 months and 21 months post-retransplant. A serum creatinine of 1.1 mg/dL was reported during the 21-month followup visit. The second patient was a 29-year-old Caucasian female simultaneous kidney-pancreas transplant recipient. BKVN was diagnosed at approximately 4 years after transplant. Severe allograft dysfunction ensued with glomerular filtration rate (GFR) falling to 13 mL/min despite therapy with intravenous cidofovir and conversion of CNI from tacrolimus to cyclosporine. Preemptive live-donor renal transplant from a 1 haplotype-mismatched biological sister was performed with simultaneous allograft nephrectomy. Antithymocyte globulin induction therapy was provided and maintenance immunosuppression consisted of prednisone, mycophenolate mofetil, and cyclosporine. The authors observed a decline in plasma BK virus levels by PCR from 50000 copies/mL prior to retransplantation to undetectable at 5 days after retransplant. Plasma BK was detected at 12 months after retransplant. The short-term favorable outcome in the case-reports by Womer et al. supports early retransplant of patients following BKVN-associated allograft failure. Consideration should be given to simultaneous graft nephrectomy during retransplant.

7. Familial renal disease

Autosomal dominant polycystic kidney disease (ADPKD) is often encountered in transplant candidates presenting with a family history of renal disease and ESRD. The requirement and optimal timing of kidney nephrectomy may pose a dilemma for the prospective patient, referring physicians, and transplant center. Skauby et al. retrospectively analyzed their single center live-donor transplant experience comparing the outcome of a consecutive series of 159 kidney transplant recipients with ADPKD [59]. After excluding 2 patients with insufficient data, 157 patients were divided into 2 groups of ADPKD patients. Group A (n=79) received live-donor kidney transplant alone whereas group B (n=78) underwent simultaneous bilateral nephrectomy (SBN) and live-donor kidney transplant. The authors observed a higher rate of intraoperative complications in group B with significantly longer operative time, a higher requirement for blood transfusion, and need for plasma products. Two patients from group B required dialysis in comparison to non in group A. However, graft survival rates at 1 year and 5 years were similar in groups A and B at 94.8% and 89.6% versus 96.1% and 90.8%, respectively. Patient survival up to 5 years was also similar between the 2 groups. Based on their study, the authors advocated the following decision algorithm. The choice to undergo SBN is dependent on the patient's personal opinion, residual renal function, presence of mass effect, propensity for renal infections, and suspicion for malignancy. When nephrectomy of native kidneys is necessary and a live donor is available, kidney transplant with SBN may be preemptively performed. In the event that plasmapheresis or anticoagulation is required during the perioperative period and nephrectomy of native kidneys is deemed necessary, bilateral nephrectomy is performed prior to the transplant.

Alport's syndrome is an X-linked disease causing ESRD and affecting predominantly male patients. Transplant candidates should be made aware of the uncommon (less than 5%) development of anti-glomerular basement membrane (anti-GBM) disease after kidney transplant. Anti-GBM disease in allograft presents as crescentic glomerulonephritis with linear fixing of IgG and C3 to the glomerular basement membrane and usually induces graft loss. Retransplant of candidates with Alport's syndrome and failed allografts due to anti-GBM disease remains challenging. Despite plasmapheresis and appropriate anti-T cell therapy, Browne et al. showed that graft loss remained unavoidable in patients with Alport posttransplant anti-GBM disease [60].

8. Hematology considerations

Blood transfusion is often necessary in the perioperative period especially in transplant recipients at risk for bleeding. Preemptive transplant candidates may also present with profound anemia due to advance uremia or lack of erythropoietin replacement therapy. Scornik et al. investigated the contribution of posttransplant blood transfusion to development of human leukocyte antigen (HLA) antibodies in 746 patients transplanted over a 6-year period [61]. Data on solid-phase HLA antibody testing was available in 199 patients. Blood transfusion was provided to 45% of the cohort and approximately 80% of the transfusion was given during the first month after transplant. The authors observed that the frequency of *de novo* antibodies was 16% in the 199 patients tested. Only 1 person developed anti-HLA antibodies in a group of 12 patients who had required transfusion of greater than 10 red cell units. In the study, non donor-specific anti-HLA antibodies were not induced by blood transfusion. Within the limitation of a single center retrospective analysis, the authors concluded that unlike pretransplant transfusion, blood transfusion in the posttransplant setting did not sensitize transplant recipients [61].

9. Endocrine considerations

Overweight is defined as a body mass index (BMI) of greater than or equal to 25 kg/m^2 whereas obesity is defined as a BMI of greater than or equal to 30 kg/m^2 [62]. Concurrent with an epidemic of obesity in the general population of developed and developing countries, the prevalence of obesity has also increased in kidney transplant candidates in recent years [63]. Severely obese transplant candidates are at risk for perioperative complications such as poor wound healing and DGF. Weissenbacher et al. retrospectively analyzed their single center data on 1132 deceased-donor transplant between 2000 and 2009 [64]. The DGF rate was 32.4% in the entire cohort. Multivariate analyses showed that BMI and dialysis vintage were independent risk factors for DGF. The authors demonstrated that the incidence of DGF was increased in obese recipients with BMI over 30 kg/m^2 at 52.6% ($P<0.0001$) when compared to non-obese kidney transplant recipients [64]. The DGF rate was 25.2%, 29.8%, and 40.9% for recipients with BMI of less than 18.5 kg/m^2, 18.5 to 24.9 kg/m^2, and 25 to 29.9 kg/m^2 respectively. In the study, DGF resulted in poor 1- and 5-year graft and patient survival.

In general, prospective transplant candidates with obesity should be referred to a transplant dietician for counseling. Eckel has reviewed the treatment option for obesity in the general population [62]. Alexander et al. studied gastric bypass procedure (GBP) in thirty morbidly obese patients who had chronic renal failure and kidney transplants [65]. Of the 30 patients, 19 patients had chronic kidney disease (12 were already on dialysis), 8 patients had GBP after kidney transplant, and 3 patients had kidney transplant following GBP. The authors observed that reduction in BMI in excess above 25 kg/m^2 at 1, 2, and 3 years after GBP was similar with or without transplantation. The reduction of BMI in excess above 25 kg/m^2 was around 70% at 1 year for the various cohorts. Among the 30 patients, only 1 had serious wound infection after removal of sutures and no other complications related to the GBP were reported. Further studies are needed in the ESRD population to determine a safe strategy for managing obesity while patients are on the transplant wait-list. Morbidly obese transplant candidates who are recalcitrant to diet and exercise may require surgical interventions to lose weight.

10. High-risk candidates

Additional preoperative preparations are warranted for high-risk transplant candidates who are predisposed to perioperative graft dysfunction (Table 4). Herein, three different clinical scenarios will be discussed that may impact early graft function and require special attention before transplant.

High-Risk Category	Treatment Options
Presensitized & highly sensitized candidate	1. Desensitization protocols including plasmapheresis, IVIG, and/or Rituximab 2. Kidney-paired donation (if living donor available) 3. Utilization of marginal donor kidneys 4. Utilization of pediatric donor kidneys
Hypercoagulable Conditions	1. Correct underlying disorder if possible 2. Begin anticoagulation perioperatively with/without heparin bridge and warfarin 3. Consider preoperative inferior vena cava filter
Chronic low blood pressure	1. Consider mineralcorticoid administration 2. Maintain aggressive volume resuscitation 3. Consider postoperative anticoagulation 4. Consider vasopressor administration

Table 4. High-Risk Kidney Transplant Candidates

Evaluation of a prospective transplant candidate with respect to the blood type and determining HLA compatibility as well as confirming a negative donor crossmatch are minimum requirements to assess the immunologic risk prior to kidney transplantation.

Crossing the ABO blood type barrier as well as transplanting highly sensitized patients with anti-donor HLA antibodies may result in hyperacute or accelerated early rejection. Hence, at the present time, transplanting an ABO incompatible or complement-dependent cytotoxicity (CDC) crossmatch positive kidney should not be undertaken without prior "desensitization". Determination of ABO compatibility between the donor and recipient is easily accomplished but must be rigorously enforced in the clinic. Characterizing a sensitized prospective transplant candidate is more complicated with recent advancement beyond the routine CDC crossmatch method to detect subtle class I and class II anti-donor HLA antibodies. Contemporary crossmatch techniques involve the use of flow cytometry-based principle to detect anti-HLA antibodies. Together with ELISA-based method, flow-cytometry, and single antigen fluorescent bead (SAFB) or Luminex platform represent new solid-phase assays in determining the degree of sensitization in the transplant candidate. These techniques have been previously reviewed [66-67]. Contrary to desensitization in the field of allergy, "desensitization" in transplantation refers to the procedure of reducing anti-donor HLA antibodies prior to engraftment. Specific protocols to desensitize patients are beyond the scope of this chapter but have been extensively published in the literature. Most centers utilize a combination of plasmapheresis, IVIG, and rituximab to desensitize and prepare patients with significant immunologic risk [68-69].

The next at-risk ESRD population going into kidney transplantation to be discussed are those predisposed to thrombosis of the allograft in the early posttransplant period. Determination of transplant candidates with thrombophilia starts with obtaining a history for hypercoagulopathy. Laboratory studies for Factor V Leiden, protein C and S, lupus anticoagulant (LA) antibodies, anticardiolipin antibodies (aCL) and anti-β_2-glycoprotein I antibodies (anti-β_2GPI) may further inform the risk of thrombosis. Antiphospholipid syndrome (APLS) is a common cause of acquired thrombophilia characterized by the presence of antiphospholipid antibodies (APA). Canaud et al. recently demonstrated the negative impact of APA in kidney transplants recipients [70]. Of a cohort of 37 patients with APA, 12 met the diagnostic criteria for APLS at the time of transplant. Of the 12 patients with APA positive APLS, 4 died early after transplant. Compared to control, patients with positive APA had more frequent early graft thrombosis and deep venous thrombosis (27% vs. 7%, $P<0.05$ and 35% vs. 14%, $P<0.05$ respectively). The authors observed that APA positive patients also had a more rapid decline in GFR at 1 year after transplant [70].

Another high-risk group of transplant candidates have consistently low blood pressure heading into the transplant procedure. Webber et al. investigated the role of low blood pressure from 993 kidney transplant recipients between 2003 and 2008. They showed using a case-control study design that an average mean arterial pressure less than or equal to 80 mmHg during the 3 months prior to kidney transplantation is a risk factor for primary nonfunction of the allograft [71].

11. Dual organ transplantation

Kidney transplantation may be performed concurrently with other solid organs such as liver, heart, and pancreas. According to the OPTN/SRTR 2006 annual report, the rate of combined pancreas-kidney transplants has remained steady over a five-year period since 2001. In contrast, multiorgan transplants involving liver-kidney and heart-kidney have substantially increased [72]. Considerations given to potential candidates for pancreas and liver transplants are listed in Table 5. Herein, evaluation of potential candidates for simultaneous pancreas-kidney as well as liver-kidney transplantation will be discussed.

An estimated 23000 pancreas transplants had been performed worldwide since the procedure was introduced four decades ago by Dr. Richard Lillehei [73]. Recently, the Centers for Medicare and Medicaid Services (CMS) approved and will cover pancreas transplant alone (PTA) procedure done on or after April 26, 2006 [72]. Patients with ESRD and insulin-dependent type I diabetes mellitus may benefit from simultaneous pancreas-kidney (SPK) or pancreas after kidney (PAK) transplantation. Because the waiting time depending on local variance may be substantial, approximately half of the wait-listed SPK candidates may die if not transplanted within 4 years of listing [74]. Therefore, if a live kidney donor is available, PAK should be considered in suitable prospective SPK candidates. In 2005, the number of active candidates on the SPK waiting list was approximately 1500 whereas it was approximately 330 for the PAK list [72]. The eligibility guidelines for pancreas transplantation were reviewed in reference [75]. The presence of insulin therapy is required and documentation of a lack of endogenous insulin production is accomplished by checking C-peptide level. A reasonably young age is one of the criteria for pancreas transplant. We reviewed our single center data on greater than 50-year-old pancreas transplant recipients and found them to also be feasible candidates [76]. Further studies are needed to establish if a strict age limit should be enforced on prospective pancreas transplant candidates. Potential pancreas transplant candidates should be evaluated for coronary artery disease (CAD) with consideration for coronary angiogram in patients with significant CAD risk factors such as smoking, presence of hypertension, and presence of peripheral arterial occlusive disease. Diabetic complications such as retinopathy, peripheral and autonomic neuropathy, microangiopathy and macroangiopathy, as well as life-threatening metabolic syndrome such as hypoglycemic unawareness must be documented during evaluation. Prospective candidate should be informed of the benefits of achieving euglycemia via pancreas transplant. The beneficial effects of pancreas transplant on retinopathy, neuropathy, nephropathy, vasculopathy, and quality of life were reviewed in reference [75]. In addition, candidates must be made aware of the 10-year survival advantage after SPK over DD kidney transplant alone (65% versus 46% respectively) [77]. For candidates awaiting pancreas transplants on the PAK list, renal allograft function should be adequate with creatinine clearance generally well above 40 mL/min. Studies investigating the risk of developing diabetes mellitus after successful pancreas transplant may provide insights into the optimal preoperative selection of pancreas transplant candidates. Dean et al. examined the outcome of 144 pancreas transplants from their center between 2001 and 2005 [78]. Posttransplant diabetes mellitus (PTDM) was diagnosed in 28 patients (19.4%) over the study period and developed at a median time of 87 days after pancreas engraftment. The presence of endogenous insulin secretion was confirmed by measuring C-peptide when PTDM was diagnosed. Of the 28 patients with PTDM, 26 became insulin dependent whereas 2 received oral hypoglycemic agents. The authors observed when comparing the PTDM group to those who did not develop diabetes mellitus that age at transplant, pretransplant hemoglobin A1c, prednisone doses or tacrolimus concentrations were similar. However, patients in the PTDM group had a higher median pretransplant BMI (29 vs. 24 kg/m^2), higher pretransplant median daily insulin requirement (69 vs. 40 units per day), higher mix of pretransplant type II diabetes mellitus (45% vs. 17%), and increased incidence of acute rejection. The authors concluded that PTDM could occur in pancreas transplant recipients despite documentation of a functioning pancreas allograft in patients with increased pretransplant BMI, elevated pretransplant insulin requirement, and increased acute pancreas rejection episodes.

Pancreas Transplant Candidate Considerations
Extent of complications of type 1 diabetes mellitus
Assess/optimize preoperative body mass index (BMI)
Review total daily insulin requirement
Previous transplants (i.e. potential locations suitable for placement of pancreas allograft)
Baseline blood pressure (chronic hypotension increases risk of pancreas allograft thrombosis)
Hypercoagulable conditions (lupus anticoagulant, anticardiolipin antibodies, anti-β_2-glycoprotein I antibodies)
Availability of a living donor for kidney transplantation
Liver Transplant Candidate Considerations
Presence of hepatorenal syndrome as cause of end-stage renal disease
Intrinsic renal disease
Renal replacement therapy dependence for >8 weeks
Model of End-stage Liver Disease (MELD) score
Hepatitis B & C virus specific considerations
Cardiovascular preoperative assessment
Rule out underlying preoperative infections
Nutritional status preoperatively (liver transplant associated with high morbidity)

Table 5. Dual Organ Transplant Considerations

The model of end-stage liver disease (MELD) was instituted on February 27, 2002. Increasingly, simultaneous liver-kidney transplants (SLK) are performed in more orthotopic liver transplant (OLT) candidates since the introduction of the MELD system [79]. In 2001, 134 recipients of SLK transplants were recorded by the SRTR. By 2007 the number of SLK transplant recipients had increased to 444 [79]. Eason et al. reviewed the SRTR database up to 2007 and identified that the MELD scores during listing and at transplant were 24 and 25 respectively for SLK candidates not on dialysis whereas for candidates on dialysis they were 27 and 31 respectively [79]. Data from SRTR between the year 2002 to 2005 showed that the unadjusted waiting list survival for SLK candidates on dialysis fared worst when compared to liver transplant alone (LTA) candidates with or without dialysis and SLK candidates not on dialysis [79]. Davis et al. recommended an algorithm when evaluating OLT candidates for possible SLK [80]. Assessment of renal function based on urinalysis, serum creatinine, and spot urine protein to creatinine as well as albumin to creatinine ratios and 24-hour urine analysis should be the initial steps taken during evaluation. Abnormal findings during the evaluation warrant further assessment based on imaging studies, kidney biopsy, and serological analysis. The key element to distinguish when evaluating potential SLK candidates is the presence of acute kidney injury (AKI) versus chronic kidney disease (CKD). Pichler investigated the etiology of renal insufficiency or persistent hepatorenal syndrome (HRS) greater than 4 weeks in 26 OLT candidates [81]. The authors observed 6 cases of MPGN, 5 cases of IgA nephropathy, 4 cases of AKI, 4 cases of focal global glomerulosclerosis, 3 cases of diabetic nephropathy, and 4 cases of normal histology [81]. Wadei et al. investigated the feasibility, value, and risk of percutaneous kidney biopsy on 44 OLT candidates with GFR of less than 40 mL/min/1.73m^2 or on renal replacement therapy [82]. Of the 44 subjects, 13 had acute tubular necrosis (ATN), 5 had MPGN, 11 had minimal findings, and 15 had advance interstitial fibrosis (≥30%)/glomerulosclerosis (≥40%) (IF/GS). Of the 15 patients with IF/GS detected on kidney biopsy, 14 candidates were listed for SLK, 1 patient was deemed not a suitable candidate for transplant. Twenty-seven patients who were listed for LTA had renal biopsy findings that showed ATN (3 cases), MPGN (2 cases), IF/GS (1 case), and minimal findings (11 cases). The biopsy complication rate in the study was 30% with 8 major complications and 5 minor complications. Seven of the 8 major complications consisted of retroperitoneal hematoma and gross hematuria, which required selective coil embolization in 5 patients. The authors reported no mortality or surgical intervention related to the biopsy [82]. Participants of a consensus conference on SLK recommended that SLK should be offered to cirrhotic patients with ESRD and symptomatic portal hypertension or hepatic vein wedge pressure gradient of ≥10 mmHg, liver failure and CKD with GFR ≤30 mL/min, AKI or HRS with serum creatinine ≥2.0 mg/dL and renal replacement therapy for ≥8 weeks, liver failure and renal biopsy showing >30% GS or IF [79].

12. Retransplant considerations

An increasingly number of candidates on the waiting list represent failed kidney transplant patients who have been recycled. These patients are potentially sensitized from their previous transplants and have unique issues to be considered during re-evaluation.

Retransplant candidates may present after a long-term history of graft function or a brief period of functioning kidney graft. It is important to determine the etiology of transplant failure especially if a prior kidney transplant biopsy is available for examination. Cases whereby recurrent disease is responsible for graft failure often presents a challenge to the candidate and the transplant center. Goldfarb-Rumyantzev et al. analyzed the USRDS database to gain insight into the role of preemptive retransplant and subsequent graft and patient outcome [83]. A total of 92844 pediatric and adult kidney transplant patients were identified between 1990 and 1999 with the follow-up period captured through end of 2000. The authors analyzed 11714 recipients who had a single retransplant during the study period. Of the 11714 recipients, 1609 received a preemptive retransplant whereas 10,105 were recipients of non-preemptive retransplant. Consistent with current findings in the clinic, the study had a high proportion of DD in recipients of non-preemptive retransplant.

The authors showed that the risk of graft failure was higher in preemptive retransplant by 36% but did not impact on recipient survival [83]. The study also revealed that prolonged prior graft survival was protective on successive patient and graft survival.

Failed kidney transplants in patients with ESRD contribute to increased morbidity and mortality [84]. The role of graft nephrectomy may pose as a clinical dilemma in early and late kidney transplant failure, which occurs less than or greater than 12 months after engraftment. The benefit of removal of a nonfunctional kidney must be weighed against the risk of sensitization especially if preemptive retransplant is being considered. Johnston et al. investigated the impact of graft nephrectomy on repeat transplant [85]. The retrospective analysis was performed utilizing USRDS database including transplants from 1995 to 2003 and preemptive repeat kidney transplants were excluded. Of the 19107 patients included in the study, 6213 patients underwent a nephrectomy whereas 12894 patients were without nephrectomy. The authors observed that transplant nephrectomy was frequently performed and twice as common in early versus late graft failure. Transplant nephrectomy appeared to be protective in patients with late graft failure but was associated with an increased risk of death in patients with early graft loss. However, nephrectomy in late graft loss was associated with an increased risk of retransplant failure whereas it was protective in patients with early graft loss. Interpretation of the study was limited by a lack of information on the indication for nephrectomy and the retrospective nature of the analysis. Marrari et al. studied the contribution of graft nephrectomy to the development of donor-specific HLA antibodies [86]. A total of 16 international histocompatibility laboratories contributed 65 cases for analysis. The authors found that the incidence of DSA reactivity determined by Luminex assay prior to and after nephrectomy was 64% vs. 87% ($p=0.0033$) for HLA-A,B mismatch category and 57% vs. 86% ($p=0.001$) for HLA-DRB1 mismatch category. The frequencies of individual reactive antigens pre- and post-nephrectomy was 49% vs. 75% ($p<0.0001$) for HLA-A,B mismatch category and 48% vs. 79% ($p=0.0001$) for HLA-DRB1 mismatch category. In contrast, the frequencies of DSA to DRB3/4/5 (65% vs. 78%, $p=0.22$) and DQ mismatches (76% vs 87%, $p=0.18$) were not significantly different before and after graft nephrectomy.

13. Conclusions

The deceased-donor kidney transplant wait-list in the US has grown from a 15000 patient list in 1990 to an approximately 55000 patient list in 2002 and is now approaching a 100000 patient list in 2012 [29]. The waiting time continues to increase since the annual transplant rate has not kept pace. In the US, only approximately 16000 kidney transplants were performed in 2009 [87]. Maintaining oversight of the ever-expanding waiting list with careful timely review of candidates is an important task for the transplant center. Because ESRD patients are at risk for cardiac events while on the waiting list, to reduce posttransplant complications, it is imperative that cardiac surveillance is updated in a timely manner. For the high-risk diabetic patient, cardiac evaluation may have to be updated on an annual basis. Prospective candidates on the list who are suitable should be identified and educated on the benefits of ECD kidney transplant. In conclusion, transplant evaluation is an important process for the transplant center to distinguish suitable candidates from ineligible ESRD patients. The goal is to anticipate and minimize posttransplant complications and to prolong kidney allograft survival.

Author details

Cheguevara Afaneh
Department of Surgery, New York Presbyterian Hospital-Weill Cornell Medical Center, New York, NY, USA

Choli Hartono
The Rogosin Institute, New York, NY, USA
Division of Nephrology and Hypertension, Department of Medicine, New York Presbyterian Hospital-Weill Cornell Medical Center, New York, NY, USA
Department of Transplantation Medicine, New York Presbyterian Hospital-Weill Cornell Medical Center, New York, NY, USA

14. References

[1] Xue JL, Ma JZ, Louis TA et al. Forecast of the Number of Patients with End-Stage Renal Disease in the United States to the year 2010. Journal of American Society of Nephrology 2001;12: 2753–2758.
[2] Wolfe RA, Ashby VB, Milford EL, et al. Comparison of Mortality in all Patients on Dialysis, Patients on Dialysis Awaiting Transplantation, and Recipients of a First Cadaveric Transplant. New England Journal of Medicine 1999;341: 1725-1730.
[3] Metzger RA, Delmonico FL, Feng S, et al. Expanded Criteria Donors for Kidney Transplantation. American Journal of Transplantation 2003;3(Suppl 4): 114-125.
[4] Kasiske BL, Cangro CB, Hariharan S, et al. The Evaluation of Renal Transplant Candidates: Clinical Practice Guidelines. American Journal of Transplantation 2001;2(Suppl 1): 5-95.
[5] British Transplantation Society: Standards for Solid Organ Transplantation in the United Kingdom: http://www.rcseng.ac.uk/surgeons/working/docs/Standards_For_Solid_Organ_Tranplantation_UK1.pdf/view (accessed 5 August 2012).
[6] Knoll G, Cockfield S, Blydt-Hansen T, et al. Canadian Society of Transplantation Consensus Guidelines on Eligibility for Kidney Transplantation. Canadian Medical Association Journal 2005;173(10): S1-S25.
[7] Bunnapradist S, Danovitch GM. Evaluation of Adult Kidney Transplantation Candidates. American Journal of Kidney Diseases 2007;5(50): 890-898.
[8] Scandling JD. Kidney Transplant Candidate Evaluation. Seminar Dialysis 2005;18(6): 487-494.

[9] Gill J, Bunnapradist S, Danovitch GM, et al. Outcomes of Kidney Transplantation From Older Living Donors to Older Recipients. American Journal of Kidney Diseases 2008;52: 541-552.
[10] Shah T, Bunnapradist S, Hutchinson I, et al. The Evolving Notion of "Senior" Kidney Transplant Recipients. Clinical Transplantation 2008;22: 794-802.
[11] Foote C, Ninomiya T, Gallagher M, et al. Survival of Elderly Dialysis Patients is Predicted by Both Patient and Practice Characteristics. Nephrology Dialysis Transplantation 2012 May [Epub ahead of print].
[12] Bunnapradist S, Danovitch GM. Kidney Transplants for the Elderly: Hope or Hype? Clinical Journal of American Society of Nephrology 2010;5: 1910-1911.
[13] Veroux M, Grosso G, Corona D, et al. Age is an Important Predictor of Kidney Transplantation Outcome. Nephrology Dialysis Transplantation 2012;27: 1663-1671.
[14] Tamura MK, Covinsky KE, Chertow GM, et al. Functional Status of Elderly Adults Before and After Initiation of Dialysis. New England Journal of Medicine 2009;361(16): 1539-1547.
[15] U.S. Renal Data System. USRDS 2008: Annual Data Report: Atlas of Chronic Kidney Disease and End-Stage Renal Disease in the United States. Bethesda, MD: National Institute of Diabetes and Digestive and Kidney Diseases, 2008.
[16] U.S. Renal Data System. USRDS 2009: Annual Data Report: Atlas of Chronic Kidney Disease and End-Stage Renal Disease in the United States. Bethesda, MD: National Institute of Diabetes and Digestive and Kidney Diseases, 2009.
[17] Schold JD, Meier-Kriesche HU. Which Renal Transplant Candidates Should Accept Marginal Kidneys in Exchange for a Shorter Waiting Time on Dialysis? Clinical Journal of American Society of Nephrology 2006;1: 532-538.
[18] Rao PS, Merion RM, Ashby VB, et al. Renal Transplantation in Elderly Patients Older Than 70 Years of Age: Results From the Scientific Registry of Transplant Recipients. Transplantation 2007;83: 1069-1074.
[19] Huang E, Poommipanit N, Sampaio MS, et al. Intermediate-Term Outcomes Associated with Kidney Transplantation in Recipients 80 Years and Older: An Analysis of the OPTN/UNOS Database. Transplantation 2010;90: 974-979.
[20] Kahn MR, Fallahi A, Kim MC, et al. Coronary Artery Disease in a Large Renal Transplant Population: Implications for Management. American Journal of Transplantation 2011;11: 2665-2674.
[21] El-Zoghby ZM, Stegall MD, Lager DJ, et al. Identifying Specific Causes of Kidney Allograft Loss. American Journal of Transplantation 2009;9: 527-535.
[22] Organ Procurement and Transplantation Network (OPTN) and Scientific Registry of Transplant Recipients (SRTR). OPTN/SRTR 2010 Annual Data Report. Department of Health and Human Services, Health Resources and Services Administration, Healthcare Systems Bureau, Division of Transplantation. American Journal of Transplantation 2012;12(Suppl 1): 22-23.
[23] Tapiawala SN, Tinckam KJ, Cardella CJ, et al. Delayed Graft Function and the Risk for Death with a Functioning Graft. Journal of American Society of Nephrology 2010;21:153-161.

[24] Cosio FG, Hickson LJ, Griffin MD, et al. Patient Survival and Cardiovascular Risk after Kidney Transplantation: The Challenge of Diabetes. American Journal of Transplantation 2008;8: 593-599.
[25] Ramanathan V, Goral S, Tanriover B, et al. Screening Asymptomatic Diabetic Patients for Coronary Artery Disease Prior to Renal Transplantation. Transplantation 2005;79: 1453-1458.
[26] Witczak BJ, Hartmann A, Jenssen T, et al. Routine Coronary Angiography in Diabetic Nephropathy Patients Before Transplantation. American Journal of Transplantation 2006;6: 2403-2408.
[27] Zlotnick DM, Axelrod DA, Chobanian MC, et al. Non-invasive Detection of Pulmonary Hypertension Prior to Renal Transplantation is a Predictor of Increased Risk for Early Graft Dysfunction. Nephrology Dialysis Transplantation 2010;25: 3090-3096.
[28] Issa N, Krowka M, Griffin M, et al. Pulmonary Hypertension is Associated with Reduced Patient Survival After Kidney Transplantation. Transplantation 2008;86: 1384-1388.
[29] Gaston RS, Danovitch GM, Adams PL, et al. The Report of a National Conference on the Wait List for Kidney Transplantation. American Journal of Transplantation 2003;3: 775-785.
[30] Engels EA, Pfeiffer RM, Fraumeni Jr JF, et al. Spectrum of Cancer Risk Among U.S. Solid Organ Transplant Recipients: The Transplant Cancer Match Study. Journal of American Medical Association 2011;306(17): 1891-1901.
[31] Tsai MK, Yang CY, Lee CY, et al. De novo Malignancy is Associated with Renal Transplant Tourism. Kidney International 2011;79: 908-913.
[32] Maisonneuve P, Agodoa L, Gellert R, et al. Cancer in Patients on Dialysis for End-Stage Renal Disease: An International Collaborative Study. The Lancet 1999;354: 93-98.
[33] Opelz G, Dohler B. Lymphomas After Solid Organ Transplantation: A Collaborative Transplant Study Report. American Journal of Transplantation 2003;4: 222-230.
[34] Sampaio MS, Cho YW, Bunnapradist S, et al. Impact of Epstein-Barr virus Donor and Recipient Serostatus on the Incidence of Post-Transplant Lymphoproliferative Disorder in Kidney Transplant Recipients. Nephrology Dialysis Transplantation 2012;27(7): 2971-2979.
[35] Naina HVK, Harris S, Dispenzieri A, et al. Long-Term Follow-Up of Patients with Monoclonal Gammopathy of Undetermined Significance after Kidney Transplantation. American Journal of Nephrology 2012;35: 365-371.
[36] Rama Ines, Grinyo JM. Malignancy After Renal Transplantation: The Role of Immunosuppression. Nature Reviews Nephrology 2010;6: 511-519.
[37] Zwald FO, Christenson LJ, Billingsley EM, et al. Melanoma in Solid Organ Transplant Recipients. American Journal of Transplantation 2010;10: 1297-1304.
[38] Ponticelli C, Glassock RJ. Posttransplant Recurrence of Primary Glomerulonephritis. Clinical Journal of American Society of Nephrology 2010;5: 2363-2372.
[39] Choy BY, Chan TM, Lai KN, et al. Recurrent Glomerulonephritis After Kidney Transplantation. American Journal of Transplantation 2006;6: 2535-2542.

[40] Pollak MR. The Genetic Basis of FSGS and Steroid-Resistant Nephrosis. Seminar in Nephrology 2003;23: 141–146.

[41] Bertelli R, Ginevri F, Caridi G et al. Recurrence of Focal Segmental merulosclerosis After Renal Transplantation in Patients with Mutations of Podocin. American Journal of Kidney Disease 2003;41: 1314-1321.

[42] Weber S, Gribouval O, Esquivel EL, et al. NPHS2 Mutation Analysis ws Genetic Heterogeneity of Steroid-Resistant Nephrotic Syndrome Low Post-Transplant Recurrence. Kidney International 2004;66: 571–579.

[43] Abbott KC, Sawyers ES, Oliver JD III, et al. Graft Loss Due to Recurrent Focal Segmental Glomerulosclerosis in Renal Transplant Recipients in the United States. American Journal of Kidney Disease 2001;237: 366-373.

[44] Krishnan N, Buchanan PM, Dzebisashvili N, et al. Monozygotic Transplantation: Concerns and Opportunities. American Journal of Transplantation 2008;8(11): 2343-2351.

[45] Cibrik DM, Kaplan B, Campbell DA, et al. Renal Allograft Survival in Transplant Recipients with Focal Segmental Glomerulosclerosis. American Journal of Transplantation 2003;3: 64–67.

[46] Savin VJ, Sharma R, Sharma M, et al. Circulating Factor Associated with Increased Glomerular Permeability to Albumin in Recurrent Focal Segmental Glomerulosclerosis. New England Journal of Medicine 1996;334: 878-883.

[47] Wei C, El Hindi S, Li J, et al. Circulating Urokinase Receptor as a Cause of Focal Segmental Glomerulosclerosis. Nature Medicine 2011;17(8): 952-960.

[48] Nozu K, Iijima K, Fujisawa M, et al. Rituximab Treatment for Posttransplant Lymphoproliferative Disorder (PTLD) Induces Complete Remission of Recurrent Nephrotic Syndrome. Pediatric Nephrology 2005;20: 1660–1663.

[49] Pescovitz M, Book BK, Sidner RA. Resolution of Recurrent Focal mental Glomerulosclerosis Proteinuria After Rituximab Treatment. England Journal of Medicine 2006;354: 1961–1963.

[50] Strologo LD, Guzzo I, Laurenzi C, et al. Use of Rituximab in Focal Glomerulosclerosis Relapses After Renal Transplantation. Transplantation 2009;88: 417-420.

[51] Fornoni A, Sageshima J, Wei C, et al. Rituximab Targets Podocytes in Recurrent Focal Segmental Glomerulosclerosis. Science Translational Medicine 2011;3(85): 85ra46.

[52] Vivarelli M, Pasini A, Emma F. Eculizumab for the Treatment of Dense-Deposit Disease. New England Journal of Medicine 2012;366(12): 1163-1165.

[53] Daina E, Noris M, Remuzzi G. Eculizumab in a Patient with Dense-Deposit Disease. New England Journal of Medicine 2012;366(12): 1161-1163.

[54] Radhakrishnan S, Lunn A, Kirschfink M, et al. Eculizumab and Refractory Membranoproliferative Glomerulonephritis. New England Journal of Medicine 2012;366(12): 1165-1166.

[55] McCaughan JA, O'Rourke DM, Courtney AE. Recurrent Dense Deposit Disease After Renal Transplantation: An Emerging Role for Complementary Therapies. American Journal of Transplantation 2012;12: 1046-1051.

[56] Stock PG, Barin B, Murphy B, et al. Outcomes of Kidney Transplantation in HIV-Infected Recipients. New England Journal of Medicine 2010;363(21): 2004-2014.
[57] Hirsch HH, Knowles W, Dickenmann M, et al. Prospective Study of Polyomavirus type BK Replication and Nephropathy in Renal-Transplant Recipients. New England Journal of Medicine 2002;347: 488-496.
[58] Womer KL, Meier-Kriesche HU, Patton PR, et al. Preemptive Retransplantation for BK Virus Nephropathy: Successful Outcome Despite Active Viremia. American Journal of Transplantation 2006;6: 209-213.
[59] Skauby MH, Oyen O, Hartman A, et al. Kidney Transplantation With and Without Simultaneous Bilateral Native Nephrectomy in Patients With Polycystic Kidney Disease: A Comparative Retrospective Study. Transplantation 2012 July [Epub ahead of print].
[60] Browne G, Brown PAJ, Tomson CRV et al. Retransplantation in Alport Post-Transplant Anti-GBM Disease. Kidney International 2004;65:675-681.
[61] Scornik JC, Schold JD, Bucci M, et al. Effects of Blood Transfusions Given After Renal Transplantation. Transplantation 2009;87:1381-1386.
[62] Eckel RH. Nonsurgical Management of Obesity in Adults. New England Journal of Medicine 2008;358: 1941-1950.
[63] Abbott KC, Glanton CW, Agodoa LY. Body Mass Index and Enrollment the Renal Transplant Waiting List in the United States. Journal of Nephrology 2003;16: 40-48.
[64] Weissenbacher A, Maximilian J, Ulmer H, et al. Recipient and Donor Body Mass Index as Important Risk Factors for Delayed Graft Function. Transplantation 2012;93: 524-529.
[65] Alexander JW, Goodman HR, Gersin K, et al. Gastric Bypass in Morbidly Obese Patients with Chronic Renal Failure and Kidney Transplant. Transplantation 2004;78: 469-474.
[66] Tait BD, Hudson F, Cantwell L, et al. Review Article: Luminex Technology for HLA Antibody Detection in Organ Transplantation. Nephrology 2009;14: 247-254.
[67] Tait BD, Hudson F, Brewin G, et al. Solid Phase HLA Antibody Detection Technology-Challenges in Interpretation. Tissue Antigens 2010;76: 87-95.
[68] Vo AA, Lukovsky M, Toyoda M, et al. Rituximab and Intravenous Immune Globulin for Desensitization During Renal Transplantation. New England Journal of Medicine 2008;359: 242-251.
[69] Montgomery RA, Warren DS, Segev DL, et al. HLA Incompatible Renal Transplantation. Current Opinion in Organ Transplantation 2012;17(4): 386-392.
[70] Canaud G, Bienaime F, Noel LH, et al. Severe Vascular Lesions and Poor Functional Outcome in Kidney Transplant Recipients with Lupus Anticoagulant Antibodies. American Journal of Transplantation 2010;10: 2051-2060.
[71] Webber A, Hambleton J, Chami A, et al. Mean Arterial Blood Pressure While Awaiting Kidney Transplantation Is Associated With the Risk of Primary Nonfunction. Transplantation 2012;93: 54-60.

[72] Andreoni KA, Brayman KL, Guidinger MK, et al. Kidney and Pancreas Transplantation in the United States, 1996-2005. American Journal of Transplantation 2007;7(Part 2): 1359-1375.
[73] Gruessner AC, Sutherland DER. Pancreas Transplant Outcomes For United States (US) and non-US Cases As Reported to the United Network for Organ Sharing (UNOS) and the International Pancreas Transplant Registry (IPTR) as of June 2004. Clinical Transplantation 2005;19: 433-455.
[74] Gruessner RW, Sutherland DE, Gruessner AC. Mortality Assessment for Pancreas Transplants. American Journal of Transplantation 2004;4: 2018- 2026.
[75] Hariharan S, Pirsch JD, Lu CY, et al. Pancreas After Kidney Transplantation. Journal of American Society of Nephrology 2002;13: 1109-1118.
[76] Afaneh C, Rich BS, Aull MJ, et al. Pancreas Transplantation: Does Age Increase Morbidity? Journal of Transplantation Epub 2011 June 4.
[77] Morath C, Zeier M, Dohler B, et al. Metabolic Control Improves Long-Term Renal Allograft and Patient Survival in Type I Diabetes. Journal of American Society of Nephrology 2008;19(8): 1557-1563.
[78] Dean PG, Kudva YC, Larson TS, et al. Posttransplant Diabetes Mellitus After Pancreas Transplantation. American Journal of Transplantation 2008;8: 175-182.
[79] Eason JD, Gonwa TA, Davis CL, et al. Proceedings of Consensus Conference on Simultaneous Liver Kidney Transplantation (SLK). American Journal of Transplantation 2008;8: 2243- 2251.
[80] Davis CL, Feng S, Sung R, et al. Simultaneous Liver-Kidney Transplantation: Evaluation to Decision Making. American Journal of Transplantation 2007;7: 1702-1709.
[81] Pichler R, Dittrich MO, Anderson AE et al. Prediction of Benefit From Simultaneous Liver–Kidney Transplantation versus Liver-Alone Transplantation: Potential Role for Native Kidney Biopsy. Journal of American Society of Nephrology 2006;17: 795A.
[82] Wadei HM, Geiger XJ, Cortese C, et al. Kidney Allocation to Liver Transplant Candidates with Renal Failure of Undetermined Etiology: Role of Percutaneous Renal Biopsy. American Journal of Transplantation 2008;8: 2618-2626.
[83] Goldfarb-Rumyantzev AS, Hurdle JF, Baird BC, et al. The Role of Pre-emptive Re-Transplant in Graft and Recipient Outcome. Nephrology Dialysis Transplant 2006;21:1355-1364.
[84] Lopez-Gomez JM, Perez-Flores I, Jofre R, et al. Presence of a Failed Kidney Transplant in Patients Who are on Hemodialysis Is Associated with Chronic Inflammatory State and Erythropoietin Resistance. Journal of American Society of Nephrology 2004;15: 2494-2501.
[85] Johnston O, Rose C, Landsberg D, et al. Nephrectomy After Transplant Failure: Current Practice and Outcomes. American Journal of Transplantation 2007;7: 1961-1967.
[86] Marrari M, Duquesnoy RJ. Detection of Donor-Specific HLA Antibodies Before and After Removal of a Rejected Kidney Transplant. Transplant Immunology 2010;22: 105-109.

[87] Organ Procurement and Transplantation Network (OPTN) and Scientific Registry of Transplant Recipients (SRTR). OPTN/SRTR 2010 Annual Data Report. Department of Health and Human Services, Health Resources and Services Administration, Healthcare Systems Bureau, Division of Transplantation. American Journal of Transplantation 2012;12(Suppl 1): 18-19.

Chapter 2

Evaluation of Potential Living Kidney Donors

Leila Kamal and David Serur

Additional information is available at the end of the chapter

http://dx.doi.org/10.5772/53682

1. Introduction

Renal transplantation is considered to be the treatment of choice for patients with ESRD. The incidence of ESRD is increasing, as a result of the increase in diabetes as well as other CKD causes. However the rise in ESRD is not matched by a rise in available kidneys for transplantation. As cadaveric kidneys have failed to meet the growing need for organs, attention has turned to organs from living donors [1].

2. History of living kidney donation and justification

2.1. First identical twin transplant

The first successful kidney transplant program was at The Peter Bent Brigham hospital in Boston. There, in December 1954, Dr. Joseph Murray performed the first successful kidney transplant between identical twins. The recipient's renal disease was presumably secondary to chronic glomerulonephritis. The opportunity of transplantation was suggested since the patient had a healthy twin brother. Cross skin grafting was performed between the 2 brothers and skin grafts survived for weeks establishing "genetic identity". Thirty days after the skin grafting, the transplant was performed; Dr. Hartwell Harrison removed the donor kidney, which was implanted in the recipient by Dr. Joseph Murray. The team performed seven more such transplants during the next four years. The patient died after eight years due to development of recurrent glomerulonephritis in the transplanted kidney [2-4].

2.2. Long-term survival of living kidney donor allografts

For recipients of a first deceased kidney in the United States, current 1-year patient and graft survival probabilities are about 95% and 88%, respectively. For recipients of a first living donor kidney, current 1-year patient and graft survival probabilities are 98% and 94%, respectively [5]. Improved immunosuppressive medications have decreased early acute rejection. However, despite the improved short term survival, graft survival half-lives have increased only very little, but are almost two-fold higher in recipients of living donors than those in patients receiving a transplant from a deceased donor (ten years for deceased donors versus 20 years for living donors).[6] The slow improvement in long term survival is related in part to chronic allograft nephropathy (CAN) as well as the nephrotoxic effect of calcineurin inhibitors. Stronger immunosuppressive regimens lead to increased incidence of malignancies and infections that may alter renal function. Immunosuppressive medications can also have unfavorable effects on blood pressure, glycemic control and lipid levels that may also lead to worsening renal function.

According to the UNOS renal transplant registry, estimated cadaveric graft half-lives were 7.9 years for the 1988-1989 (2- year) cohort, 9.2 years for the 1994-1995 cohort, and 11.6 years for the 1998-1999 cohort, despite the concurrent greater use of organs from older and less optimal deceased donors. Estimated living donor graft half-lives were 12.5 years for the 1988-1989 cohort, 15.8 years for the 1994-1995 cohort, and 19.3 years for the 1998-1999 cohort [7].

Graft survival in living transplants may be favorably affected by the relatively low delayed graft function rates (4 % vs. 24 % in cadaveric transplants) [8].

2.3. Insufficient supply of cadaveric allografts, Limiting waitlist time

As the incidence of ESRD is rising, kidney transplantation has failed to keep pace. Despite all the efforts to increase deceased kidney donation, there is still a shortage of deceased kidneys leading to increasing times on the waiting list. This implies increased workload for the transplantation centers, to ensure that patients on the waitlist remain fit enough to be able to receive a transplant [5]. Efforts have been made to use deceased organs that might have formerly not been used. Examples of this are the increased use of Expanded Criteria Donor (ECD) kidneys as well as use of donation after cardiac death (DCD) organs [6].

This organ shortage has also created a number of ethical and social dilemmas that vary across different countries of the world. The prevalence of kidney transplant from living donors varies widely around the globe. Factors such as the availability of deceased donors, the role of the government, the attitude of local physicians towards the risks of living donation, the level of awareness and education about ESRD and transplantation among the general population all affect the rates of donation. The proportion of kidney transplant from living kidney donors is less than 15 % in most European countries, except for the United Kingdom, where it has reached 47% in the last few years [9]. This proportion is only 3.3% in Finland, 8% in France, 12% in Belgium, compared to 49.5% in the USA [10]. In Spain, efficient identification of deceased renal donors has kept the waiting time short and living donors account for less than 5% of all kidney transplants. In Japan, social and cultural barriers have limited deceased donor transplantation and living donors account for 80% of kidney transplants [11]. In other countries like Egypt and Pakistan, living donor kidney transplant is the sole method of transplant available.

Transplantation increases the survival of patients with renal failure when compared to dialysis. One study of United States Renal Data System (USRDS) data compared outcomes in patients on the transplant waiting list (who were continuing to receive dialysis) versus those who had received a kidney transplant. It found that, after 3 to 4 years of follow-up, transplantation reduced the risk of death overall by 68 % [1]. Transplantation conferred a survival benefit in almost all subgroups. In addition, over the long term, it is more cost-efficient than dialysis. Thus, transplantation remains the optimal therapy for patients with ESRD [5].

3. Team approach to donor selection and evaluation

3.1. Medical

3.1.1. Amsterdam Forum Guidelines

In April 2004, renal transplant physicians and surgeons met in Amsterdam, The Netherlands, for the International Forum on the Care of the Live Kidney Donor. The participants included over 100 experts in transplantation from more than 40 countries [12]. The main purpose of this forum was to develop an international consensus on the standards of care for the living kidney donor and to emphasize the concern of the transplant community for the welfare of the donor. It also formed an alliance with the World Health Organization (WHO) to implement these standards of care, in continuation to the Madrid WHO conference on organ donation and transplantation that was held in October 2003. The forum emphasized the low operative risk of renal transplantation that has a perioperative mortality rate of 0.03% [13]. It also stressed the importance of long-term safety of this procedure noting the absence of accelerated loss of renal function and lack of appearance of hypertension in healthy donors post nephrectomy. The forum elaborated in detail about the acceptance criteria of donors with hypertension, obesity, dyslipidemia, low-normal renal function, hematuria, proteinuria, stone disease and other factors.

3.1.2. General medical evaluation and informed consent

The medical evaluation starts with a general assessment that includes a detailed history and physical examination, age appropriate medical screening, and a determination of contraindications to kidney donation such as active malignancy, active infection, transmissible conditions among other conditions that will be discussed in detail below.

Elements of the living donor evaluation vary across different transplant centers. Some of the major components of the general medical evaluation are outlined in table 1 [14].

Donor age:

Almost all transplant centers preclude individuals younger than 18 years old from donating and consider the age of 18–21 years as a relative contraindication to donation. Young donors with even what seems like mild or borderline risk factors should be evaluated more stringently as they have many years ahead of them to potentially develop medical conditions that may harm the remaining kidney such as diabetes and hypertension [14]. In fact, the OPTN (**Organ Procurement and Transplantation Network**) data showed that most

Blood group, HLA typing, crossmatch
Urinalysis and urine culture
24 hour urine collection for protein and creatinine clearance
CBC, Prothrombin time, Partial thromboplastin time
Comprehensive metabolic panel (electrolytes, albumin, alkaline phosphatase, transaminases, Calcium, phosphorus, bilirubin)
Infectious screen: HIV, hepatitis B and C, Epstein-Barr virus, cytomegalovirus, herpes simplex virus, RPR, tuberculosis (PPD, quantiferon) and if indicated, screen for toxoplasma, trypanosoma, malaria, West Nile.
Human chorionic gonadotropin quantitative pregnancy test in women younger than 55 years
Fasting blood glucose and lipid profile
Hemoglobin A1c, glucose tolerance test as clinically indicated
ECG, CXR
Echocardiography, cardiac stress testing if clinically indicated
Age appropriate cancer screening:
mammogram, pap smear for women
PSA for men
colonoscopy
Renal imaging: CT angiogram or Magnetic resonance angiogram

Table 1. Living donor medical evaluation [14]

of the donors who were later listed on the transplant list donated between the ages of 18 and 34 years and developed ESRD more than 15 years after donating [15]. In a 2007 survey of US transplant centers, 21% of the centers list the age of 65 as an upper limit to exclude donation, while 60% don't set an upper age limit for donation [16]. Donation from well selected older donors (>60 years old) appears to be safe and has good short and long term outcomes. Well selected older donors have no difference in perioperative outcomes when compared to younger donors [17,18].

Informed consent:

Living donor transplantation creates a conflict between the duty to do no harm and the duty to respect the donor's autonomy [19]. A fundamental part of the donor evaluation is informed consent. The elements of the informed consent process include a careful assessment of the donor's capacity to make medical decisions and understand the information provided. The donor should be informed in detail about:

- the different elements of the donor evaluation process
- the surgical procedure and the recovery period
- the potential medical or psychosocial risks to the donor
- the short and long-term follow-up care requirements
- the quality of life after donation
- the availability of alternative treatments for the transplant recipient
- the recipient's risks, recurrent disease, and chances for survival

- national and center-specific outcomes for recipients and living donors
- the possibility that the donor's medical evaluation could reveal conditions that the transplant program must report to governmental authorities, such as infection with the human immunodeficiency virus
- the possibility that future health problems related to the donation may not be covered by the donor's insurance and the ability to obtain health disability or life insurance may be affected
- the donor's right to opt out of donation at any time during the donation process.

(*adapted from The living donor advocate: a team approach to educate, evaluate, and manage donors across the continuum [20]*)

3.1.3. Hypertension

Hypertension (HTN) has been considered as a risk factor for chronic kidney disease (CKD). Screening for hypertension in a potential donor includes blood pressure (BP) measurement on three separate occasions [12]. Other experts advocate the use of ambulatory blood pressure monitoring (ABPM) [21].

Hypertension, defined by JNC7 as Systolic BP > 140 mm and/or Diastolic BP > 90 mm Hg or an average daytime blood pressure > 135/85 on ABPM, is a relative contraindication for renal transplantation. Most renal transplant centers exclude potential donors with BP greater than 140/90 by ABPM from donation. The prospective donor should have a mean awake BP less than 135/85 mm Hg and a BP less than 120/75 mm Hg when asleep.

On the other hand, the association of HTN with CKD has been argued in other studies. The RHEDY Study examined 1856 patients with primary HTN, with an average age of 47 years. Microalbuminuria and macroalbuminuria were detected, respectively, in 22.7 and 0.7% of the entire population. Systolic BP and abdominal obesity were two important determinants of microalbuminuria. However, only 5.2% of patients had simultaneously albuminuria and a reduced estimated GFR, implying a weak relation to one another [22].

Renal outcomes of kidney donors who were hypertensive at baseline were found to be favorable in some studies. Gil Thiel reported 18 donors who were hypertensive at the time of nephrectomy. The renal function, assessed by the creatinine clearance, of the 18 donors who were hypertensive at nephrectomy, was no different than the 75 normotensive donors [23]. In a report from Stegall from the Mayo clinic, 24 donors had hypertension, as defined by awake ABPM>135/85 mm Hg and/or office BP>140/90 mm Hg before donation. Hypertensive donors were older (53.4 vs. 41.4 years, P<.0001). The GFR (determined by iothalamate clearance) of the 24 hypertensive donors was not statistically different than 150 normotensive donors prior to nephrectomy or at 1 year postdonation. None of the subjects had albuminuria [24].

The following consensus guidelines regarding hypertensive donors were adopted at the Amsterdam Forum on the Care of the Live Kidney Donor [12]:

- Patients with a BP > 140/90 mmHg by ABPM are generally not acceptable as donors.

- BP should preferably be measured by ABPM, particularly among older donors (≥50 years and/or those with high office BP readings.
- Some patients with easily controlled hypertension who meet other defined criteria (e.g., >*50* years of age, GFR ≥ 80 mL/min/1.73m^2, and urinary albumin excretion < 30 mg/day) may represent a low-risk group for development of kidney disease after donation and may be acceptable as kidney donors.
- In cases with borderline high BP, and/or abnormalities suggesting cardiomegaly, or left ventricular hypertrophy on chest radiograph or electrocardiogram, an echocardiogram may be considered to evaluate for cardiac hypertrophy.

Patients with borderline BP and/or easily controlled hypertension can be considered for donation if they meet the following criteria [12]:

- more than 50 years of age
- not African American
- urine albumin excretion<30mg/day
- no signs of end organ damage
- GFR>80ml/min/1.73m^2

3.1.4. Nephrolithiasis

Nephrolithiasis affects 12% of the population and is increasing in prevalence [25]. The routine evaluation of kidney donor should include screening for kidney stones. The risk of kidney donation in a stone former includes the risk of stone recurrence and development of obstructive uropathy as well as urinary tract infections that may lead to worsening kidney function. Most stones are calcium containing stones, and carry a 50% recurrence risk at 5-10 years [26]. Patients with nephrolithiasis should be screened for metabolic abnormalities that predispose to stone formation.

Burgher et al conducted a retrospective evaluation of 300 male patients, 62.8 years old on average, who were followed for a mean of 3.26 years for asymptomatic renal calculi. Mean stone diameter was 10.8mm. 77% of patients experienced disease progression, with 26% requiring surgical intervention. Stone size, blood and urine uric acid level were associated with increased risk of growth. Small (<4mm), non uric acid, upper-pole calculi in patients with normal metabolic profile had the slowest progression [25].

After unilateral nephrectomy for pyelonephritis in patients with stone disease, the overall risk for stone recurrence is about 30% over a mean follow up of 5 years. In this study, the kidney function remained normal over the 5 year follow up period [27].

According to the Amsterdam forum,[12] an asymptomatic potential donor with history of a single stone may be suitable for kidney donation if:

- No hypercalcuria, hyperuricemia, metabolic acidosis, hypocitraturia, cystinuria or hyperoxaluria

- No urinary tract infection
- Multiple stones or nephrocalcinosis are not evident on computed tomography (CT) scan

Asymptomatic potential donor with *current single stone* may be suitable if [12]:

- The donor meets the criteria shown previously for single stone formers, and
- Current stone is <1.5 cm in size or potentially removable during transplant
- No evidence of nephrocalcinosis on imaging

Stone formers who should not donate are those with [12]:

- Nephrocalcinosis on X ray
- Multiple stone in one kidney or bilateral stone disease; and
- Stone types that have high recurrence rates and are difficult to prevent, such as:
    - Cystine stones that have a high rate of recurrence
    - Struvite stones or infection stones, which would be difficult to eradicate in an immunosuppressed host
    - Stones associated with inherited or other systemic disorders, such as primary or enteric hyperoxaluria, distal renal tubular acidosis, sarcoid and inflammatory bowel disease
    - Recurrence while on appropriate treatment

Spiral CT is the imaging technique of choice to detect stones or nephrocalcinosis. Age is an important clinical parameter that predicts recurrence since a stone detected in a person older than 50 years is unlikely to recur, whereas stone recurrence is higher in subjects aged 25-35 years [28].

3.1.5. Obesity

Obesity is defined by a BMI greater than 30kg/m^2. Obesity has been regarded as a risk factor for surgical complications, diabetes, glomerular disease (focal segmental glomerulosclerosis) with proteinuria, hypertension and ESRD in prospective living donors [29]. The relative risk for developing ESRD is threefold for a BMI between 30 and 35 kg/m^2 and nearly fivefold for a BMI of 35–40 kg/m^2 [30].

Obesity was shown to have a positive correlation with the development of proteinuria and renal insufficiency in patients who had previously undergone nephrectomy and who had normal renal function and no proteinuria at the time of the nephrectomy. Praga et al conducted a cross-sectional study in 73 patients who had undergone unilateral nephrectomy with normal kidney function at the time of nephrectomy. Indications for nephrectomy were stones, renal mass, pyelonephritis, hydronephrosis or tuberculosis. The group of patients who developed proteinuria and renal insufficiency at follow up had a mean BMI of 31 at the time of nephrectomy in comparison with a BMI of 24 in the group who did not have any proteinuria or renal insufficiency. The time elapsed between nephrectomy and onset of proteinuria was 10.1 +/- 6.1 years. The time elapsed between proteinuria appearance and the onset of renal insufficiency was 4.1 +/- 4.3 years [31].

On the other hand, a retrospective analysis of 553 kidneys donors showed that obese (BMI>35) vs. non obese (BMI<25) donors had a similar peri-operative complications except for more wound infections (9% vs. 94%) and longer operative time (mean increase 19 minutes) in the obese group. Both groups had similar GFR at 1 year and no blood pressure elevation or proteinuria at 1 year follow up [32].

About 50% of transplant centers in the USA exclude potential donors with BMI more than 35, and 10% exclude donors with BMI above 30kg/m^2 [26]. The Amsterdam Forum on the Care of the Live Kidney Donor [12] suggested that patients with a BMI > 35 kg/m^2 should be discouraged from donating, especially when other comorbid conditions are present and encouraged to adopt healthy lifestyle and to lose weight.

3.1.6. Diabetes

Diabetes Mellitus is defined as having fasting plasma glucose level of at least 126mg/dl or a plasma glucose level of at least 200mg/dl 2 hours after a 75 grams glucose challenge, confirmed by a repeat testing on a different day (see table 2).

	Prediabetes	**Diabetes**
Fasting plasma glucose (mg/dl)	100-125 (impaired fasting glucose: IFG)	≥ 126
2 hr plasma glucose after 75g glucose load (mg/dl)	140-199 (impaired glucose tolerance: IGT)	≥200
Hemoglobin A1c	5.7-6.4%	≥6.5%

Table 2. Diagnostic criteria for Diabetes and Prediabetes

All potential living donors should have a fasting plasma glucose testing. Those with fasting plasma glucose between 100 and 125 mg/dl and patients with risk factors for diabetes (BMI>30, parent or first degree relative with diabetes, history of gestational diabetes, delivery of large birth weight baby (>9lbs), BP>140/90, dyslipidemia, vascular disease, history of alcohol abuse, polycystic ovary syndrome, acanthosis nigricans), should have an oral glucose tolerance test (OGTT). Donors younger than 40 years old with a second-degree relative with type 2 diabetes should also undergo an OGTT [26].

Single kidney diabetic patients have higher proportion of albuminuria and lower GFR than single kidney non diabetic patients and diabetic patients with 2 kidneys [33]. Most transplantation centers regard established diabetes mellitus as a contraindication to living donation. According to International Amsterdam forum on living donor care, individuals with a history of diabetes or fasting blood glucose of ≥126 mg/dl on at least two occasions (or 2-h glucose with OGTT ≥ 200mg/dl) should be precluded from donating [12].

Prediabetes is viewed as a relative contraindication to living donation. Prospective donors with prediabetes (IFG, IGT) should be assessed on an individual basis. A study by Okamoto of 44 donors with impaired glucose tolerance concluded that these patients had equal survival compared to a non-diabetic cohort at 5, 10, and 20 years. None of these prediabetic donors had chronic kidney disease or required diabetic medications at mean follow-up point of 7 years [34]. Individuals with prediabetes should be counseled about lifestyle modifications, healthy diet, exercise, and smoking cessation. They should be counseled about the risk of progression to overt diabetes. Experts recommend against donation in patients who have impaired glucose tolerance and additional risk factors, as listed above. Patients with impaired fasting glucose in the high range have a high risk of progression to diabetes and are discouraged from donation.

3.1.7. Inheritable diseases

When evaluating related living donors, special attention should be given to evaluate for potential inherited renal diseases. An extensive family history of renal disease manifestations, as well as extrarenal manifestations, namely hearing and ocular abnormalities and biopsy documentation of recipient's renal disease provide critical information in the decision-making process of kidney donation [35].

APKD

Autosomal dominant polycystic kidney disease (ADPKD) is the most common hereditary renal disease, occurring in 1 in 400–1,000 live births, and accounting for more than 5% of cases of ESRD in Europe and North America. 85 % of the cases are secondary to a mutation in PKD1 gene on chromosome 16, which encodes polycystin1 and progress to ESRD at a mean age of 54 years. The remaining 15% of the cases are caused by a mutation in PKD2 gene, located on chromosome 4, that encodes for polycystin 2 and manifest with ESRD at the age of 74 [36].

The diagnosis of ADPKD is made based on age-specific criteria. In families of unknown genotype, the presence of 3 or more (unilateral or bilateral) renal cysts is sufficient for establishing the diagnosis in individuals aged 15 to 39 years, two or more cysts in each kidney is sufficient for individuals aged 40 to 59 years, and four or more cysts in each kidney is required for individuals ≥60 years. Conversely, fewer than two renal cysts in at-risk individuals aged ≥40 years are sufficient to exclude the disease [37].

In at risk individuals aged more than 30 years, absence of cysts by ultrasound excludes diagnosis of ADPKD in 98% of cases. In at risk individuals less than 30 years, a negative ultrasound does not rule out the disease; more sensitive imaging is needed such as CT Scanning and T2 weighted MRI which are more sensitive in detecting small cysts (<2-3mm). In potential donors aged <30 years, a negative renal ultrasound scan does not exclude type 2 ADPKD; however, a negative renal ultrasound scan and a negative CT scan may be adequate to exclude type 1 ADPKD in such donors [35]. When results of imaging are equivocal, genetic testing is available. This includes linkage analysis and gene sequencing. Linkage analysis requires multiple affected and unaffected family members. However, in clinical practice, it is difficult to elucidate an extensive family history of ADPKD. In that case, direct PKD gene sequence analysis would be required and is the most commonly used genetic testing. Because of the high prevalence of polymorphisms, the diagnosis is established unequivocally by gene sequencing in only about 40–60% of all cases [38].

The failure to confirm or exclude the diagnosis of ADPKD has broad implications for both the donor and recipient, especially when the prospective donor is a young family member, in whom ultrasonography is less likely to be helpful. Huang et al [39] attempted to provide a diagnostic strategy that is based on genetic testing of live kidney donors at 50% risk for ADPKD in whom renal imaging studies are inconclusive. First, if genetic linkage analysis is not feasible, then the prospective recipient undergoes PKD gene sequencing. If a PKD gene mutation is identified then directed genetic testing of the donor is done. A donor is ineligible if the genetic test is positive. If the mutation is not found in the donor, then the diagnosis of ADPKD is excluded and transplantation can proceed. If the recipient's genetic test is indeterminate, then genotyping of the donor is not performed and donation is deferred. This strategy is likely to increase the number of renal transplants from living related donors who would otherwise have been excluded by their indeterminate renal imaging. It can also uncover undiagnosed ADPKD. On the other hand, the diagnostic sensitivity of direct sequencing is relatively low, especially for the PKD1 gene, because it is highly polymorphic. The test is expensive and adds to the cost of pretransplant evaluation. In summary, living donation is contraindicated in potential donors aged <30 years old for whom imaging techniques do not show cysts but for whom genetic tests show positive results for mutated PKD genes, although no data exist on the risk of ESRD in such individuals [35]. It is considered safe to proceed with kidney donation if imaging studies and genetic studies exclude ADPKD.

Alport's syndrome

In approximately 85% of patients, Alport syndrome is inherited as an X linked disease and is caused by mutations in the COL4A5 gene, which encodes the α5 chain of type IV collagen. De novo mutations occur in 10% of cases of X linked Alport syndrome. In 15% of the cases, the transmission is autosomal recessive, and is caused by mutations affecting COL4A3 or COL4A4 located on chromosome 2. The autosomal dominant form of Alport syndrome is very rare and is caused by heterozygous mutations in COL4A3 or COL4A4 genes. Affected individuals can also have sensironeural hearing loss and ocular abnormalities. Sensorineural hearing loss is the most common extrarenal manifestation and the progression of hearing loss often parallels the progression of renal disease. Anterior lenticonus, a conical protrusion of the lens in the anterior chamber, develops progressively and mainly occurs in male patients. The most common renal manifestation is hematuria.

Prospective donors with a family history of Alport's should be assessed by a urinalysis, estimation of glomerular filtration rate, a vision test and a hearing test. Male siblings aged >20 years without hematuria are very unlikely to have the disease and are suitable donors. Sisters of affected male recipients with X linked disease have a 50% risk of being carriers, unless the disease in the brother is caused by a neomutation. Gross et al reported the long term outcomes of six heterozygous mothers with microhematuria who had donated a kidney to their affected children. Three of the women developed new onset hypertension and two developed proteinuria over a mean follow up time of 6.7 years. Renal function declined significantly in four of the donors [40]. A female relative without hematuria, has a low risk for being a carrier and is a suitable donor. Female relatives with proteinuria should be excluded from donation. Female relatives with persistent microhematuria are most likely carriers. Up to 25% of female carriers of X-linked Alport mutations develop renal failure and they should not donate [41]. Genetic analysis of COL4A5 genotype is not useful for determining the suitability of women for kidney donation given the absence of correlation between the genotype and the phenotype in women [35].

Thin Basement Membrane Disease

Thin basement membrane disease (TBMD) affects around 1% of the general population. Approximately 50% of patients have a heterozygous mutation in COL4A3 or COL4A4 genes. Although the long term prognosis of the majority of patients with thin basement membrane nephropathy is excellent, some patients develop proteinuria and progressive renal failure, especially those with documented heterozygous mutations in COL4A3 or COL4A4 genes [35]. The clinical course of TBMD is generally benign. However, the duration of most longitudinal studies has been too short to reflect prognosis. One study reported that 7% of patients with biopsy-proven TBMD had renal dysfunction with a serum creatinine level greater than 1.2mg/dl. Risk factors for progression are proteinuria, hypertension and abnormal renal function [42]. Other coexistent glomerular lesions, found in about 5% of patients with TBMN, namely IgA nephropathy, amongst others, can explain the abnormal renal function in these patients [43].

Donation from patients with TBMD remains controversial, given the lack of long term studies that address the outcomes of kidney donation in these patients. Patients with hypertension, proteinuria, or abnormal kidney function should not donate. Careful assessment of the potential donor's family history and extrarenal manifestations of Alport syndrome should be done. Patients with isolated glomerular hematuria must be assessed thoroughly for atypical features and, when these are present, a renal biopsy is advised to detect possible Alport syndrome and any other disease such as IgA glomerulonephritis. A kidney biopsy, however, might not distinguish between TBMD and early Alport's syndrome [44]. Atypical features include episodic gross hematuria that is uncommon in TBMD, but common in IgA nephropathy and Alport's. A family history of renal failure is common in IgA nephropathy and Alport's but not in TBMD [45]. Prospective donors should be counseled that, although TBMD has a benign course in general, renal failure may occur and long term risks remain unknown.

Systemic lupus erythematosus (SLE)

SLE occurs in about 12% of first degree relatives of patients with SLE. Prospective donors should be screened for ANA (antinuclear antibody), complement levels and abnormal urinary findings. Antiphosholipd antibody testing is suggested if the medical history is positive for deep vein thrombosis, stroke, pulmonary embolism, fetal loss, thrombocytopenia, hemolytic anemia, or livedo reticularis. Family member of a patient with SLE who has a positive ANA has a 40 fold increased risk of SLE and should not donate [45].

3.2. Evaluation of renal function

3.2.1. Glomerular Filtration Rate (GFR)

The most common approach to estimating GFR is with a 24-hour urine for creatinine clearance. This is the method used by approximately 90% of transplant centers in US, with the remaining programs using a radioactive isotope or iodinated tracer [16]. Creatinine based estimation equations are not reliable in the donor population, who have normal kidney function and should not be used. However, inadequate collection, low protein diet, low muscle mass and other factors may lead to low creatinine clearances in those with actually normal kidney function. Radionuclide methods, including iodine 124-iothalamate or technetium 99m-diethylenetriamine are used if the 24-hour creatinine clearance is borderline. The general cutoff for most centers is GFR of 80 mL/min/1.73 m^2, although as many as 20% of U.S. transplant centers would accept a creatinine clearance as low as 60 ml/min/1.73m^2 [12]. Some centers take into account the normal decline in GFR with aging at a rate of 4-5ml/min/1.73m^2 per decade of life starting the age of 20, allowing for kidney donation at lower limits of GFR.

3.2.2. Proteinuria

Proteinuria should be assessed with a 24-hour urine collection. Spot urine protein to creatinine ratio may underestimate the level of proteinuria. Most programs use protein>300 mg/day in a 24-hour urine collection as the cutoff to exclude donation [12,16]. Special attention should be made to transient causes of proteinuria, such as fever, urinary tract infections and exercise. When abnormal, the collection should be repeated to confirm the persistence of proteinuria.

3.2.3. Hematuria

Urinalysis is indicated in all prospective donors. Microscopic hematuria, defined as more than 3-5 RBC/HPF, needs further evaluation. Menstruation in premenopausal women should be ruled out as well as urinary tract infection. Persistent hematuria, confirmed on more than one urinalysis, deserves more investigation. Medical history should look carefully for a family history of TBMD, Alport's, ADPKD. The concomitant presence of proteinuria or RBC casts or dysmorphic RBCs is suggestive of underlying glomerular disease. Patients with persistent isolated hematuria should have urine cytology and urological workup including cystoscopy. They should also be screened for nephrolithiasis by a CT urogram (routinely performed as part of CT angiogram; discussed next). African American patients should be screened for sickle cell disease. In the absence of any specific abnormalities, a kidney biopsy may be indicated looking for Alport's, IgA nephropathy, among other pathologies [12,46]. If a full evaluation for persistent isolated hematuria is negative, most centers proceed with donation, since the risk for progressive renal disease is small. However, a survey of US transplant centers showed that 21% of programs automatically exclude potential donors with greater than 10 RBC/HPF, regardless of work-up [16].

3.2.4. Pyuria

In the presence of pyuria, urinary tract infections and prostatitis in men should be ruled out. If pyuria is persistent, renal tuberculosis should be ruled out with 3 morning urine acid-fast bacilli cultures. If these tests are negative, a renal biopsy should be considered to rule out interstitial nephritis or chronic pyelonephritis. Donation is contraindicated if there is evidence of renal tuberculosis, or interstitial nephritis or pyelonephritis [45].

3.3. Radiologic Evaluation of potential allografts

CT-based imaging is routinely used to evaluate the potential donor's anatomy. The 64 slice multidetector CT (MDCT) urogram and angiogram has become the gold standard imaging technique and has replaced the traditional arteriography and intravenous urography.

MDCT can provide assessment of the renal vein and artery, ureteral structure, renal parenchymal lesions, renal cystic diseases, stones, and surrounding anatomic variant. In addition, MDCT can measure kidney volume, a more sensitive index of size than length as available from sonography [47].

The left kidney is preferred for laparoscopic living donor nephrectomy because of its relative technical ease of removal and flexibility afforded by the longer left venous pedicle. MDCT permits detection of vascular abnormalities and variants. A right donor nephrectomy may be performed if complex vascular anatomy (e.g., multiple arteries or veins) is present in the left kidney. Preoperative imaging also helps identify the lower quality kidney (i.e., with incidental findings such as a small stone or hemorrhagic cyst), which is usually chosen in living donor transplantation [48].

MDCT detects asymmetry in the size of the kidneys, in which case a renal scan (MAG3) may be needed and the lower functioning kidney would be chosen for donation. The urogram phase of MDCT can delineate the presence of stones and abnormalities in the collecting system, such as ureteral diverticulum, calyceal diverticulum, hydronephrosis and ureteropelvic junction obstruction, ureteral duplication that may alter the surgical approach. Up to 30% of kidneys evaluated by MDCT have incidental renal finding such as renal cysts or calyceal calcifications. Patients with multiple stones, large single stone (>1.5cm), nephrocalcinosis or medullary sponge kidney are excluded from donation. [26,45] MDCT can also detect the amount of perirenal fat. This information is useful to determine if donors with higher BMI are amenable to a laparoscopic nephrectomy [26].

Donation is usually contraindicated if the following are present [45]:

- parenchymal abnormalities, including significant unilateral atrophy, or horseshoe kidney, presence of 2 or 3 cysts in each kidneys or complex or septated cyts, or angiomyolipoma
- vascular abnormalities: significant atherosclerotic disease, fibromuscular dysplasia

Compared to MRI/MRA, MDCT has greater accuracy, is faster, and more cost effective. MRA has inferior resolution in evaluating the renal vein anatomy. It is useful in patients with iodinated contrast allergy [49].

3.4. Surgical evaluation

3.4.1. Workup and evaluation

Potential donors should have a careful assessment of their perioperative risk for cardiovascular and pulmonary complications as well as thrombotic complications.

Unstable coronary syndromes, decompensated heart failure, significant arrhythmias and severe valvular disease are contraindications to live kidney donation. Most of the intermediate predictors (mild angina, previous myocardial infarction, compensated or prior heart failure, diabetes mellitus) are also contraindications to donation. Other, minor predictors warrant further testing [12]. Cardiovascular testing includes a transthoracic echocardiography if the history is positive for chest pain, palpitations, dizziness, syncope or SOB and/or the physical exam reveal a murmur.

A holter monitoring is indicated if history of arrhythmia, syncope, dizziness, or palpitations. Some transplant centers perform cardiac stress testing in prospective donors if they have one or more risk factors for coronary artery disease (age> 45 years old in men, and more than 55 in women, family history of premature coronary artery disease, hypertension, smoking).[26,45] However, the American College of Cardiology and the American Heart Association (ACC/AHA) guidelines published in 2007, recommended stress testing only in high risk patients with poor functional capacity, who are scheduled for vascular surgery and only when such testing would change the management [50]. In most instances, when evaluating prospective donors, cardiac stress testing does not appear to be indicated.

Pulmonary function testing (PFT)

Pulmonary function testing (PFT) is not routinely indicated unless the history and physical examination suggest lung disease, in which case further testing, including PFT is indicated. Moderate to severe pulmonary disease is a contraindication to living donation (Forced expiratory volume (FEV1) or forced vital capacity (FVC) less than 70% of predicted or FEV1: FVC ratio less than 65% on PFTs). Patients with asthma who are well controlled, and with a peak flow measurement less than 80% predicted, can be considered on an individual basis for live kidney donation [51].

Smoking cessation

Smokers have a higher risk of pulmonary and wound infections after surgery than nonsmokers. Observational evidence suggests a benefit to smoking cessation before surgery [52]. Abstinence of smoking for only 12 hours can greatly reduce carboxyhemoglobin concentrations, improve oxygen content and reverse negative inotropic and arrhythmic effects. Polycythemia and increased blood viscosity take a few days to reverse. Sputum production declines 6 weeks after smoking cessation. Amsterdam forum guidelines recommend smoking cessation at least 4 weeks prior to donation.

Alcohol abstinence

An increase in postoperative morbidity is reported for alcohol abusers who drink at least five drinks (more than 60 g ethanol) a day. Observational evidence in other clinical suggest that alcohol withdrawal is recommended for at least 1 month before surgery [53].

Hypercoagulability

Persons with personal history of one or more venous thrombosis or recurrent miscarriage or with a family history of thrombotic disease should be screened for hypercoagulable disorders. These include activated protein C resistance associated with factor V Leiden mutation, lupus anticoagulant, anticardioplin antibody, prothrombin gene mutation (FII-20210), hyperhomocystenemia. Factor V-Leiden is the most common hereditary blood coagulation disorder, present in 3–8% of the healthy white population [54]. The odds ratio of a venous thrombolic event is 11 times greater in women taking oral contraceptives who have the Factor V Leiden mutation than for those who do not [55]. Some experts suggest that oral contraceptives and hormone replacement therapy should be withheld for 3 months prior to an elective surgery, given the high incidence of factor V Leiden in the population. A history of thrombotic disorders and presence of risk factors for future events (such as lupus anticoagulant, anticardiolipin antibody, abnormal activated protein C resistance ratio) as well as disorders requiring chronic anticoagulation are contraindications for kidney donation. However, a person with heterozygous factor V leiden mutation and without previous thrombotic episodes is not necessarily excluded from donation [12,26,45].

3.5. Psychosocial evaluation

Every prospective donor should undergo a psychosocial evaluation. This evaluation is especially important for unrelated donation. The psychiatric evaluation should be performed by a psychiatrist or mental health professional who has no personal and clinical relationship with the recipient. The evaluation should address the protection of donor's confidentiality and should be performed in the absence of the recipient or recipient's advocates. If translation is needed, translators should be unknown to recipient and donor.

The evaluation would start by obtaining standard background information, such as donor's educational level, living situation, religious beliefs, cultural background, and employment history.

- The main elements of the psychosocial evaluation include the following:
- The donor's ability to make a decision should be assessed carefully, by evaluating for any underlying psychiatric disorders and any history of substance abuse. The donor should demonstrate a full capacity to give informed consent.
- The evaluation should assess the donor's accurate knowledge of recipient's health benefits, and the accurate understanding of the donation process, and its physical and

mental consequences, including short term surgical complications and long term effects of donation on health outcomes.

- The evaluation process should explore the nature of the relationship of the donor with the recipient, if any, and whether the donation was imposed by some expectations or perceived obligations on the part of either the donor or the recipient.
- The evaluation should assess the donor's motivation and inform the donor about the available option of not donating and the other treatment options available for the recipient. The prospective donor's rationale and reasoning for donating should be explored. The evaluation should exclude coercion, secondary gain (monetary or other personal gain, such as stabilizing self-image or dealing with a psychological conflict).
- The interview should inquire about the employment status of the donor and the availability of family support resources during the operative recovery period. The donor should have adequate financial and social support.
- The outcomes of transplantation should be explored, these include increased self-esteem after a successful transplantation and resentment and depression after an unsuccessful transplantation. In case of altruistic donation, the donor may experience depression because s/he may not witness and enjoy the positive outcome of the donation [45,56,57].

The major psychosocial contraindications for live donation include [57]:

- active psychiatric illness or substance use
- the presence of major financial stressors that could either have a coercive effect on the donor's decision to donate, or interfere with the need for medical care after donation
- evidence that the prospective donor has experienced pressure or coercion from others to donate
- a limited understanding or capacity to understand the donor's or the recipient's risks and benefits from kidney donation
- ambivalence about proceeding with the donation

3.5.1. Financial aspects

The economic impact of donation should be discussed with the prospective donor. The medical expenses are usually covered by the recipient's insurance, or, in certain circumstances, by the Transplant Centers Organ Acquisition Fund. The expenses include:

- the donor evaluation
- the actual donation surgery
- the post operative care

Other non medical expenses such as travel and lodging expenses are not covered by the recipient's insurance.

The act of donation should not preclude the donor from obtaining medical insurance or increase the cost of insurance [45]. In the USA, the organ donor leave act was created in 1999 and entitles the donor for 30 days of paid leave (Organ Donor Leave Act of 1999). However, it is recommended that the prospective donor obtain health and life insurance prior to donation.

The donor should be financially stable and free of financial hardship. The evaluation should explore the ability of the donor to cover financial obligations for expected and unexpected donation-related expenses. The donor should be able to afford time away from work mainly for unplanned extended recovery time [56].

Paid donation

Despite the legal constraints, paid donation and commercialism are common in many parts of the world. In the USA, the Uniform Anatomical Gift Act was created in 1968 in order to establish an ethical system that regulated the availability of organs for transplantation. Further advances were made in 1984 by the National Organ Transplant Act, which established the nationwide computer registry operated by the United Network for Organ Sharing. The same act prohibits buying or selling of organs in the United States. Similar laws have been enacted in other countries around the world. The Declaration of Istanbul on Organ Trafficking and Transplant Tourism strictly condemns all forms of organ trade [58]. It should be mentioned that other experts argue that the donors should be allowed to have monetary compensation and that the donors are entitled to use their bodies as they see fit. To address this issue and the concern of the short supply of kidneys available for donation, a regulated system of living unrelated paid donor kidney transplantation was legally adopted in Iran in 1988 [59]. However, most of the donors are poor and uneducated and follow up studies have shown that their lives have not improved after compensation for donation. Several types of regulated models offering indirect incentives or compensation for organ donations, such as health insurance, life insurance, disability coverage, or social benefits, have been proposed to encourage organ donations in developed countries [60]. Paid donation carries significant risks of exploitation of the poor. It poses significant health risks both for the donor and the recipient, including infectious complications, as well as other surgical and medical complications that, in part, are due to poor donor screening and evaluation [61].

4. Risks to donor

4.1. Surgical complications

Open nephrectomy is now largely replaced by laparoscopic surgical techniques that account for more than 50% of donor nephrectomy procedures in the USA [62]. Compared to open nephrectomy, laparoscopic procedure provides shorter hospital stays (2 to 4 days compared with 3 to 7 days), less incisional discomfort, minimal surgical scar and better cosmetic appearance and an earlier return to work (12 to 21 days compared with 30 to 60 days) [63].

Traditionally, laparoscopic nephrectomy (LN) is performed through 3 to 5 small incisions and has become the standard of care in most academic centers. Newer techniques are available; these include single port technique that has been shown to improve cosmetic results and lead to faster recovery [64-66].

Other new techniques include robotic assisted laparoscopic nephrectomy that allows the surgeon to dissect more meticulously and prevent bleeding more easily, along with shorter hospital stays [67].

Conversion to open nephrectomy occurs in approximately 2% of procedures [63]. The perioperative mortality reported for living kidney donors including both open and laparoscopic methods is 0.03% [13,62], although in a recent survey, all reported deaths were after laparoscopic nephrectomy [68].

The risk of perioperative and postoperative complications from unilateral laparoscopic nephrectomy is 10-15% [69]. These include, but are not limited to, bleeding, infection, bowel injury, hernia, and postanaesthesia depression.

Matas at al [68] surveyed 234 kidney transplant programs to determine living donor morbidity and mortality for open nephrectomy, hand-assisted LN, and non-hand-assisted LN between 1999 and 2001:

- 52% of nephrectomies were done by open procedure, 21 % by hand-assisted Laparoscopic nephrectomy, and 27% via non-hand-assisted LN
- 2 donors (0.02%) died from surgical complications, both after laparoscopic nephrectomy
- Reoperation was necessary in 0.4% of the open cases, 1.0% of the hand-assisted LN cases, and 0.9% of the non-hand-assisted LN cases
- Complications not requiring reoperation were reported in 0.3% -1% of the cases without statistical difference between the groups
- Readmission rate was higher for LN (1.6%) vs. open (0.6%) donors, mainly secondary to gastrointestinal symptoms, (nausea, vomiting, ileus, constipation)

With more experience, the reported complications of laparoscopic nephrectomy have decreased, after an initial steep learning curve. The morbidity of the laparoscopic procedure has decreased with more experience, and the mortality rate remains low.

A 2008 meta-analysis evaluated 73 studies that included 3751 and 2843 patients who had undergone laparoscopic surgery and open nephrectomy, respectively. Compared with open nephrectomy, the laparoscopic surgery group had a significantly shorter hospital stay and a quicker recovery. Both groups had similar rates of delayed allograft function and allograft loss [70].

While operative time is longer in laparoscopic nephrectomy (3-4 hours versus 2-3 hours in open nephrectomy), both procedures have similar recipient outcomes, graft function, rejection rate and graft survival [70,71].

4.2. Life expectancy

The survival of donors appears to be similar to that of the controls in the general population [8]. A Swedish study analyzed survival of 430 living donors. After 20 years of follow-up, 85% of donors were alive, whereas the expected survival rate was 66%. The better survival among donors is likely due to the selection process involved in donor work-up. Patients with health issues are ruled out. Mortality pattern was similar to that in the general population, the most common causes of death being cardiovascular diseases and cancer [72].

4.3. Likelihood of renal disease in donor

4.3.1. Renal function and proteinuria

Unilateral nephrectomy is followed by a compensatory increase in the GFR in the remaining kidney to achieve about 70%-80% of prenephrectomy GFR within days to weeks after nephrectomy. Some proposed that the degree of compensation may be better in younger patients [73]. The detrimental effect of kidney hyperfiltration and hypertrophy are more pronounced when nephron number is reduced in infancy than when nephron number is reduced later in life [74]. This has been shown in many studies, including the study of 56 world war II soldiers, who had a unilateral nephrectomy at an average age of 25 years old, and who were reassessed 45 years following nephrectomy and compared to veterans with 2 kidneys. Mortality, prevalence of HTN and proteinuria were equal in both groups. 10 subjects had autopsy examinations and glomerular sclerosis was not increased [75].

Studies examining renal outcome in donors are heterogeneous and frequently lack a control group. However, long term follow up studies, more than 30 years after nephrectomy, did not show an accelerated decline of renal function. The decline in renal function seemed to parallel the age related decline of healthy individuals with 2 kidneys.

A study of 3,698 kidney donors from 1963 through 2007 showed that mortality of kidney donors was comparable to the general population. From 2003 till 2007, kidney function of 255 donors was assessed by iohexol clearance and urinary albumin to creatinine ratio. The mortality was comparable to the general population. 85.5% of the donors had an iohexol GFR >60 mL/min/1.73 m^2. Hypertension was noted in 32% of the donors, albuminuria (defined as urine albumin/creat ratio above 0.02) in 12.7%, and none of the donors with albuminuria had an iohexol GFR lower than 45 ml per minute per 1.73 m^2. Importantly, the prevalence of hypertension and albuminuria in kidney donors were similar to those in controls who were matched for age, sex, race or ethnic group, and body-mass index. There was no excess risk of ESRD in donors. Factors linked to a reduced GFR in donors are the same as those that have been observed in the general population, namely, age and obesity [8].

In this study, a longer time since donation, however, was independently associated with albuminuria. This may be attributable to single nephron hyperfiltration, secondary to reduced renal mass but does not seem to be associated with higher risk of renal dysfunction.

In a review that summarizes 48 studies that included a total of 5000 donors on average, kidney donation resulted in small increases in urinary albumin, which increased with the time after donation (three studies totaling 59 controls and 129 donors; controls 83mg/day, donors 147mg/day, weighted mean difference 66mg/day, 95% confidence interval (CI) 24–108) [76]. Whether the hyperfiltration injury that is reflected by the albuminuria leads to a progressive deterioration in kidney function has been the subject of many debates.

In this same review, after an average of 7 years after donation, the average 24 h urine protein was 154 mg/day and the average GFR was 86 ml/min. Ten years after nephrectomy, donors had a GFR that was 10 ml/ min lower compared to controls. In addition approximately 12% of donors developed a GFR less than 60 ml/min during follow-up. However, after the initial decrement in GFR from the nephrectomy, there was no evidence of an accelerated loss in GFR over that anticipated with normal aging [76].

4.3.2. Hypertension

Although some studies show that the prevalence of HTN among donors is identical to that observed in the general population [77], other studies did reveal that the incidence of hypertension increases after kidney donation [78,79].

However, in most of these studies, this increase in arterial pressure is statistically significant but clinically irrelevant and most of the donors do not reach values to be considered as hypertensive [80]. In a metanalysis done by Boudville et al [79] in 2006, the authors described an increase of 5 mmHg in the 5–10 years following the kidney donation.

However, racial disparities should be taken into account as it has been suggested recently that non-Caucasian donors could have a higher risk of HTN. This has been shown in a retrospective analysis of the prevalence of Diabetes, HTN and CKD among 4650 donors compared to the prevalence patterns in the 2005-2006 National Health and Nutrition Examination Survey (NHANES) for the general population. Compared to white donors, AA and hispanic donors were found to have increased risk of HTN, diabetes and CKD. The absolute prevalence of diabetes among all donors did not exceed that in the general population, but the prevalence of hypertension exceeded NHANES estimates in some subgroups. End-stage renal disease was identified in less than 1% of donors but was more common among black donors than among white donors [81]. These findings emphasize the importance of increased attention to health outcomes among demographically different donors and the need for close medical follow up.

4.4. The need for transplantation of previous living kidney donors

The UNOS database has recorded since 1987 an incidence of about 0.04% of living donors who have been listed for kidney transplantation, similar to the 0.03% incidence in the general US population. In the follow up study by Ibrahim et al of 3698 donors, 11 donors developed ESRD, at a rate of 180 cases per million per year, compared to the rate of 268 per million persons per year in the white population in USA. Three of the 11 donors had the same cause of ESRD as their sibling recipients, suggesting unrecognized familial renal disease or risk factors.

Upon review of the OPTN (Organ Procurement and Transplantation Network) database, as of February 2002, a total of 56 previous living donors have been identified as having been listed for deceased donor kidney transplant. The majority of these patients originally donated a kidney to a sibling (86%); five patients donated to a parent, and three patients donated to a child, highlighting again the possible role of unrecognized familial risk factors for kidney disease [82].

According to the UNOS/OPTN database between 1993 and 2005, African-Americans constitute 40% of the donors on the waiting list for transplant, although they represent only 14% of the whole living kidney donor population, emphasizing the fact that AA might be at greater risk for ESRD after kidney donation [15].

The Amsterdam forum proposed the current UNOS policy for live kidney donors that assigns an allocation priority for a deceased donor kidney if the previous live kidney donor subsequently become a candidate for a kidney transplant later in life. However, there was no consensus to develop such a policy internationally [12].

5. Non directed donation

As of January 2009, biologically unrelated donors constituted about 40% of the living donors in the USA. Most of these donors were emotionally related and have an apparent, strong and deep relationship with the recipient (spouse, close friend, significant other, adopted sibling). Prospective donors with a much more casual relationship with the recipient (coworkers, members of faith community) or with little or no relationship to donors (solicited through internet, media…) are becoming increasingly common and about half of unrelated donors fall into this category.

Non directed donors, also called altruistic donors, or 'Good Samaritan Donors' donate their kidney to a completely unknown recipient, whom the donor might never meet. They represent about 1.5% of all living donors in the USA as of January 2009. This practice is not allowed in some countries in Europe and South America because of the fear that the donor might be selling his/her kidney.

Generally, the recipient is a patient on the deceased donor list, with a compatible blood group, the most waiting time and a negative crossmatching. The nondirected donors play an important role in kidney paired donation and living donor exchange programs. The evaluation process of nondirected donors has a strong emphasis on the psychosocial aspects of the donation, exploring any false perceptions or covert depression. Nondirected donors might be at a greater risk for depression or regret since they might not be able to enjoy the positive psychological gain that comes from seeing the recipient benefit from their altruism [26,57].

6. Paired kidney donation

Patients with potential donors who are incompatible due to ABO differences or positive crossmatch can still reap the benefits of living donation through kidney paired donation (KPD). A simple "two-way" exchange, or swap, can be arranged between two incompatible pairs or a more complicated combination can be achieved using many pairs in many different hospitals. Such a large exchange is often initiated by a non-directed donor. This concept of KPD was first suggested by Felix Rapaport in 1986 and in 1991, the first kidney exchange was performed in South Korea. The next year, the first KPD transplants were performed in the USA in 2000. As of the third quarter of 2010, over 1000 KPD transplants have been performed in the USA [57,83].

Author details

Leila Kamal and David Serur
Department of Medicine, Division of Nephrology & Hypertension, and the Rogosin Institute, NewYork-Presbyterian Hospital/Weill Cornell Medical College, New York, NY, USA

7. References

[1] Truog RD: The ethics of organ donation by living donors. N Engl J Med 2005;353:444-446.
[2] Merrill JP, Murray JE, Harrison JH, Guild WR: Successful homotransplantation of the human kidney between identical twins. J Am Med Assoc 1956;160:277-282.
[3] Murray JE: The first successful organ transplants in man. J Am Coll Surg 2005;200:5-9.
[4] Lytton B: The early history of kidney transplantation at yale (1967-1985): A personal memoir. Yale J Biol Med 2005;78:173-184.
[5] Magee CC, Pascual M: Update in renal transplantation. Arch Intern Med 2004;164:1373-1388.
[6] Collins AJ, Foley R, Herzog C, Chavers B, Gilbertson D, Ishani A, Kasiske B, Liu J, Mau LW, McBean M, Murray A, St Peter W, Xue J, Fan Q, Guo H, Li Q, Li S, Peng Y, Qiu Y, Roberts T, Skeans M, Snyder J, Solid C, Wang C, Weinhandl E, Zaun D, Zhang R, Arko C, Chen SC, Dalleska F, Daniels F, Dunning S, Ebben J, Frazier E, Hanzlik C, Johnson R, Sheets D, Wang X, Forrest B, Constantini E, Everson S, Eggers P, Agodoa L: Excerpts from the united states renal data system 2007 annual data report. Am J Kidney Dis 2008;51:S1-320.
[7] Cecka JM: The unos renal transplant registry. Clin Transpl 2001:1-18.
[8] Ibrahim HN, Foley R, Tan L, Rogers T, Bailey RF, Guo H, Gross CR, Matas AJ: Long-term consequences of kidney donation. N Engl J Med 2009;360:459-469.
[9] Martin PY, Hazzan M: [how far to promote renal transplantation from living kidney donors?]. Nephrol Ther;7:519-520.
[10] Davis CL, Cooper M: The state of u.S. Living kidney donors. Clin J Am Soc Nephrol;5:1873-1880.
[11] Okamoto M, Akioka K, Nobori S, Ushigome H, Kozaki K, Kaihara S, Yoshimura N: Short- and long-term donor outcomes after kidney donation: Analysis of 601 cases over a 35-year period at japanese single center. Transplantation 2009;87:419-423.
[12] Delmonico F: A report of the amsterdam forum on the care of the live kidney donor: Data and medical guidelines. Transplantation 2005;79:S53-66.
[13] Davis CL: Living kidney donors: Current state of affairs. Adv Chronic Kidney Dis 2009;16:242-249.
[14] Kher A, Mandelbrot DA: The living kidney donor evaluation: Focus on renal issues. Clin J Am Soc Nephrol;7:366-371.
[15] Gibney EM, King AL, Maluf DG, Garg AX, Parikh CR: Living kidney donors requiring transplantation: Focus on african americans. Transplantation 2007;84:647-649.
[16] Mandelbrot DA, Pavlakis M, Danovitch GM, Johnson SR, Karp SJ, Khwaja K, Hanto DW, Rodrigue JR: The medical evaluation of living kidney donors: A survey of us transplant centers. Am J Transplant 2007;7:2333-2343.

[17] Dols LF, Kok NF, Roodnat JI, Tran TC, Terkivatan T, Zuidema WC, Weimar W, Ijzermans JN: Living kidney donors: Impact of age on long-term safety. Am J Transplant;11:737-742.
[18] Jacobs SC, Ramey JR, Sklar GN, Bartlett ST: Laparoscopic kidney donation from patients older than 60 years. J Am Coll Surg 2004;198:892-897.
[19] Petrini C: Ethical issues with informed consent from potential living kidney donors. Transplant Proc;42:1040-1042.
[20] Rudow DL: The living donor advocate: A team approach to educate, evaluate, and manage donors across the continuum. Prog Transplant 2009;19:64-70.
[21] Textor SC, Taler SJ, Larson TS, Prieto M, Griffin M, Gloor J, Nyberg S, Velosa J, Schwab T, Stegall M: Blood pressure evaluation among older living kidney donors. J Am Soc Nephrol 2003;14:2159-2167.
[22] Cerasola G, Mule G, Nardi E, Cusimano P, Palermo A, Arsena R, Guarneri M, Geraci C, Cottone S: Clinical correlates of renal dysfunction in hypertensive patients without cardiovascular complications: The redhy study. J Hum Hypertens;24:44-50.
[23] Leichtman A, Abecassis M, Barr M, Charlton M, Cohen D, Confer D, Cooper M, Danovitch G, Davis C, Delmonico F, Dew MA, Garvey C, Gaston R, Gill J, Gillespie B, Ibrahim H, Jacobs C, Kahn J, Kasiske B, Kim J, Lentine K, Manyalich M, Medina-Pestana J, Merion R, Moxey-Mims M, Odim J, Opelz G, Orlowski J, Rizvi A, Roberts J, Segev D, Sledge T, Steiner R, Taler S, Textor S, Thiel G, Waterman A, Williams E, Wolfe R, Wynn J, Matas AJ: Living kidney donor follow-up: State-of-the-art and future directions, conference summary and recommendations. Am J Transplant;11:2561-2568.
[24] Textor SC, Taler SJ, Driscoll N, Larson TS, Gloor J, Griffin M, Cosio F, Schwab T, Prieto M, Nyberg S, Ishitani M, Stegall M: Blood pressure and renal function after kidney donation from hypertensive living donors. Transplantation 2004;78:276-282.
[25] Burgher A, Beman M, Holtzman JL, Monga M: Progression of nephrolithiasis: Long-term outcomes with observation of asymptomatic calculi. J Endourol 2004;18:534-539.
[26] Danovitch G: Medical and surgical aspects of kidney donation, ed 2005. 2005.
[27] Lee YH, Huang WC, Chang LS, Chen MT, Yang YF, Huang JK: The long-term stone recurrence rate and renal function change in unilateral nephrectomy urolithiasis patients. J Urol 1994;152:1386-1388.
[28] Worcester E, Parks JH, Josephson MA, Thisted RA, Coe FL: Causes and consequences of kidney loss in patients with nephrolithiasis. Kidney Int 2003;64:2204-2213.
[29] Chertow GM, Hsu CY, Johansen KL: The enlarging body of evidence: Obesity and chronic kidney disease. J Am Soc Nephrol 2006;17:1501-1502.
[30] Hsu CY, McCulloch CE, Iribarren C, Darbinian J, Go AS: Body mass index and risk for end-stage renal disease. Ann Intern Med 2006;144:21-28.
[31] Praga M, Hernandez E, Herrero JC, Morales E, Revilla Y, Diaz-Gonzalez R, Rodicio JL: Influence of obesity on the appearance of proteinuria and renal insufficiency after unilateral nephrectomy. Kidney Int 2000;58:2111-2118.
[32] Heimbach JK, Taler SJ, Prieto M, Cosio FG, Textor SC, Kudva YC, Chow GK, Ishitani MB, Larson TS, Stegall MD: Obesity in living kidney donors: Clinical characteristics and outcomes in the era of laparoscopic donor nephrectomy. Am J Transplant 2005;5:1057-1064.

[33] Silveiro SP, da Costa LA, Beck MO, Gross JL: Urinary albumin excretion rate and glomerular filtration rate in single-kidney type 2 diabetic patients. Diabetes Care 1998;21:1521-1524.

[34] Okamoto M, Suzuki T, Fujiki M, Nobori S, Ushigome H, Sakamoto S, Yoshimura N: The consequences for live kidney donors with preexisting glucose intolerance without diabetic complication: Analysis at a single japanese center. Transplantation;89:1391-1395.

[35] Niaudet P: Living donor kidney transplantation in patients with hereditary nephropathies. Nat Rev Nephrol;6:736-743.

[36] Hateboer N, v Dijk MA, Bogdanova N, Coto E, Saggar-Malik AK, San Millan JL, Torra R, Breuning M, Ravine D: Comparison of phenotypes of polycystic kidney disease types 1 and 2. European pkd1-pkd2 study group. Lancet 1999;353:103-107.

[37] Pei Y, Obaji J, Dupuis A, Paterson AD, Magistroni R, Dicks E, Parfrey P, Cramer B, Coto E, Torra R, San Millan JL, Gibson R, Breuning M, Peters D, Ravine D: Unified criteria for ultrasonographic diagnosis of adpkd. J Am Soc Nephrol 2009;20:205-212.

[38] Blumenfeld JD: Pretransplant genetic testing of live kidney donors at risk for autosomal dominant polycystic kidney disease. Transplantation 2009;87:6-7.

[39] Huang E, Samaniego-Picota M, McCune T, Melancon JK, Montgomery RA, Ugarte R, Kraus E, Womer K, Rabb H, Watnick T: DNA testing for live kidney donors at risk for autosomal dominant polycystic kidney disease. Transplantation 2009;87:133-137.

[40] Gross O, Weber M, Fries JW, Muller GA: Living donor kidney transplantation from relatives with mild urinary abnormalities in alport syndrome: Long-term risk, benefit and outcome. Nephrol Dial Transplant 2009;24:1626-1630.

[41] Jais JP, Knebelmann B, Giatras I, De Marchi M, Rizzoni G, Renieri A, Weber M, Gross O, Netzer KO, Flinter F, Pirson Y, Dahan K, Wieslander J, Persson U, Tryggvason K, Martin P, Hertz JM, Schroder C, Sanak M, Carvalho MF, Saus J, Antignac C, Smeets H, Gubler MC: X-linked alport syndrome: Natural history and genotype-phenotype correlations in girls and women belonging to 195 families: A "european community alport syndrome concerted action" study. J Am Soc Nephrol 2003;14:2603-2610.

[42] Savige J, Rana K, Tonna S, Buzza M, Dagher H, Wang YY: Thin basement membrane nephropathy. Kidney Int 2003;64:1169-1178.

[43] Savige J: Thin basement membrane nephropathy and coincidental renal biopsy lesions. Nephrology (Carlton) 2004;9:52.

[44] Ierino FL, Kanellis J: Thin basement membrane nephropathy and renal transplantation. Semin Nephrol 2005;25:184-187.

[45] Pham PC, Wilkinson AH, Pham PT: Evaluation of the potential living kidney donor. Am J Kidney Dis 2007;50:1043-1051.

[46] Sachdeva M, Bhaskaran M, Molmenti EP, Dalton D, Mattana J: Approach to the pretransplant evaluation of the living kidney donor. J Transplant;2011:245738.

[47] Chen CH, Shu KH, Cheng CH, Wu MJ, Yu TM, Chuang YW, Huang ST, Hung SW: Imaging evaluation of kidney using multidetector computerized tomography in living-related renal transplantation. Transplant Proc;44:7-10.

[48] Raman SS, Pojchamarnwiputh S, Muangsomboon K, Schulam PG, Gritsch HA, Lu DS: Surgically relevant normal and variant renal parenchymal and vascular anatomy in preoperative 16-mdct evaluation of potential laparoscopic renal donors. AJR Am J Roentgenol 2007;188:105-114.

[49] Singh AK, Sahani DV: Imaging of the renal donor and transplant recipient. Radiol Clin North Am 2008;46:79-93, vi.
[50] Fleisher LA, Beckman JA, Brown KA, Calkins H, Chaikof EL, Fleischmann KE, Freeman WK, Froehlich JB, Kasper EK, Kersten JR, Riegel B, Robb JF: 2009 accf/aha focused update on perioperative beta blockade incorporated into the acc/aha 2007 guidelines on perioperative cardiovascular evaluation and care for noncardiac surgery: A report of the american college of cardiology foundation/american heart association task force on practice guidelines. Circulation 2009;120:e169-276.
[51] Smetana GW: Preoperative pulmonary evaluation. N Engl J Med 1999;340:937-944.
[52] Thomsen T, Villebro N, Moller AM: Interventions for preoperative smoking cessation. Cochrane Database Syst Rev:CD002294.
[53] Tonnesen H, Rosenberg J, Nielsen HJ, Rasmussen V, Hauge C, Pedersen IK, Kehlet H: Effect of preoperative abstinence on poor postoperative outcome in alcohol misusers: Randomised controlled trial. BMJ 1999;318:1311-1316.
[54] De Stefano V, Martinelli I, Mannucci PM, Paciaroni K, Chiusolo P, Casorelli I, Rossi E, Leone G: The risk of recurrent deep venous thrombosis among heterozygous carriers of both factor v leiden and the g20210a prothrombin mutation. N Engl J Med 1999;341:801-806.
[55] Sidney S, Petitti DB, Soff GA, Cundiff DL, Tolan KK, Quesenberry CP, Jr.: Venous thromboembolic disease in users of low-estrogen combined estrogen-progestin oral contraceptives. Contraception 2004;70:3-10.
[56] Dew MA, Jacobs CL, Jowsey SG, Hanto R, Miller C, Delmonico FL: Guidelines for the psychosocial evaluation of living unrelated kidney donors in the united states. Am J Transplant 2007;7:1047-1054.
[57] Delmonico FL, Dew MA: Living donor kidney transplantation in a global environment. Kidney Int 2007;71:608-614.
[58] The declaration of istanbul on organ trafficking and transplant tourism. Kidney Int 2008;74:854-859.
[59] Ghods AJ, Savaj S: Iranian model of paid and regulated living-unrelated kidney donation. Clin J Am Soc Nephrol 2006;1:1136-1145.
[60] Jafar TH: Organ trafficking: Global solutions for a global problem. Am J Kidney Dis 2009;54:1145-1157.
[61] Bruzzone P, Berloco PB: Ethical aspects of renal transplantation from living donors. Transplant Proc 2007;39:1785-1786.
[62] Najarian JS, Chavers BM, McHugh LE, Matas AJ: 20 years or more of follow-up of living kidney donors. Lancet 1992;340:807-810.
[63] Davis CL, Delmonico FL: Living-donor kidney transplantation: A review of the current practices for the live donor. J Am Soc Nephrol 2005;16:2098-2110.
[64] Afaneh C, Sheth S, Aull MJ, Leeser DB, Kapur S, Del Pizzo JJ: Laparoendoscopic single-site nephrectomy in obese living renal donors. J Endourol;26:140-146.
[65] Leeser DB, Wysock J, Gimenez SE, Kapur S, Del Pizzo J: Single port donor nephrectomy. J Vis Exp
[66] Wang GJ, Afaneh C, Aull M, Charlton M, Ramasamy R, Leeser DB, Kapur S, Del Pizzo JJ: Laparoendoscopic single site live donor nephrectomy: Single institution report of initial 100 cases. J Urol;186:2333-2337.

[67] Hubert J, Renoult E, Mourey E, Frimat L, Cormier L, Kessler M: Complete robotic-assistance during laparoscopic living donor nephrectomies: An evaluation of 38 procedures at a single site. Int J Urol 2007;14:986-989.

[68] Matas AJ, Bartlett ST, Leichtman AB, Delmonico FL: Morbidity and mortality after living kidney donation, 1999-2001: Survey of united states transplant centers. Am J Transplant 2003;3:830-834.

[69] Hadjianastassiou VG, Johnson RJ, Rudge CJ, Mamode N: 2509 living donor nephrectomies, morbidity and mortality, including the uk introduction of laparoscopic donor surgery. Am J Transplant 2007;7:2532-2537.

[70] Nanidis TG, Antcliffe D, Kokkinos C, Borysiewicz CA, Darzi AW, Tekkis PP, Papalois VE: Laparoscopic versus open live donor nephrectomy in renal transplantation: A meta-analysis. Ann Surg 2008;247:58-70.

[71] Shokeir AA: Open versus laparoscopic live donor nephrectomy: A focus on the safety of donors and the need for a donor registry. J Urol 2007;178:1860-1866.

[72] Fehrman-Ekholm I, Elinder CG, Stenbeck M, Tyden G, Groth CG: Kidney donors live longer. Transplantation 1997;64:976-978.

[73] Krohn AG, Ogden DA, Holmes JH: Renal function in 29 healthy adults before and after nephrectomy. JAMA 1966;196:322-324.

[74] Hayslett JP: Effect of age on compensatory renal growth. Kidney Int 1983;23:599-602.

[75] Narkun-Burgess DM, Nolan CR, Norman JE, Page WF, Miller PL, Meyer TW: Forty-five year follow-up after uninephrectomy. Kidney Int 1993;43:1110-1115.

[76] Garg AX, Muirhead N, Knoll G, Yang RC, Prasad GV, Thiessen-Philbrook H, Rosas-Arellano MP, Housawi A, Boudville N: Proteinuria and reduced kidney function in living kidney donors: A systematic review, meta-analysis, and meta-regression. Kidney Int 2006;70:1801-1810.

[77] El-Agroudy AE, Sabry AA, Wafa EW, Neamatalla AH, Ismail AM, Mohsen T, Khalil AA, Shokeir AA, Ghoneim MA: Long-term follow-up of living kidney donors: A longitudinal study. BJU international 2007;100:1351-1355.

[78] Gossmann J, Wilhelm A, Kachel HG, Jordan J, Sann U, Geiger H, Kramer W, Scheuermann EH: Long-term consequences of live kidney donation follow-up in 93% of living kidney donors in a single transplant center. Am J Transplant 2005;5:2417-2424.

[79] Boudville N, Prasad GV, Knoll G, Muirhead N, Thiessen-Philbrook H, Yang RC, Rosas-Arellano MP, Housawi A, Garg AX: Meta-analysis: Risk for hypertension in living kidney donors. Ann Intern Med 2006;145:185-196.

[80] Delanaye P, Weekers L, Dubois BE, Cavalier E, Detry O, Squifflet JP, Krzesinski JM: Outcome of the living kidney donor. Nephrol Dial Transplant;27:41-50.

[81] Lentine KL, Schnitzler MA, Xiao H, Saab G, Salvalaggio PR, Axelrod D, Davis CL, Abbott KC, Brennan DC: Racial variation in medical outcomes among living kidney donors. N Engl J Med;363:724-732.

[82] Ellison MD, McBride MA, Taranto SE, Delmonico FL, Kauffman HM: Living kidney donors in need of kidney transplants: A report from the organ procurement and transplantation network. Transplantation 2002;74:1349-1351.

[83] Wallis CB, Samy KP, Roth AE, Rees MA: Kidney paired donation. Nephrol Dial Transplant;26:2091-2099.

Chapter 3

Medical Management of the Kidney Transplant Recipient

Dhaval Patel and Jun Lee

Additional information is available at the end of the chapter

http://dx.doi.org/10.5772/54099

1. Introduction

Once a patient receives kidney transplant, critical attention should be paid to ensure patient's hemodynamic stability, they should be monitored for any side effects of the new medications and prevent infections that may jeopardize the renal allograft and patients' general health. Medical problems such as diabetes and hypertension that may be medical complications of transplant immunosuppression need to be managed appropriately. This chapter will go over the medical management of the kidney transplant recipient.

2. Early post operative management

2.1. Assessing fluid status

There are two broad goals to assess fluid status: the transplanted kidney needs to receive adequate perfusion and make adequate amounts of urine.

When patients' are admitted for kidney transplant, it is preferred to have the patient about 1kg above their dry weight (1). This is to decrease the risk for hypotension intra-operatively, and ensure that the patients are somewhat hypervolemic and there is enough mean arterial pressure to perfuse the new transplanted kidney at the end of the surgery. Post transplant, it is important to assess urine output on hourly basis to ensure that patients are not oliguric, i.e., urine output should at least be greater than 0.5ml/kg/hr or 500ml/24hrs. Patient's pre-transplant urine output should be known and be accounted for when assessing for urine output adequacy post-transplant. Initial blood pressure and volume status on clinical exam should dictate fluid replacement. If the patient is hypovolemic, patient should be given isotonic saline in 500ml to 1L boluses until mean arterial pressure of at least 65 mm hg can be established. Most patients are hypervolemic. In that scenario, it is not necessary to replace all of the urine output.

There are many different protocols for replacement and maintenance fluids. In general, there is no evidence that crystalloids are better than colloids. Replacement fluid should also account for any other body fluid losses such as in nasogastric tube output. Half normal saline can be used for replacement fluid as urinary sodium after kidney transplant initially tends to be between 60 and 80 mEq/L (1). Maintenance fluids should account for insensible losses which can range in from 500cc to 1500cc in a 24 hour period for surgical patients (3). Typically the maintenance fluid used is 5% dextrose in water at the rate of at least 30cc/hr (1). For cases where electrolyte replacement is needed such as in potassium, this should be carefully given monitoring for any risk of hyperkalemia if patient is oliguric and preferably through a separate intravenous line. Electrolytes including potassium, phosphate, calcium and magnesium should be checked at least every 6 hours (1).

2.2. Delayed & slow graft function

The consensus definition of delayed graft function (DGF) is lacking, though, it is generally agreed upon that if dialysis is needed within first 7 days of transplant that constitutes delayed graft function (2). Delayed graft function, in reality, is acute kidney injury in transplanted kidney and should be worked up as any other acute kidney injury with attention paid to the special circumstance that is kidney transplant and differential diagnosis broadened accordingly to include acute rejection as well as acute ischemic tubular necrosis.

The long waiting list of patients awaiting kidney transplant and shortage of donors has necessitated accepting expanded criteria donors (ECD) and donation after cardiac death donors (DCD). Not surprisingly, incidence of DGF has increased to 21% for the years 1998-2008 from 14% during 1985-1992 (6,7,9). DGF increases the risk of graft rejection, transplant glomerulopathy and ultimately, decreases the long-term allograft survival (4,11,12). Long-term patient survival after DGF is not known, but it is likely that patients who suffer graft failure compared to patients with functioning grafts may have decrease survival rates. Besides ECD and DCD kidneys, there are several other risk factors for DGF. Donor specific risk factors include: donor age >60, cold ischemia time >15 hours, warm ischemia time > 45 minutes, Non T-cell antibody induction, female gender and obese donor (5, 7, 8, 9, 10, 13, 14, 15, 16). Recipient risk factors include: maintenance hemodialysis prior to transplantation, obesity, diabetes, male gender, age > 55, African-American race, small-for-size organ and prior immune sensitizing events such as blood transfusions, pregnancy and previous transplant (7, 10, 15, 16, 17). Machine perfusion technique for preservation of organ also seems to decrease the risk for DGF in ECD kidneys (7). The underlying mechanisms including molecular pathways and cytogenetic mechanisms are being established and may aid future prevention as well as treatment measures for DGF. For now, focus remains on prevention with controlling for risk factors as well as trying to avoid intra-operative and post-operative hypovolemic states and hypotensive conditions. If patient does have DGF, patient is supported with preventing further nephrotoxicity from all measures and providing dialysis until allograft kidney function recovers.

Indications for dialysis should be dictated by clinical circumstances but persistent acidosis, hyperkalemia especially with EKG changes suggestive of destabilization of cardiac membrane and volume overload that is resistant to high doses of diuretics. Both intermittent hemodialysis and peritoneal dialysis can be used. When hemodialysis is used, close attention should be paid to patient's blood pressure and unless need for hypervolemic status, ultrafiltration should be avoided. Peritoneal dialysis can be used, though, dwelling volumes may need to be as low as 500ml in order to avoid worsening pain (1). Preferably hemodialysis should be performed, unless peritoneal dialysis catheter is readily available.

There is a subset of transplanted patients that do not require dialysis within the first 7 days, but the serum creatinine is very slow to decrease. This group of patients can be defined as having intermediate graft function or slow graft function (18). The risk factors and the graft outcomes are likely similar to DGF, though less severe (18). This can possibly be explained by lesser severity kidney injury or lesser degree of baseline clinical or subclinical kidney dysfunction in the allograft (18).

2.3. Immunosuppression

Every transplant center has their own immunosuppressive protocol which serves as guides for therapy based on type of transplant (kidney vs. kidney-pancreas) and patient's risk group determined by pre-formed antibodies, sensitization status, age and race (2). Low-risk group patients such as two-haplotype match may require less immunosuppression. African-Americans, on the other hand, have been shown to require higher doses of immunosuppression.

There are two phases to immunosuppression. Acute rejection risk is highest from time zero to first few months after transplantation (2). The immunosuppresion induced at time zero is called induction phase. Maintenance immunosuppression is also introduced early-on, however, this therapy is maintained for the rest of the patient's transplant life and constitutes the post-induction phase, the maintenance phase.

Both phases of immunosuppression are described in a separate chapter in this textbook and will not be further discussed here

2.4. Infection prophylaxis

All patients undergoing kidney transplant should received prophylaxis for infection as immunocompromised state post-transplant puts this group of patient at high risk of life-threatening common and uncommon infections. Any infection subsequently also increases risk of allograft failure through primary (e.g. ATN secondary to sepsis) or secondary mechanisms (e.g.. allograft rejection).

The following antimicrobial therapy should be given peri-operatively (1,2):

1. Standard antibiotic pre-operative prophylaxis per center based guidelines should be used. Prophylaxis should be against common skin and urinary tract pathogens. Cefazolin 1 or 2 grams based on body weight, generally, is the preferred agent.

2. Also, bactrim should be introduced as prophylaxis against for UTI, sepsis, nocardia and pneumocystis jiroveci pneumonia (pjp). One single strength tablet daily is the general recommendation. Dosing should be done renally and adjusted to patient's creatinine clearance. For UTI prophylaxis, patients allergic to bactrim can use any other oral quinolone such as levaquin. In that scenario, patients should also get atovaquone 1500mg daily for pneumocystis jiroveci. Pentamidine monthly nebulized is another option if atovaquone cannot be tolerated. Dapsone 100mg daily may be used for same prophylaxis, though G6PD status must be checked. Any such prophylaxis should be continued for one year for pjp prophylaxis.
3. CMV status should be checked for both donor and recipient. CMV negative recipients from CMV positive donors are at highest risk for CMV disease as are patients receiving OKT3 or other t-cell depleting agents. CMV positive recipients are at risk for reactivation. All such patients should receive valganciclovir 900mg daily or three times weekly adjusted to renal function for 6 months. Alternatively, ganciclovir 1000mg three times daily or valacyclovir 2g four times daily can be used. All donor and recipient CMV negative patients should receive Acyclovir 400mg twice daily for 3 months.
4. During induction phase, oral or topical antifungal agents such as clotrimazole or nystatin are used. Systemic antifungal agents are not recommended in uncomplicated renal transplant.

3. Early post-transplant follow-up: First three months

3.1. Immunosuppression

The risk of acute rejection and allograft loss is highest in the first three months, so immunosuppression should be at its highest levels in this time period. The topic of immunosuppression has been reviewed in a separate chapter.

4. Long-term follow-up

4.1. Immunosuppression

All patients should be maintained on 2 or 3 drug regimen as long as the patient has functional graft. Target drug levels may be lowered after the first three months.

4.2. Patient and graft survival

Graft survival (i.e., patient survival with a functioning graft) has steadily improved. Graft survival for deceased donor kidneys in 2009 was 94.4% at 6 months; for transplants in 2008, 92.0% at 1 year; for transplants in 2006, 81.9% at 3 years; for transplants in 2004, 70.0% at 5 years; and for transplants in 1999, 42.7% at 10 years (19). Graft survival for living donor transplants in 2009 was 97.7% at 6 months; for transplants in 2008, 96.5% at 1 year; for transplants in 2006, 90.9% at 3 years; for transplants in 2004, 82.5% at 5 years; and for transplants in 1999, 59.6% at 10 years (19). While one-year graft survival has improved significantly, there is much room for improvement in 10-year graft survival.

The rate of late graft failure is traditionally measured by the graft half-life conditional on 1-year survival, defined as the time to when half of grafts surviving at least 1 year are still functioning. Graft half-lives for deceased and living donor kidneys have increased (19). For deceased donor kidneys, the half-life increased 45%, from 10.1 years for transplants in 1991 to 14.7 years for transplants in 2007 (19). For living donor kidneys, the half-life increased 68.2%, from 15.8 years for transplants in 1991 to 26.6 years for transplants in 2007 (19). Remarkably as per the 2010 Scientific Registry of Transplant Recipients/Organ Procurement and Transplantation Network annual report, the half-life of a deceased donor kidney in 2007 (14.7 years) is less than the half-life of a living donor kidney in 1991 (15.8 years). This suggests there is substantial room to improve the rate of late graft failure, at least for recipients of deceased donor kidneys.

The number of patients with a functioning kidney graft has doubled, from 68,200 in 1998 to 144,180 in 2009 (19).

Besides donor type, DGF and presence of HLA-antibodies also reduces the short-term graft survival. Long-term graft survival is also reduced by DGF, history of known HLA antibodies, HLA mismatching, cold ischemia time and insufficient immunosuppression. Inadequate renal mass for body size, CMV seropositivity, ongoing renal injuries, medical non-compliance, poorly managed hypertension, hyperlipidemia and recurrent or de novo glomerular disease are some of the other risk factors portending shorter graft survivial.

The most common causes of death in kidney transplant recipients include death from cardiovascular disease followed by infection, malignancy and other miscellaneous causes. The miscellaneous causes, such as pulmonary embolus, brain hemorrhage, colon or peptic ulcer perforation etc. can contribute 1-2% each to annual death rate (20). Death from cardiovascular disease remains the leading cause of mortality. It accounts for 40-55% of all deaths in transplant recipients (20). This includes congestive heart failure, coronary artery disease, cerebrovascular disease, and peripheral vascular disease. Renal transplant recipients have up to 10 times the rate of cardiac death and 50 times the annual rate of fatal or nonfatal cardiovascular events as the general population (21). Nearly 40% of patients have experienced a cardiovascular event at 36 months after renal transplantation, with congestive heart failure and myocardial infarction being the most common events (22, 23)). The prevalence of cerebrovascular events, though less than dialysis patients, is still high in patients who have undergone renal transplantation, and the risk of cerebral hemorrhage is higher than in the general population (24, 25). Finally, incidence of peripheral arterial disease is lower in renal transplant recipients, though *de novo* peripheral arterial disease increases the relative risk for death by almost twofold (26).

There are also other risk factors that impact survival of transplant recipients. Survival is superior with an allograft from a living donor compared to those who receive a kidney from a deceased donor, including both standard criteria and extended criteria donors. Older patients who undergo renal transplantation have a higher mortality rate than younger recipients. The presence of systemic disorders, particularly vascular disease, is associated with poorer long-term patient survival after renal transplantation. Survival of diabetic patients after renal transplantation (75 to 80 percent at five years) is lower than that reported in nondiabetic patients. It is still better than diabetic patients on dialysis whose 5-year survival is estimated to be 30% (2).

Perhaps, the most important predictor of graft survival is renal function. 1-year creatinine of less than 1.5mg/dl and change of less than 0.3mg/dl portends excellent long-term graft survival (5). Higher creatinine values at one year signal poor long-term graft outcome.

Despite all of these, patient and graft survival has improved significantly in the recent decade, which likely reflects our improved ability to manage patient and graft related risk factors.

5. Management of medical co-morbidities

5.1. Hypertension

Immediate post transplant hypertension is common and most commonly reflects pain, although, could also reflect overzealous volume resuscitation (27). If patient is volume overloaded, he or she should be diuresed. Controlling pain likely needs to be done simultaneously as sometimes early-on it is difficult to determine the causative etiology of hypertension. Moderately elevated blood pressure should be tolerated as it will help to maintain adequate renal perfusion to the transplanted kidney. However, if blood pressure is greater than 180mm hg despite best pain control in euvolemic patient, a dihydropyridine calcium channel blocker such as nifedipine can be used (28). This will allow for dual benefit of ameliorating some of the afferent arteriolar vasoconstriction induced calcineurin inhibitors. Alternatively, an alpha blocker such as clonidine can be used if pain is difficult to control and blood pressure remains high, i.e., there is excessive sympathetic stimulation. Blood pressure should not be lowered below 110 mm hg. If patient is not taking medications orally, labetalol or hydralazine can be used for intravenous administrations.

Chronic hypertension is a risk factor for CVD and affects graft survival in the long-term (27). In the era of CNIs, roughly 60-90% of patients seem to be afflicted with hypertension (29). The etiology of hypertension is likely multifactorial and management needs to be more nuanced. Goal blood pressure as defined by KDOQI guidelines should be <130/80 mm Hg (30). The same medications used for hypertension control in general population may be beneficial in renal transplant population as well.

KDOQI establishes five points for the evaluation and management of hypertension in renal transplant patients (30). First, patients should be evaluated for chronic kidney disease, cardiovascular disease and any cardiovascular risk factors. Second, diet and lifestyle changes should be part of all therapy including sodium intake <2.4g/day, weight loss if BMI is >25kg/m^2, exercise, moderate alcohol intake and smoking cessation. Third, risk factors for cardiovascular disease should be managed concurrently such as diabetes and hyperlipidemia. Fourth, systolic blood pressure should be managed to less than 130 mm Hg with anti-hypertensive medications. Fifth, for patients with spot urinary protein-to-creatinine ratio >500-1000mg/g a lower blood pressure goal may be advisable, an ACE inhibitor or ARB should be added or dose should be increased, ACE inhibitor or ARB may need to be used in combination and if still needed another antihypertensive medication should be added as needed to lower proteinuria.

Since calcium channel blockers are used early in transplant, they can be considered first-line therapy (29). ACE inhibitors are second line therapy and have been shown safe to use 6-12 weeks after transplant. For de novo initiation, it is recommended that therapy be started at least 6 weeks post-transplant (29). A recent randomized study comparing nifedipine and lisinopril demonstrated improved kidney outcomes (lower creatinine and improved GFR at 2 years) with the use of nifedipine (28). However, the study had limited follow-up, and it cannot be determined whether the improved GFR with calcium-channel blockers reflects the short-term hemodynamic effects of these agents or a long-term protective effect. Post transplant patients with hypertension and a compelling indication for an ACE inhibitor or an ARB should be restarted on therapy as soon as the graft is functional, the serum creatinine level is <2.5 mg/dL, and the potassium level is <5.5 mEq/L. If the patient has proteinuria, ACE inhibitor or ARB can be used as long as the reduction in GFR is less than 30% over 4 months. Since ACE inhibitor or ARB can potentiate hyperkalemia caused by CNIs, close attention should be paid to patient's potassium. Finally, tailoring of therapy for hypertension should be ultimately based on patient's risk factors as disucussed below.

Heart failure patients can be treated with thiazide diuretics (assuming adequate function of the transplant kidney), beta-blocker, ACE inhibitor or an ARB. Post-MI patients can be treated with beta-blocker and ACE inhibitor. Patients with cardiovascular risk factors can be treated with same anti-hypertensive medications as heart failure patients. Patient with diabetes may benefit from added anti-proteinuric effect of non-dihydropyridine calcium channel blocker such as verapamil. Verapamil can increase the levels of CNIs and levels need to monitored more closely. Patients with CKD, previous stroke and post transplant erythrocytosis may benefit from ACE inhibitor. ARB can be used as an alternative in cases of CKD and post-transplant erythrocytosis. All of the above indications for specific anti hypertensive regimens for various clinical entities have nicely been summarized by Dunn et al. as well (29).

Renal artery stenosis in allograft is a rare cause of hypertension and should be thought of when blood pressure is persistently elevated despite multiple pharmacologic interventions, patient has flash edema and/or sudden elevations in blood pressure. It usually occurs 3 months to 2 years after transplant, but early occurrences can happen post-transplant (31). Reported incidence is variable between 1 and 23%. Risk factors for renal artery stenosis include deceased donor kidney, delayed graft function, obese patients, severe atherosclerotic disease, CMV infection, difficulties with surgical technique when harvesting the graft or when transplanting the graft in the recipient (31). In this scenario, a Doppler renal ultrasound can be ordered which has 100% specificity and sensitivity when peak systolic velocity is greater than or equal to 2.5m/sec (2). MRI may be needed and should be pursued after discussing risks and benefits of nephrogenic systemic fibrosis with the patient. Stenting or surgery may be necessary if patient does have renal artery stenosis.

5.2. Diabetes

New-onset diabetes after transplant (NODAT) or pre-transplant diabetes is associated with increased CVD risk, especially NODAT. Diabetes is also associated with increased mortality (87% relative risk) and increased graft failure (63% relative risk) (35). Other complications seen in non-transplant patients such as retinopathy, nephropathy and infections especially in immunocompromised state as well as neuropathy resulting in diabetic ulcers can occur. It is estimated that about 30% of patients can have new diagnosis of diabetes post-transplant and another 1/3rd can have impaired glucose tolerance by 1 year post-transplant (32). Risk factors for NODAT are same those for developing diabetes in non-transplant patients including age, obesity, African American race and Hispanic ethnicity, family history and impaired glucose tolerance (2). Tacrolimus more than cyclosporine has been associated with NODAT, perhaps due to its higher toxicity to pancreatic islet cells (34). Furthermore, a strong association has been demonstrated between HCV status and the development of diabetes after kidney transplantation, particularly in patients receiving tacrolimus-based immunosuppression from the time of transplantation (33).

According to 2003 International Consensus Guidelines and subsequent updates, diabetes mellitus after transplantation may be diagnosed at any time after transplantation by any of the following (35, 36):

- Symptoms of diabetes plus random plasma glucose ≥200 mg/dL (11.1 mmol/L). Symptoms include polyuria, polydipsia, and unexplained weight loss.
- Fasting plasma glucose ≥126 mg/dL (7.0 mmol/L). Fasting is defined as no caloric intake for at least eight hours.
- Two-hour plasma glucose ≥200 mg/dL (11.1 mmol/L) during an oral glucose tolerance test with 75g of anhydrous glucose dissolved in water according to WHO guidelines.

Impaired fasting glucose and/or impaired glucose tolerance is diagnosed by:

- Fasting plasma glucose between 100 and 125 mg/dL (5.6 and 6.9 mmol/L) or a two-hour plasma glucose between 140 and 199 mg/dL (7.8 and 11.0 mmol/L) during an oral glucose tolerance test, respectively, according to ADA guidelines.

Management of diabetes includes screening for risk factors, monitoring for biochemical evidence of impaired glucose tolerance/NODAT, modifying immunosuppression as needed and treating diabetes mellitus aggressively.

Stepwise approach to evaluation and management is recommended by International Consensus Guidelines for renal transplant patients (35). Pre-Transplant patients should be screened for diabetes. Post-transplant HbA1c should be checked every 3 months for the 1st year and a HbA1c <7.0 should be targeted, even if insulin is required. Immunosuppresion modulation must be weighed against the risk of rejection and avoided if at all possible. If modulated, glucocorticoids dosage can be reduced first, followed by decreasing dosing of tacrolimus and switching to cyclosporine if still needed. Dietitian, ophthalmologist, endocrinologist and podiatrist should be involved early in management of diabetic patients.

Microalbuminuria should be treated with ACEI or ARB. Non-pharmacologic management should be given a chance including diet, exercise before pharmacologic approach is accepted. Other risk factors including lipids should be managed appropriately as CVD risk factor.

Once decision has been made to initiate oral therapy, oral agent may be alpha-glucosidase inhibitor (e.g., acarbose), biguanide (metformin is the most commonly used biguanide), a meglitinide (e.g., repaglinide), a sulfonylurea, or a thiazolidinedione (e.g., rosiglitazone) (35). Metformin is contraindicated in women with cr >1.5mg/dl and in men with cr >1.4mg/dl for concern of lactic acidosis (23). Sulfonylureas are safe in general to use, but glyburide is should be avoided in patients with GFR <50ml/min/1.73m^2 (23). Acarbose should be avoided with cr <2mg/dl (23). Repaglinide should be started at 0.5 mg with meals if GFR <40 mL/min/1.73 m2 and titrated carefully (23). Thiazolidinediones do not require any dose adjustment. Other medication such as exetanide, an incretin mimetic should be avoided if gfr <30ml/min/1.73m^2 (23). Dipeptidyl Peptidase-4 inhibitor, sitagliptin needs to be dosed renally (23).

As a complication of pre-existing diabetes if patients do develop diabetic ketoacidosis, they should be managed in intensive care unit. Algorithm is available from American Diabetic Association for management and should be closely followed. Volume resuscitation and insulin drip should be initial treatment. Many liters of normal saline may be required especially in post-op setting. Close eye should be kept on magnesium, potassium and phosphorous and they should be repleted aggressively. Subcutaneous insulin can be switched to once anion gap closes with 3-4 hours overlap with insulin drip.

5.3. Dyslipidemia

Dyslipidemia is common after kidney transplant. Although causative association between kidney transplant and cardiovascular disease (CVD) remains unproven, kidney transplant is considered to be coronary heart disease equivalent risk (37). Accordingly, hyperlipidemia should be managed aggressively.

Elevations in total cholesterol with low-density lipoprotein (LDL) are common, and triglycerides can be elevated often as well (23, 37). High-density lipoprotein (HDL) is usually normal. Cyclosporine, rapamycin and steroids have the greatest effect on serum lipid levels in dose-related fashion (23, 37). Other traditional risk factors as diabetes, obesity, smoking, hypertension, genetic factors and physical inactivity are also of equivalent importance. KDOQI has published guidelines for management of dyslipidemia in CKD patients which should be followed for transplant patients as well. Given the benefits of lowering CVD risk in general population and high risk of CVD in transplant population, the same risk reduction steps in terms of managing dyslipidemia should be taken for the transplant population. Goal LDL should be less than 100mg/dl (38). Therapeutic lifestyle changes (TLC) should be applied above 100mg/dl of LDL which include goals for intervention to minimize traditional risk factors. Patients should be counseled in smoking cessation with any necessary pharmacotherapy and psychotherapy, controlling blood pressure as detailed previously, reducing saturated and trans fats, taking daily 81mg aspirin, at least 30minutes of walking at least 5 days a week or running 15 mins for 3 days a week, weight loss of at least 10% in 1st year and managing diabetes as discussed previously (23, 37). If TLC fails to lower LDL below in 100mg/dl, statins should be added to TLC. If the LDL level is 130mg/dl of more, TLC and statins should be initiated simultaneously. Careful attention should be paid to introduction of statins to cyclosporine-based medication regimen. Cyclosporine increases AUC of all statins and especially with fluvasatin can cause rhabodmyolysis (23, 38). A good rule of thumb is this scenario is to use half of the recommended dose of statins with cyclosporine and tacrolimus (23, 37). Bile acid sequestrants such as cholestyramine are not typically recommended because they interfere with absorption of immunosuppressive medications, unless patients have severe coronary disease, have failed maximal medical management and risk of mortality from ischemic heart disease outweighs risk of rejection.

Triglycerides (TGs) should be below 500mg/dl and may need pharmacotherapy above these levels to reduce the risk of pancreatitis in addition to TLC (37). Consideration should also be given, in cases where maximal medical management has failed to lower LDL below recommended levels, to changing the immunosuppressive protocol to one that is less likely to cause high LDL levels, if this can be done without causing undue risk to graft (37).

Non-HDL cholesterol, which is calculated as total cholesterol minus HDL cholesterol may be a better predictor of coronary mortality and may be a surrogate for the major atherogenic protein, apolipoprotein B (38). Lowering non-HDL cholesterol to less than 130mg/dl may ultimately require a combined approach to reduce LDL and TG. If LDL is less than 100mg/dl or more but TGs are 200mg/dl and non-HDL is 130mg/dl or more, treatment of non-HDL to levels below 130mg/dl should be pursued with statin and fibrate or nicotinic acid (37).

The overall prevalence of dyslipidemia during the first year after transplantation is >50% (23). This high prevalence of dyslipidemia justifies screening and monitoring. In all adults, complete lipid profile should be checked (23, 37):

- 2-3 months after transplantation, or
- 2-3 months after change in treatment, or other conditions known to cause dyslipidemias, and
- At least, annually thereafter

5.4. Obesity

Obesity in adults is defined, as it is in major guidelines for the general population, as body mass index (BMI) ≥30 kg/m^2 (23). Because some individuals may have BMI ≥30 kg/m^2 that is not due to excess body fat, it is recommended that the definition of obesity in adults include waist circumference ≥102 cm (≥40 in.) in men and ≥88 cm (≥35 in.) in women (23).

Weight gain is common after renal transplant and can be associated with steroid usage (38). Hyperphagia as a side effect of steroid usage also contributes. Obesity contributes dyslipidemia, hypertension, CVD and diabetes mellitus in transplant patients. Risk factors for weight gain post-transplant include female gender, African American race and young age (38). Obesity is also a risk factor for DGF (See Delayed Graft Function) and obese renal transplant recipients suffers more surgical complications, including wound infections, delayed wound healing, lymphoceles and perinephric hematomas (1,38, 39). Longer surgical times and hospital stays are also reported in obese transplant recipients (38). Obesity is also a risk factor for decreased pancreas and kidney graft survival in combined pancreas-kidney transplant recipients (1).

Is it beneficial to lose weight before transplantation? DOPPS found that in dialytic population higher BMI (30-34.9 kg/m^2) is associated with lower mortality (42); higher mortality is associated with malnutrition (38). Weight loss also remains a difficult goal to achieve in dialytic population. Should the obese patients be excluded from transplant? Evidence has shown that when obese patients are transplanted their mortality rate is lower than the dialytic population (38).

Obesity in transplant patients should be managed with diet, exercise and nutritional counseling. A nutritionist should be involved in management. Small, uncontrolled trials in KTRs suggest that diet and other behavior modifications are safe and help reduce weight over the short term (40, 41). There is no evidence that any one diet is more effective than any other. A reasonable goal is to create a caloric deficit of 500–1000 kcal/day (23). Diets of 1000–1200 kcal/day for women and 1200–1500 kcal/day for men can be effective with increased physical activity in maintaining sustained weight loss (23).Weight loss medications have not been studied in renal transplant patients and as such Orlistat should not be given with cyclosporine as it interferes with its bioavailability and absorption. In cases of morbid obesity, patients may choose to undergo gastric bypass. This procedure may be safe in transplant patients, though, experience is limited (38). Absorption and metabolism of immunosuppressive medications may be altered after gastric bypass. Cyclosporine, tacrolimus, sirolimus and mycophenolic acid levels have been noted to be altered in gastric bypass patients and requires specific levels for those medications to be followed up (43). Gastric bypass also increases risk for hyperoxaluria and oxalate nephropathy, and when undergoing gastric bypass patients should be advised against risks for oxalate nephrolithiasis and secondary CKD (38). When patients develop oxalate nephropathy, reversal of bypass needs to be considered (38).

5.5. Smoking

Given smoking's pleotropic detrimental effects on almost every organ in our body and association with CVD as well as post-transplant cancer, intense efforts should be made to help patients quit smoking. This should include asking at each visit, advising to quit, providing psychiatric and non-psychiatric counseling as needed, initiating pharmacotherapy as needed and helping patients set up target dates to quit smoking. Studies have shown that the patients more likely to quit smoking have been more likely than not been counseled by their physicians. Even counseling for 3 min or less is effective (44). The '5 As' of counseling include: (i) ask about tobacco use, (ii) advise to quit through clear and personalized messages, (iii) assess willingness to quit, (iv) assist quitting and (v) arrange follow-up and support (44). A number of pharmacological approaches are available to promote smoking abstinence. All nicotine replacement therapies such as lozenges, gum, inhaler, spray and patch are safe to use (23). Varenicline, a partial agonist of nicotinic receptor can also be used in transplant recipients (23). Bupropion increases cyclosporine levels and they should be monitored (23).

5.6. Cardiovascular disease

So far we have discussed the traditional risk factors of CVD. Non-traditional risk factors such as homocysteine, uremia, left ventricular hypertrophy and graft dysfunction also have a significant role to play (21).There is a complex interplay between traditional and non-traditional risk factors causing CVD in kidney transplant patients. The strongest risk factor for cardiac risk is pre-existing CVD prior to transplant. All risk factors as discussed thus far should be managed aggressively whether patient has pre-existing CVD or new-onset CVD. Allograft dysfunction also contributes to CVD risk, whether this is mediated to systemic inflammation or through secondary hypertension, hyperlipidemia and albuminuria is unclear. Homocysteine levels are known to be significantly high in patients who experience cardiovascular events and are associated with higher mortality (45, 46). However, the causal effect of high homocysteine levels on CVD has not been established. High dose folic acid as well as vitamin B6 and B12 can effectively reduce homocysteine levels. When this reduction was achieved using folic acid, vitamin b6 and vitamin b12 in a randomized control trial, it did not reduce the all-cause mortality, ESRD or composite outcome which included cardiovascular death and myocardial infarction among other things (47). Another risk factor that increases CVD risk is anemia and this will be discussed next.

5.7. Anemia

World Health Organization defined anemia in 1968 as <13g/dl for men and <12g/dl for women which was based on observations from international nutritional studies (48). Since then there have been multiple attempts at re-defining anemia. Dependent on cut-off level of hemoglobin used for defining anemia, prevalence in post-transplant population varies roughly between 10% and 40% (49-53). Anemia is associated with worse patient and graft survival, higher rates of acute rejection and may further exaggerate left ventricular hypertrophy which is associated with higher cardiovascular mortality.

The belief that enough erythropoietin production with new allograft will resolve any degree of anemia in patients with CKD is not always fully realized (49). There can be many reasons for this phenomenon. In the early-post transplant period, anemia can be related to blood loss from surgery. Later on though the anemia may be related to decline in kidney function and secondary loss of erythropoietin production or from bone marrow suppression from immunosuppressants (50-53). However, other traditional and non-traditional risk factors need such as iron deficiency anemia with or without gastrointestinal bleeding, folate or vitamin b12 deficiency, hemolysis, parvovirus or other viral infections and medications need to be investigated and treated appropriately (50-53). Iron deficiency anemia is under-recognized and under-treated in post-transplant patients. Up to 60% of patients without initial iron deficiency can become iron-deficiency by 6 months (2). Since iron deficiency is associated with cardiovascular mortality independent of anemia timely recognition and treatment is important. Iron repletion can be estimated by ferritin 200mg/dl and transferrin saturation above 20%. Parvovirus infection which can cause refractory anemia can be treated with intravenous immunoglobulin and by lowering immunosuppression (1). Azathioprine, mycophenolic acid and sirolimus can also cause anemia, and the doses of these medications may need to be reduced (1). Other medications such as ACEIs, ARBs, ganciclovir or trimethoprim-sulfamethoxazole also cause anemia and need to be kept in mind when cause is being investigated (1). When no cause is found, iron stores are adequate, allograft function is impaired and meets indications for treatment as they are stated by KDOQI guidelines for CKD patients, epoetin alfa and aranesp should be administered (1).

5.8. Thrombotic microangiopathy

As a related cause of anemia, thrombotic microangiopathy (TMA) needs to included in differential diagnosis for causes of hemolysis. TMA is a histology manifestation of several clinical conditions such as TTP-HUS, antibody-mediated rejection (AMR) or toxicity of CNI. TMA may manifest itself limited to allograft or there might be evidence of systemic hemolysis such as increased lactate dehydrogenase, positive direct COOMBs test, increase indirect bilirubin, low haptoglobin and increase reticulocyte index with evidence of fragmented RBCs on peripheral smear. Thrombocytopenia accompanies systemic evidence of TMA. 15% of transplant patients have evidence of TMA and 3% show evidence of TTP (1). Treatment includes substitution of the calcineurin inhibitor with an alternative agent; belatacept and plasmapheresis may be utilized for management. If AMR is suspected, it should be treated accordingly; steroids should be pulsed, rituximab or bortezomib may also be used along with IVIG. Use of bortezomib may be limited by degree of thrombocytopenia. Another potential treatment if all else fails is eculizumab, which remains experimental.

5.9. Erythrocytosis

Post-transplant erythrocytosis (PTE) occurs in 8-15% of recipients (2). It is defined as a hemoglobin concentration greater than 17 g/dL and/or hematocrit greater than 51 percent that occurs following transplantation, persists for more than 6 months and occurs in the absence of another underlying cause (2). Most often PTE occurs within the first 8-24 months after transplantation (2). PTE appears predominantly in patients without native kidney nephrectomy and in those, who had an adequate erythropoiesis prior to transplantation, as evidenced by no or limited use of ESA while on dialysis (54). The pathogenesis of PTE is not well understood and multiple hormonal systems as well as growth factors such as erythropoetin, Insulin-like growth factor-1, serum-soluble stem cell factor (sSCF), rennin-angiotensin system and endogenous androgens have been implicated (2, 55-59). Endogenous erythropoietin appears to play the central role. Persistent erythropoietin secretion from the diseased and chronically ischemic native kidneys does not conform to the normal feedback. However, erythropoietin levels in most PTE patients still remain within the "normal range," indicating that erythrocytosis finally ensues by the contributory action of additional growth factors on erythroid progenitors, such as angiotensin II, androgens, sSCF and insulin-like growth factor 1 (IGF-1) (55-57, 59). 25% of all patients with PTE may see resolution without any treatment. 60% of patients experience symptoms which can include lethargy, dizziness, plethora, headache among other things (2). 10% to 20% patients experience both venous and arterial thromboembolic events (2). Secondary causes should be excluded: pulmonary disease, erythroleukemia, renal cancer, and hepatitis B or C (2). It is recommended that the hemoglobin be maintained at <17.5 g/dl by ACE inhibitors or ARB even if the patient is normotensive (2, 60). Phlebotomy is used for patients with PTE who do not respond to treatment with an ARB or ACE inhibitor (60, 61). It is also used in conjunction with ACE inhibitors or ARBs for patients who present with hemoglobin greater than 18.5 gm/dL (60, 61). Relapse of PTE is common if therapy is discontinued (2, 60).

5.10. Reproductive Issues

5.10.1. Men

After renal transplantation about 2/3rd of men experience improved libido and sexual function. Males with CKD can experience hypogonadism (63). Balance is restored in hypothalamic-pituitary axis (HPA) after transplantation; however, the degree of pathologic injury to testis determines the reversibility of sexual function (1). Histologically, seminiferous tubular destruction and germinal cell aplasia can be seen (64). Consequently, sperm motility improves but not sperm count or morphology (65). Both sirolimus and cyclosporine can impair biosynthesis of testosterone (1, 66-67). Azathioprine doesn't seem to alter male fertility. It should be kept in mind that beta-blockers and alpha-blockers can induce infertility in transplant patients and calcium channel blockers may cause reversible functional defects in sperm (62). Male patients should be asked about their sexual function and referred to urology as necessary. There are no contraindications to use of agents such as sildenafil for erectile dysfunction in kidney transplant recipients.

5.10.2. Women

Female infertility in CKD results from altered HPA axis with high FSH, LH and prolactin levels. The normal hormonal balance is restored within a year after transplantation (1). Since 1958 over 14000 pregnancies have been reported in renal transplant recipients (69).

5.10.3. Family planning

Pregnancy in transplant patients should be considered high-risk. It used to be that the patients were told to wait 2 yrs after transplant before planning pregnancy (1). Now, guidelines are provided by American Society of Transplantation to help counsel patient (69). Patients can safely plan pregnancy as long as the following conditions are met (68, 69).

a. Graft function is optimal, defined as a serum creatinine <1.5 mg/dL, (132 micromol/L) with <500 mg/24 h protein excretion
b. There are no concurrent fetotoxic infections, such as CMV
c. The patient is not on known teratogenic or fetotoxic medications
d. The immunosuppressive regimen is stable at maintenance levels

A recent meta-analysis covering 50 studies, 4706 pregnancies and 3570 kidney transplant patients, provides the proof as to why pregnancies in these patient population is deemed high-risk (71). According to that meta-analysis, complications of preeclampsia (27.0%), gestational diabetes (8.0%), Cesarean section (56.9%) and preterm delivery (45.6%) were higher than the general US population (3.8%, 3.9%, 31.9% and 12.5%, respectively). Pregnancy outcomes were more favorable in studies with lower mean maternal ages; obstetrical complications were higher in studies with shorter mean interval between kidney transplant and pregnancy. The overall post-transplant live birth rate was 73.5% compared to 66.7% for general US population; similarly, the overall post-transplant miscarriage rate of 14.0% was lower than 17.1%. Transplant recipients usually deliver late preterm (34-36 weeks), roughly 30-50% pregnancies experience intra-uterine growth restriction to some degree and on average give birth to low birth weight babies (~2.5 grams) (70-72). Pregnancy doesn't increase the risk of rejection (71). In the above mentioned study rejection rate was 4.2% in over 2400 pregnant patients studied for rejection (72). Pregnancy also doesn't increase the risk of graft loss (69, 71).

Patients can be counseled that there are no increase risks of birth defects from taking prednisone, azathioprine, and cyclosporine or tacrolimus during pregnancy (2). For azathioprine, no fetal anomalies have been noted at doses equal to or less than 2 mg/kg while in case of cyclosporine dose elevations may be required due to increase volume of distribution during pregnancy (1). Blood levels should be followed when CNIs are used. MMF and sirolimus should be discontinued 6 months before pregnancy, substituted with alternative agents and patients should be monitored closely for rejection during this time period (2). All pregnancies should be planned.

For the patients who are counseled contraception, barrier contraception is the best modality. The American Society of Transplantation Consensus conference suggested the use of progestin-only oral contraceptives and estrogen/progestin formulations providing blood pressure is adequately controlled (69). Also, for patients taking hormonal contraception, CNI levels should be monitored and patients should be advised on the risk of thromboembolism (2).

5.10.4. Pregnancy

The incidence of hypertension in pregnant kidney transplant patients is four-fold higher than uncomplicated pregnancies. About 30% of pregnancies experience pregnancy-induced hypertension (1). Cyclosporine may add to this burden of hypertension. Methyldopa, hydralazine and labetalol can be safely used to negotiate hypertension during pregnancy (1). ACEIs and ARBs are contraindicated during pregnancy and should be stopped as soon as the patient becomes pregnant (1).

Rejection can occur during pregnancy; given hyperfiltration during pregnancy, it can be difficult to diagnose based on creatinine. Once suspected, kidney allograft can be biopsied using real-time renal ultrasound. Rejection can be treated with steroids. Safety of antilymphocyte globulins or rituximab is unknown in pregnancy. IVIG has been used and has not reported to have adverse effects (2).

To decrease the risk of rejection during perinatal period from stress of labor, stress-dosing of hydrocortisone 100mg every 6-8 hours should be considered (1).

All immunosuppressive medications enter maternal-fetal circulation to varying degrees. There is lack of data on pharmacokinetics and pharmacodynamics for various immunosuppressants making it difficult to predict about *intra utero* medication exposure. The placenta metabolizes prednisone to prednisolone; therefore, only low levels have been detected in the fetal circulation (1). Azathioprine is a prodrug that is rapidly metabolized to 6-mercaptopurine. This moiety does pass into the fetus and a relative fetal lack of the enzyme inosine pyrophosphorylase prevents it from being transformed into its active form thioinosinic acid (72). CNI readily cross the placenta and enter the fetal circulation (1, 73). In one study, it was found that cyclosporine in fetal blood was able to inhibit T cell function to the same degree as that found in maternal serum (73). Much less is known about the maternal–fetal transport of MMF and sirolimus. Although there appear to be no obvious congenital abnormalities associated with *in utero* exposure to conventional immunosuppressive agents, long-term follow-up of exposed children is needed.

During breast feeding this exposure may continue to the infant. It is not known whether this exposure constitutes a risk to the infant. Currently according to the consensus from American Society of Transplantation, breast feeding is not contraindicated. The American Academy of Pediatrics supports breastfeeding for mothers who are taking prednisone and advises against it for those who are taking cyclosporine (74). There are no specific American Academy of Pediatrics recommendations for mothers who are taking azathioprine or tacrolimus (74)

5.11. Adherence

Nonadherence is associated with high risk of rejection and allograft loss (23). Kidney transplant recipients show most nonadherence with regards to their immunosuppression, as compared to recipients of other organs (23).

Adherence can be defined as 'the extent to which the patient's behavior matches the agreed-upon prescriber's recommendations'(23). Non adherence is defined by KDIGO as deviation from the prescribed medication regimen sufficient to adversely influence the regimen's intended effect' (23). These definitions are derived from a consensus conference on adherence (75). Non adherence can be at the time of transplant or subsequently. It can be complete or partial and encompasses non compliance with timing of medications (23). It is estimated that non adherence to long-term medication is as high as 50% in developed countries and higher in developing countries (76). Risk factors for nonadherence include nonadherence behavior prior to transplantation, psychiatric illness, personality disorders, poor social support, substance abuse and other high-risk behavior, adolescence, high education level, time since transplantation, lack of adequate follow-up with transplant specialists, inadequate pretransplant education, multiple adverse effects from medications, complex medication regimens, expensive medications and poor access to healthcare (23, 75, 77).

Ongoing patient education and psychosocial support remains two important cornerstones for treating patient nonadherence. The following are some approaches that are more likely to promote adherence and have been divided into two arms: A) education and medical interventions and behavioral and B) psychosocial approaches. Combination of these interventions produces the best results (79-80).

A. Examples of education and medical interventions (23, 77):

1. Ensure that patients know their medications by name, dosage and reason for prescription; reinforce these points during every clinic visit.
2. Inform patients about the adverse effects of drugs.
3. Provide written instructions for each change in medication dose or frequency.
4. Reduce the number and frequency of medications. If possible, medications should be given once daily
5. Ensure the patients understand that they need to continue taking immunosuppressive agents even if the transplanted organ is functioning well.
6. Help establish a system to remind patients to take their medications such as pill boxes or electronic devices that help remind the patient when to take their medications
7. Inquire about problems during every clinic visit, and address specific patient concerns.
8. Monitor compliance with laboratory work, clinic visit and prescription refills.
9. Monitor patients with highest risk of nonadherence (i.e., poorly educated, low family income, patients with history of nonadherence) and provide all possible interventions available

Concomittantly, behavioral strategies and psychosocial approaches also need to be part of the interventions as education and medical interventional strategies are unlikely to suffice on their own.

B. Examples of behavioral and psychosocial approaches (23, 77):

1. Provide positive support feedback for adherence
2. Encourage patient to demonstrate a track record of medication adherence and knowledge.
3. Encourage individual team members to develop rapport with patient.
4. Identify and involve a backup support system (family or friends).
5. Treat depression, anxiety or other psychological issues.

Ultimately there is no single strategy that works for all patients and all of the above approaches need to be individualized to the patient at hand (23). A transplant pharmacist involvement can also improve adherence at 1-year with medication regimens (80, 81)

5.12. Screening

There are as such no randomized control trials to assess risks and benefits of screening for specific health issues.

The following recommendations for cancer screening are based on American Transplantation Society and European Best Practices Guidelines for renal transplantation (82-86):

A. Breast: Annual or biennial mammography for all women older than 50 yr. Women between 40 and 49 could still undergo screening, but no evidence for or against screening at this age
B. Cervical: Annual pap smear and pelvic exam once sexually active
C. Colorectal: Annual FOBT or 5-year flexible sigmoidoscopy for patients older than 50 years
D. Prostate: Annual Digital Rectal Exam and PSA levels in all male transplant recipients older than 50
E. Hepatocellular: No firm guidelines, but alpha-fetoprotein and ultrasound can be performed every 6 months in patients at high risk
F. Skin: Monthly-self exam and annual or biennial exam by dermatologists
G. Renal: No firm recommendation. Some physicians choose to do ultrasound of native kidneys on a regular basis.
H. PTLD: Patients should be screened for EBV antibodies prior to or at the time of transplantation

For oral health, again, there are no specific recommendations, but certain general management strategies have been agreed upon by dentists.

- Routine dental exam should be avoided until 6 months after transplant. For emergency dental exams, it may be preferred to manage these patients in a hospital setting. Annual or biennial dental exam with a dentist should be pursued for long-term dental care.
- All routine dental procedures will need antibiotic prophylaxis and the choice of antibiotics should be made after consuting with patient's transplant physician.
- The most common *oral manifestations* in transplant patients are: viral, bacterial and fungal infections, gingival hyperplasia due to cyclosporine and higher risk in developing oral malignancy, and patients should be screened for them on routine dental exams (87).

Transplant patients should not be given a live vaccine. The following vaccines are recommended for transplant patients (1):

i. Haemophilus Influenza b: Recommended before and after transplant
ii. Hepatitis B: Recommended before and after transplant
iii. Human Papillomavirus: Recommended before and after transplant
iv. Influenza, injected: Recommended before and after transplant
v. Measles, mumps and rubella (MMR): Recommended only before, but not after transplant

vi. Meningococcal (conjugated or polysaccharide): Recommended before and after transplant for adults with asplenia, terminal complement deficiencies, first-year college students living in dormitories and other patients identified to be at-risk
vii. Pneumococcal (conjugated or polysaccharide); Recommended before and after transplant
viii. Tetanus, Diphtheria, Acellular Pertussis (Td/Tdap): Recommended before and after transplant
ix. Varicella: Recommended only before, but not after transplant
x. Zoster: Recommended only before, but not after transplant

Author details

Dhaval Patel and Jun Lee
Department of Medicine, Division of Nephrology, NewYork-Presbyterian Hospital/Weill Cornell Medical College, New York, NY, USA

6. References

[1] Danovitch, G. Handbook of Kidney Transplantation. 5th edition. Philadelphia: Lippincott Williams & Wilkins. 2009.
[2] Uptodate, Inc. https://www.uptodate.com. (Accessed July 20, 2012)
[3] Fuge WW, Hogg BM. The Insensible Losses In Surgical Patients. Ann. Surg. 1938; 108:1-14.
[4] Yarlagadda SG, Coca SG, Formica RN Jr, Poggio ED, Parikh CR. Association between delayed graft function and allograft and patient survival: A systematic review and meta-analysis. Nephrol Dial Transplant 2009; 24: 1039–1047.
[5] Hariharan S, McBride MA, Cherikh WS, Tolleris CB, Bresnahan BA, Johnson CP. Post-transplant renal function in the first year predicts long-term kidney transplant survival. Kidney Int 2002; 62: 311–318.
[6] United Network of Organ Sharing Database. https://www.unos.org. (Accessed July 21, 2012).
[7] Siedlecki A, Irish W, Brennan DC. Delayed Graft Function in Kidney Transplant. Am.J. Transplant. 2011; 11: 2279-2296
[8] Pretagostini R, Lai Q, Poli L, Levi Sandri GB, Travaglia D, Rossi M. Predicitive Characteristics of Delayed Graft Function After Expanded And Standard Criteria Donor Kidney Transplantations. Transplant Proc. 2009; 41:1149-51
[9] Ojo AO, Wolfe RA, Held PJ, Port FK, Schmouder RL. Delayed Graft function: Risk factors and implications for renal allograft survival. Transplantation 1997; 63: 968–974.
[10] Koning OH, Ploeg RJ, van Bockel JH, Groenewegen M, van der Woude FJ, Persijn GG, et al. Risk factors for delayed graft function in cadaveric kidney transplantation: A prospective study of renal function and graft survival after preservation with University of Wisconsin solution in multi-organ donors. European Multicenter Study Group. Transplantation 1997; 63: 1620–1628.

[11] Shoskes DA, Cecka JM. Deleterious effects of delayed graft function in cadaveric renal transplant recipients independent of acute rejection. Transplantation 1998; 66: 1697–1701.
[12] Shoskes DA, Cecka JM. Effect of delayed graft function on short and long-term kidney graft survival. Clin Transplant 1997; 297–303.
[13] McLaren AJ, Jassem W, Gray DW, Fuggle SV, Welsh KI, Morris PJ. Delayed graft function: Risk factors and the relative effects of early function and acute rejection on long-term survival in cadaveric renal transplantation. Clin Transplant 1999; 13: 266–272.
[14] Giral M, Bertola JP, Foucher Y, Villers D, Bironneau E, Blanloeil Y, et al. Effect of brain-dead donor resuscitation on delayed graft function: Results of a monocentric analysis. Transplantation 2007; 83: 1174–1181.
[15] Doshi MD, Garg N, Reese PP, Parikh CR. Recipient risk factors associated with delayed graft function: A paired kidney analysis. Transplantation 2011; 91: 666–671.
[16] Meier-Kriesche HU, Arndorfer JA, Kaplan B. The impact of body mass index on renal transplant outcomes: A significant independent risk factor for graft failure and patient death. Transplantation 2002; 73: 70–74.
[17] Parekh J, Bostrom A, Feng S. Diabetes mellitus: A risk factor for delayed graft function after deceased donor kidney transplantation. Am J Transplant 2010; 10: 298–303.
[18] Johnston O, O'kelly P, Spencer S, Donohoe J, Walshe JJ, Little DM, et al. Reduced graft function (with or without dialysis) vs immediate graft function—a comparison of long-term renal allograft survival. Neph. Dial. Transplant. 2006; 21: 2270–2274
[19] SRTR-Scientific Registry of Transplant Recipients. http://www.srtr.org/annual_reports/2010. (Accessed July 27, 2012).
[20] Briggs JD. Causes of death after renal transplantation. Nephrol Dial Transplant 2001; 16:1545.
[21] Liefeldt L, Budde K. Risk factors for cardiovascular disease in renal transplant recipients and strategies to minimize risk. Transpl International 2010; 23:1191-1204
[22] Shirali AC, Bia MJ. Management of cardiovascular disease in renal transplant recipients. Clin J Am Soc Nephrol 2008; 3: 491-504.
[23] Kidney Disease: Improving Global Outcomes (KDIGO) Transplant Work Group. KDIGO clinical practice guideline for the care of kidney transplant recipients. Am J Transplant 2009; 9(Suppl. 3): S1-155.
[24] Lentine KL, Rocca Rey LA, Kolli S, Bacchi G, Schnitzler MA, Abbott KC, et al. Variations in the risk for cerebrovascular events after kidney transplant compared with experience on the waiting list and after graft failure. Clin J Am Soc Nephrol 2008; 3: 1090-101.
[25] Abedini S, Holme I, Fellström B, Jardine A, Cole E, Maes B, et al. Cerebrovascular events in renal transplant recipients. Transplantation 2009; 87: 112-7.
[26] Snyder JJ, Kasiske BL, Maclean R. Peripheral arterial disease and renal transplantation. J Am Soc Nephrol 2006; 17: 2056-68.
[27] Opelz G, Wujciak T, Ritz E. Association of chronic kidney graft failure with recipient blood pressure: collaborative transplant study. Kidney Int 1998;53:217-22

[28] Midtvedt K, Hartmann A, Foss A, Fauchald P, Nordal KP, Rootwelt K et al. Sustained improvement of renal graft function for two years in hypertensive renal transplant recipients treated with nifedipine as compared to lisinopril. Transplantation 2001; 72:1787-1792

[29] Dunn BL, Teusink AC, Taber DJ, Hemstreet BA, Uber LA, Weimert NA. Management of Hypertension in Renal Transplant Patients: A Comprehensive Review of Nonpharmacologic and Pharmacologic Treatment Strategies. Ann Pharmacother July/August 2010; 44: 1259-1270

[30] K/DOQI Clinical Practice Guidelines on Hypertension and Antihypertensive Agents in Chronic Kidney Disease. http://www.kidney.org. (Accessed on July 31, 2012).

[31] Bruno S, Remuzzi G, Ruggenenti P. Transplant Renal Artery Stenosis. J.Am.Soc.Neph, 2004; 15 :134-141

[32] 2011 USRDS Annual Report. http://www.USRDS.org. (Accessed August 14, 2012).

[33] Bloom RD, Rao V, Weng F, Grossman RA, Cohen D, Mange KC. Association of hepatitis C with post transplant diabetes in renal transplant patients on tacrolimus. J Am Soc Nephrol 2002; 13: 1374-80.

[34] Kasiske BL, Snyder JJ, Gilbertson D, Matas AJ. Diabetes Mellitus After Kidney Transplantation In The United States. Am. J. Transplant 2003; 3: 178-185

[35] Davidson J. Diabetes after transplantation: revised guidelines; target early treatment. Diabetes Voice 2005; 5: 25-27.

[36] Davidson J, Wilkinson A, Dantal J, Dotta F, Haller H, Hernández D et al. New-onset diabetes after transplantation: 2003 International consensus guidelines. Proceedings of an international expert panel meeting. Barcelona, Spain, 19 February 2003. Transplantation 2003; 75: SS3-24

[37] Kasiske B, Cosio FG, Beto J, Bolton K, Chavers BM, Grimm R Jr et al. Clinical practice guidelines for managing dyslipidemias in kidney transplant patients: a report from the Managing Dyslipidemias in Chronic Kidney Disease Work Group of the National Kidney Foundation Kidney Disease Outcomes Quality Initiative. Am J Transplant 2004; 4 Suppl 7:13-53

[38] Potluri K, Hou S. Obesity in kidney transplant recipients and candidates. AJKD July 2010;56: 143-156.

[39] Singh D, Lawen J, Alkhudair W. Does pretransplant obesity affect the outcome in kidney transplant recipients? Transplant Proc, 2005;37: 717–720.

[40] PatelMG. The effect of dietary intervention onweight gains after renal transplantation. J Ren Nutr 1998; 8: 137–141.

[41] Lopes IM, Martin M, Errasti P, Martinez JA. Benefits of a dietary intervention on weight loss, body composition, and lipid profile after renal transplantation. Nutrition 1999;15: 7–10.

[42] Leavey SF, McCullough K, Hecking E, Goodkin D, Port FK, Young EW. Body mass index and mortality in 'healthier' as compared with 'sicker' hemodialysis patients: results from the Dialysis Outcomes and Practice Patterns Study (DOPPS). Nephrol Dial Transplant, 2001; 16 : 2386–2394.

[43] Alexander JW, Goodman HR, Gersin K, Cardi M, Austin J, Goel S et al. Gastric bypass in morbidly obese patients with chronic renal failure and kidney transplant. Transplantation (2004); 78: 469–474.
[44] Counseling to prevent tobacco use and tobacco-caused disease. In, Rockville,MD, US Preventive Services Task Force. Agency for Healthcare Research and Quality. 2003; 1–5
[45] Ducloux D, Motte G, Challier B, Gibey R, Chalopin JM.. Serum total homocysteine and cardiovascular disease occurrence in chronic, stable renal transplant recipients: a prospective study. J Am Soc Nephrol 2000; 11:134-7.
[46] Winkelmayer WC, Kramar R, Curhan GC, Chandraker A, Endler G, Födinger M et al. Fasting plasma total homocysteine levels and mortality and allograft loss in kidney transplant recipients: a prospective study. J Am Soc Nephrol 2005; 16:255-60.
[47] Bostom AG, Carpenter MA, Kusek JW, Levey AS, Hunsicker L, Pfeffer MA et al. Homocysteine-lowering and cardiovascular disease outcomes in kidney transplant recipients: primary results from the Folic Acid for Vascular Outcome Reduction in Transplantation trial. Circulation 2011; 123:1763-70.
[48] World Health Organization. Nutritional anemias: Report of a WHO Scientific Group. World Health Organ Tech Rep Ser 1968; 405: 5-37.
[49] Chadban SJ, Baines L, Polkinghorne K, Jefferys A, Dogra S, Kanganas C, *et al.* Anemia after kidney transplantation is not completely explained by reduced kidney function. Am J Kidney Dis 2007; 49: 301-309.
[50] Mix TCH, Kazmi W, Khan S, Ruthazer R, Rohrer R, Pereira BJG. *et al.* Anemia: a continuing problem following kidney transplantation. Am J Transplant 2003; 3: 1426-1433.
[51] Winkelmayer WC, Chnadraker A, Brookhart MA, Kramar R,Sunder-Plassmann Gl. A prospective study of anemia and long-term outcomes in kidney transplant recipients. Nephrol Dial Transplant 2006; 21:3559.
[52] Molnar MZ, Mucsi I, Macdougall IC, Marsh JE, Yaqoob M, Main J, *et al.* Prevalence and management of anaemia in renal transplant recipients: data from ten European centres. Nephron Clin Pract 2010; 117: c127-134.
[53] Moore LW, Smith SO, Winsett RP, Acchiardo SR, Gaber AO. Factors affecting erythropoietin production and correction of anemia in kidney transplant recipients. Clin Transplant 1994; 8: 358-64.
[54] Frei D, Guttmann RD, Gorman P. A matched-pair control study of postrenal transplant polycythemia. Am J Kidney Dis 1982; 2: 36
[55] Gaston RS, Julian BA, Curtis JJ. Post-transplant erythrocytosis: an enigma revisited. Am J Kidney Dis 1994; 24: 1.
[56] Kessler M, Hestin D, Mayeux D, Mertes PM, Renoult E. Factors predisposing to post-renal transplant erythrocytosis. A prospective matched-pair control study. Clin Nephrol 1996; 45: 83.
[57] Vlahakos DV, Marathias KP, Agroyannis B, Madias NE. Post-transplant erythrocytosis. Kidney Int 2003; 63: 1187-94.
[58] Kiberd BA. Post-transplant erythrocytosis: a disappearing phenomenon? Clin Transplant 2009; 23: 800.

[59] Malyszko J, Oberbauer R, Watschinger B.. Anemia and Erythrocytosis in patients after kidney transplantation. Transplant Int. 2012 Oct; 25 (10):1013-23

[60] Abbud-Filho M, Adams PL, Alberu, J, Cardella C, Chapman J, Cochat P, et al. A report of the Lisbon conference on the care of the kidney transplant recipient. Transplantation Apr. 2007; 83: S1-22.

[61] Barenbrock M, Spieker C, Rahn KH, Zidek W. Therapeutic efficiency of phlebotomy in post transplant hypertension associated with erythrocytosis. Clin Nephrol 1993 Oct; 40: 241-3.

[62] Benoff S, Cooper GW, Hurley I, Mandel FS, Rosenfeld DL, Scholl GM, et al. The effect of calcium ion channel blockers on sperm fertilization potential. Fertil Steril. 1994; 62: 606–617.

[63] Anantharaman P, Schmidt RJ. Sexual function in chronic kidney disease. Adv Chronic Kidney Dis. 2007; 14:119–125.

[64] Zeyneloglu HB, Oktem M, Durak T. Male infertility after renal transplantation: Achievement of pregnancy after intracytoplasmic sperm injection. Transplant Proc. 2005;37: 3081–3084.

[65] Akbari F, Alavi M, Esteghamati A, Mehrsai A, Djaladat H, Zohrevand R et al. Effect of renal transplantation on sperm quality and sex hormone levels. BJU Int. 2003 Aug; 92 : 281-3.

[66] Tondolo V, Citterio F, Panocchia N, Nanni G, Favi E, Brescia A, et al. Gonadal function and immunosuppressive therapy after renal transplantation. Transplant Proc. 2005 May;37 : 1915-7.

[67] Kaczmarek I, Groetzner J, Adamidis I, Landwehr P, Mueller M, Vogeser M. Sirolimus impairs gonadal function in heart transplant recipients. Am J Transplant. 2004 Jul;4:1084-8.

[68] McKay DB, Josephson MA. Pregnancy after Kidney Transplantation CJASN 2008 Mar;3 Suppl 2: S117-25.

[69] McKay DB, Josephson MA, Armenti VT, August P, Coscia LA, Davis CL, et al. Reproduction and transplantation: report on the AST Consensus Conference on Reproductive Issues and Transplantation. Am J Transplant 2005 Jul;5:1592-9.

[70] Davison JM, Bailey DJ. Pregnancy following renal transplantation. J Obstet Gynaecol Res 2003; 29:227–233

[71] Deshpande, N. A., et al. Pregnancy Outcomes in Kidney Transplant Recipients: A Systematic Review and Meta-Analysis. Am J Transplant 2011; 11: 2388–2404.

[72] Saarikoski S, Seppla M: Immunosuppression during pregnancy: Transmission of azathioprine and its metabolites from the mother to the fetus. Am J Obstet Gynecol 1973; 115:1100– 1106.

[73] Flechner SM, Katz AR, Rogers AJ, Van Buren C, Kahan BD: The presence of cyclosporine in body tissues and fluids during pregnancy. Am J Kidney Dis. 1985 Jan;5:60-3.

[74] American Academy of Pediatrics Committee on Drugs: The transfer of drugs and other chemicals into human milk. Pediatrics 1994; 93:137–150.

[75] Fine RN, Becker Y, De Geest S, Eisen H, Ettenger R, Evans R et al. Nonadherence consensus conference summary report. Am J Transplant. 2009 Jan;9:35-41.
[76] Butler JA, Roderick P, Mullee M, Mason JC, Peveler RC. Frequency and impact of nonadherence to immunosuppressants after renal transplantation: A systematic review. Transplantation. 2004 Mar 15;77:769-76
[77] Morrissey PE, Flynn ML, Lin S. Medication noncompliance and its implications in transplant recipients. Drugs 2007;67:1463-81.
[78] Peterson AM, Takiya L, Finley R. Meta-analysis of trials of interventions to improve medication adherence. Am J Health Syst Pharm 2003 Apr 1;60:657-65.
[79] Roter DL, Hall JA, Merisca R, Nordstrom B, Cretin D, Svarstad B. Effectiveness of interventions to improve patient compliance: A meta-analysis. Med Care 1998 Aug;36:1138-61.
[80] Claxton AJ, Cramer J, Pierce C. A systematic review of the association between dose regimens and medication compliance. Clin Ther 2001 Aug;23:1296-310.
[81] Chisholm MA, Mulloy LL, Jagadeesan M and DiPiro, JT. Impact of clinical pharmacy services on renal transplant patients' compliance with immunosuppressive medications. Clinical Transplantation. 2001; 15: 330–336.
[82] EBPG Expert Group on Renal Transplantation: European best practice guidelines for renal transplantation. Section IV: Long-term management of the transplant recipient. IV. 6.1. Cancer risk after renal transplantation. Post-transplant lymphoproliferative disease (PTLD): Prevention and treatment. Nephrol Dial Transplant 2002. 17[Suppl 4]:31– 33, 35–36
[83] EBPG Expert Group on Renal Transplantation: European best practice guidelines for renal transplantation. Section IV: Long-term management of the transplant recipient. IV. 6.3. Cancer risk after renal transplantation. Solid organ cancers: Prevention and treatment. Nephrol Dial Transplant. 2002 17[Suppl 4]:32,34– 36,
[84] EBPG Expert Group on Renal Transplantation: European best practice guidelines for renal transplantation. Section IV: Long-term management of the transplant recipient. IV. 6.2. Cancer risk after renal transplantation. Skin cancers: Prevention and treatment. Nephrol Dial Transplant 2002 17[Suppl 4]:31– 36.
[85] Kasiske BL, Vazquez MA, Harmon WE, Brown RS, Danovitch GM, Gaston RS, et al.: Recommendations for the outpatient surveillance of renal transplant recipients. American Society of Transplantation. J Am Soc Nephrol. 2000 11[Suppl 15]:S1– S86.
[86] Wong G, Chapman JR, Craig JC. Cancer screening in renal transplant recipients: what is the evidence? Clin J Am Soc Nephrol. 2008 Mar;3 Suppl 2:S87-S100.
Carlos FL, Gavaldá EC, Sarrión PMG. Dental management in transplant patients. J Clin Exp. Dent. 2011;3(1):e43-52. http://www.medicinaoral.com/odo/volumenes/v3i1/jcedv3i1p43.pdf (Accessed September 28, 2012).

Chapter 4

Surgical Management of the Kidney Transplant Recipient

Cheguevara Afaneh, Meredith J. Aull, Anthony Watkins,
Sandip Kapur and Jim Kim

Additional information is available at the end of the chapter

http://dx.doi.org/10.5772/54145

1. Introduction

The early postoperative course and management can have a significant impact on the long-term success of a kidney transplant recipient. Several factors affect long-term outcomes including the occurrence of delayed graft function (DGF), episodes of acute rejection (AR), surgical complications, and overwhelming infections, especially sepsis [1-3]. Certain medications, including calcineurin inhibitors (CNI), also have potential for nephrotoxic effects, which can later lead to transplant glomerulopathy [4]. Furthermore, recipient characteristics, such as sensitization status, and donor characteristics, such as donation after cardiac death (DCD) donors and expanded criteria donors (ECD) can all affect long-term outcomes [5]. Although basic postoperative surgical principles are applied, there are certain parameters that need to be closely monitored, especially as it pertains to fluid management, blood pressure control, and immunologic status. Early detection of graft dysfunction is paramount in determining reversibility from both medical and surgical complications. Recognizing the technical limitations during surgery can also help prevent potentially devastating mechanical complications. Thus, appropriate initial management and mitigation of various risk factors is extremely important in the long-term success of the kidney transplant patient.

2. Surgical procedure

Technical variations exist for kidney transplant, such as in the retroperitoneal exposure or implantation of the ureter, but the basic surgical procedure will be described in this section. The right iliac fossa has traditionally been described as the initial choice for implantation, but previous operations, quality of vessels, or other recipient factors may make the left side more approachable. In the case of polycystic kidney disease, where the native kidneys need to be removed, a midline incision is made.

2.1. Backtable kidney preparation

The kidney is kept cold in an ice slush bath during the preparation, which involves dissecting the renal artery and vein from the surrounding tissue. The ureter is identified and retracted away so as to avoid injury when removing extraneous fat and tissue from the kidney and hilum. Attention must be directed to protecting the blood supply to the ureter by avoiding the so-called "golden triangle" at the inferior pole of the kidney. Multiple renal arteries may also require repair and a Carrel patch may or may not be preserved depending on the degree of aortic plaque seen. In the case of a right kidney, the renal vein may require lengthening, which can be accomplished by utilizing the attached IVC.

2.2. Surgical exposure

An oblique curvilinear incision is made in the right or left lower quadrant of the abdomen, extending from near the pubic symphysis to above the anterior superior iliac spine of the iliac crest. Muscle layers can be directly divided, lateral to the rectus sheath, or split along the fibers of the external and internal obliques and transversalis. The peritoneum is identified and retracted superiorly and medially to expose the retroperitoneum. Self-retaining retractors can be placed to facilitate subsequent exposure of the psoas and iliac vessels.

2.3. Operative procedure

The common or external iliac artery and vein are identified and dissected. Lymphatics that course along the length of the vessels need to be meticulously tied or cauterized to prevent occurrence of lymphoceles. Vascular flow is controlled proximally and distally with vascular clamps and the kidney is brought into the surgical field. A venotomy is first made in the recipient iliac vein and an end-to-side anastomosis with the renal vein is created with 5-0 or 6-0 monofilament non-absorbable suture. Similarly, an arteriotomy is then made and the arterial anastomosis is completed in an end-to-side fashion. The clamps are released sequentially, with the vein before the artery, and the kidney is perfused. Once hemostasis is attained, the urinary tract is reconstructed. The bladder, which should be irrigated with antibiotic solution prior to start of the procedure, can be filled by way of a three-way Foley catheter or instilled with the antibiotic solution at the start of the operation. The kidney is positioned in the retroperitoneum and an area on the bladder is identified for implantation of the ureter. The layers of the bladder are carefully dissected and a cystostomy is created. The transplant ureter is cut to length and the anastomosis is done with or without a stent using monofilament absorbable suture. One technique described for ureteroneocystostomy is the Lich-Gregoir technique, which involves an anastomosis between the ureteral and bladder mucosa with a myotomy closure over the ureter. The abdominal wall is then reapproximated and closed in layers.

3. Early postoperative course

3.1. Renal and fluid management

The initial management of the kidney transplant recipient involves proper fluid management, focusing on volume status and electrolyte balance. Assessing volume status is multifaceted and includes monitoring urine output, central venous pressure, heart rate, and blood pressure. Attention to daily weights and total input-output tabulations can help dictate fluid management, especially regarding the use of diuretics postoperatively. A decrease in urine volume can result from hypovolemia, obstruction, acute tubular necrosis (ATN), urinary leak, or in the most severe case, vascular thrombosis.

Recipients of living donor kidney transplants have brisk urine output immediately or within minutes of implantation. Fluids may need to be replaced adequately to avoid a negative fluid balance within the first 24 hours. This can potentially compromise blood flow to the new kidney. Deceased donor allografts, in comparison, not make significant urine amounts initially. Fluid and furosemide challenges should be considered; however, if there has been little to no response after several attempts, then fluids should be administered judiciously in consideration of overall volume status from a respiratory, cardiovascular, and renal standpoint. The goal of fluid resuscitation in the early postoperative period focuses on maintaining good perfusion to the transplanted allograft.

Changes in urine output should be assessed in an objective and systematic manner. First, the foley should be assessed for patency and flushed, as patients may have mild hematuria leading to clot formation. If hypovolemia is suspected, then a fluid challenge with crystalloid or albumin should be administered [6]. Failure to respond to a fluid challenge and increases in serum creatinine should prompt assessment of the graft with Duplex ultrasonography (DUS), which can be used to assess perfusion to the allograft, rule out hydronephrosis and evaluate perinephric fluid collections. Significant, but less dramatic decreases in urine output should raise clinical suspicion for renal artery or vein thrombosis, which would warrant surgical re-exploration if caught in a timely fashion. Patients with little to no response to fluid challenges should also be administered a furosemide challenge. Patients who fail to respond to fluid or furosemide without any structural or vascular abnormalities on DUS may have ATN, which can be confirmed with a biopsy.

3.2. Cardiovascular and pulmonary assessment

Assessment and maintenance of adequate blood pressure control is imperative to the success of the kidney transplant. Because the transplanted kidney is an end-organ, it is susceptible to injury during episodes of hypotension, which can lead to ATN. Careful attention to the choice of induction therapy being administered, such as rabbit antithymocyte globulin (rATG), is important as the side effect profile includes fever, dyspnea, respiratory distress, and hypotension [7]. If other causes of respiratory distress or hypotension have been excluded, the rate of rATG administration may need to be slowed or even stopped temporarily or permanently. Basiliximab, an interleukin-2 receptor antagonist

(IL2RA), has fewer side effects and can be administered as an alternative under different immunosuppression protocols.

The use of calcium channel blockers has been shown to be beneficial in kidney transplantation. Intra-arterial administration of calcium channel blockers, such as verapamil, improves renal blood flow as well as augments immunosuppression [8]. Postoperative administration of oral calcium channel blockers has also been implemented, as there is evidence that the incidence of DGF is decreased [9]. In a large systematic review and meta-analysis of randomized controlled trials, the use of calcium channel blockers has been shown to decrease the risk of graft loss and improved post-transplant glomerular filtration rates (GFR) [10]. Furthermore, in the early transplant period, the use of calcium channel blockers have been shown to be superior to angiotensin-converting enzyme inhibitors with regards to avoiding nephrotoxicity, improving GFR, improving hemoglobin levels, minimizing the incidence of hyperkalemia, and minimizing proteinuria post-transplant [10].

Respiratory complications can lead to poor outcomes. As previously stated, the use of rATG may lead to respiratory distress as capillary leak can occur. Acute respiratory failure post-transplant can compromise allograft outcomes [11,12]. The leading cause of respiratory failure is typically bacterial pneumonia [12]. Patients with prolonged intensive care hospitalizations are at risk of invasive fungal and opportunistic infections, especially in the setting of intense perioperative immunosuppression. These infections have been linked to increased mortality [13]. Appropriate chemoprophylaxis with trimethoprim-sulfamethoxazole for *Pneumocystis jiroveci* pneumonia may be beneficial and potentially mitigate the infectious risks [14].

4. Assessment of graft function

4.1. Early graft dysfunction

Early complications leading to graft dysfunction can be separated into two categories: medical or surgical. Marginal donors, including ECD and DCD allografts, have the highest rate of medical and surgical complications [15,16]. Various medical and surgical complications resulting in early graft dysfunction are listed in Table 1. The following sections will discuss the most common culprits in each category. Hypovolemia has been discussed in a previous section.

4.2. Primary non-function

Primary non-function (PNF), defined as the lack of adequate allograft function by the third month post transplant, has a reported incidence between 1-8% [17-19]. Typically, patients at risk of PNF include highly sensitized patients and those on renal replacement therapy for a prolonged duration of time prior to transplantation. Acute rejection and surgical complications are the most common causes of PNF [19]. The use of histidine-tryptophan-ketoglutarate (HTK) solution has also been implicated as a cause of PNF in deceased donor renal transplants [17]. A recent study suggests that a mean arterial blood pressure less than or equal to 80 mm Hg approximately 3 months before kidney transplantation is a risk factor for PNF [18]. Certain donor factors, such as prolonged cold ischemia time, have also been associated with PNF [20]. Patients with PNF have poorer overall patient survival, compared to patients with immediate graft function, probably as a result of returning to renal replacement therapy at an earlier time.

Common Causes of Early Graft Dysfunction	
Medical	**Surgical**
Delayed graft function	Hemorrhage
Hypovolemia	Urinary obstruction
Acute rejection	Vascular thrombosis
Drug-induced nephrotoxicity	Hematuria
Infection	Arterial stenosis
Disease recurrence	Extrinsic obstruction

Table 1. Common causes of early graft dysfunction stratified by medical or surgical causes.

4.3. Immunologic events

4.3.1. Hyperacute rejection

Hyperacute rejection occurs in the setting of ABO incompatible transplants or in the setting of a positive lymphocytotoxic crossmatch, where the incidence is approximately 85%. Some antibodies may have lower binding affinity to receptors or fail to bind any complement. Once this process has occurred, treatment involves immediate removal of the allograft. Some protocols utilizing plasmapheresis have been used with modest results [21], but graft survival remains poor. The emergence of kidney-paired donation and chains has circumvented the need for transplantation across ABO blood groups [22]. Renal scan typically demonstrates no perfusion and pathology reveals microvascular thrombosis, thus necessitating a transplant nephrectomy. With the advent of modern immunologic testing prior to transplant, hyperacute rejection remains a rare occurrence.

4.3.2. Accelerated vascular rejection

Accelerated vascular rejection is an early aggressive form of acute rejection that may occur in sensitized recipients with a high panel-reactive antibody or patients with a previous transplant, despite a negative T cell crossmatch. This type of rejection occurs as early as postoperative day 2 or can be as late as postoperative day 5. Anti-rejection treatment modalities generally fail to be effective in these patients. Histology reveals fibrin deposition and endothelitis. These patients are typically treated similar to antibody-mediated rejection episodes with plasmapheresis, intravenous immunoglobulin, and/or antibody-depleting agents [23].

4.3.3. Acute rejection

Acute rejection can occur at any time in the early post-transplant period. The most common time point, however, is 5 to 7 days post-transplant. Acute cellular rejection remains the most common type of rejection episode. The incidence of acute rejection is highest in the first 6 months post-transplant, with overall acute rejection rates between 10-20%. The immunologic profiles of the donor and recipient as well as the use of different immunosuppression protocols are important in stratifying acute rejection risk. Signs and symptoms of acute rejection include fever, elevated serum creatinine, increasing weight, and graft tenderness. Transplant biopsy remains the gold standard for diagnosis. Histological changes in acute rejection include tubulitis and interstitial infiltrates, with or without arteritis [24].

Treatment of acute cellular rejection depends on the severity. First-line therapy includes a steroid pulse. In more severe cases of acute rejection, an antibody-depleting agent, such as rATG should be administered in addition to a steroid pulse. CNI levels should be monitored closely in the setting of acute rejection, as nephrotoxicity is more common. Moreover, in the setting of antibody-depleting therapy, patients should be monitored closely for infectious complications [25]. Graft survival is negatively impacted by episodes of acute rejection [26].

5. Technical complications

5.1. Vascular

5.1.1. Renal artery thrombosis

Renal artery thrombosis is a rare event. Technical issues, such as arterial kinking or intimal dissection, are the usual culprits. The majority of these events occur in the first few days following transplantation. Sudden cessation of urine production should raise the suspicion for vascular compromise. Risk factors for this devastating condition include the use of pediatric donors less than or equal to 15 kg without an aortic patch as well as kidneys from donors less than 5 years of age [27,28]. However, use of pediatric donors less than 10 kg has also been successfully reported without an increased rate of arterial thrombosis [29]. The diagnosis must be made promptly, as the allograft can only tolerate 30-60 minutes of warm ischemia before the allograft has irreversible injury. Even in ideal situations, recovery from ischemic injury may still be impossible. A high-index of suspicion is necessary to ensure prompt and adequate treatment of this condition with emergent re-operation. In cases where the recipient had previously made urine at baseline, the diagnosis becomes even more difficult. The diagnosis is made with DUS, which demonstrate lack of color flow (Figure 1).

When multiple renal arteries are present on the donor allograft, reconstruction may be necessary during implantation. Most authors have reported no difference in vascular complications or graft survival [30]. However, thrombosis of some minor branches supplying superior or inferior poles can lead to partial infarction of the renal allograft. Patients may present with elevated serum creatinine or hypertension. Subsequent angiogram will demonstrate a wedge perfusion defect of the allograft. Patients may then present with urine leak if caliceal infarction is present. In such circumstances, the patient may benefit from nephrostomy tube placement for complete urinary decompression as well as percutaneous drain placement in the event of urinoma development.

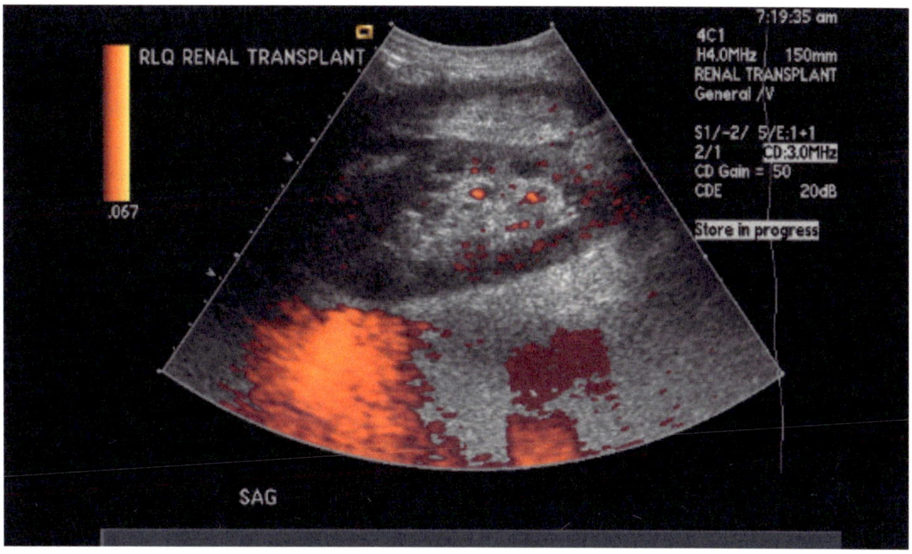

Figure 1. Doppler ultrasound demonstrates global hypoperfusion of the transplanted kidney consistent with renal artery thrombosis on postoperative day 1.

5.1.2. Renal vein thrombosis

Renal vein thrombosis is also an uncommon, but potentially devastating, complication. The usual causes include injuries to the donor renal vein that was narrowed after repair of an injury or twisting of the vein on the renal pedicle. Previously, the use of right-sided living donor renal allografts was associated with an increased risk of renal vein thrombosis due to the short length. However, we have not seen this in our large series of right-sided donors, even with modern procurement techniques, such as laparoendoscopic single-site surgery [31,32]. Patients present with gross hematuria, decreased urine output and engorgement of the graft due to venous outflow obstruction. DUS will show parvus tardus and reversal of diastolic flow in the renal artery. Immediate repair is necessary if there is to be any chance of salvaging the allograft.

5.1.3. Hemorrhage and hematoma

Most postoperative hematomas are small and insignificant. They are usually incidentally found on a post-transplant DUS. Larger and more clinically significant hematomas may occur in the setting of antiplatelet therapy or anticoagulation for patients with risk factors for venothromboembolic events (Figure 2). Patients with clinically significant hematomas will present with swelling from the incision, pain over the graft, and an acute drop in hemoglobin values. The hematoma will continue to increase in size until it ultimately impinges on the vascular pedicle of the allograft, which can lead to thrombosis or hydronephrosis. Postoperatively, patients may show signs of bruising in dependent regions of the wound, flank and groin.

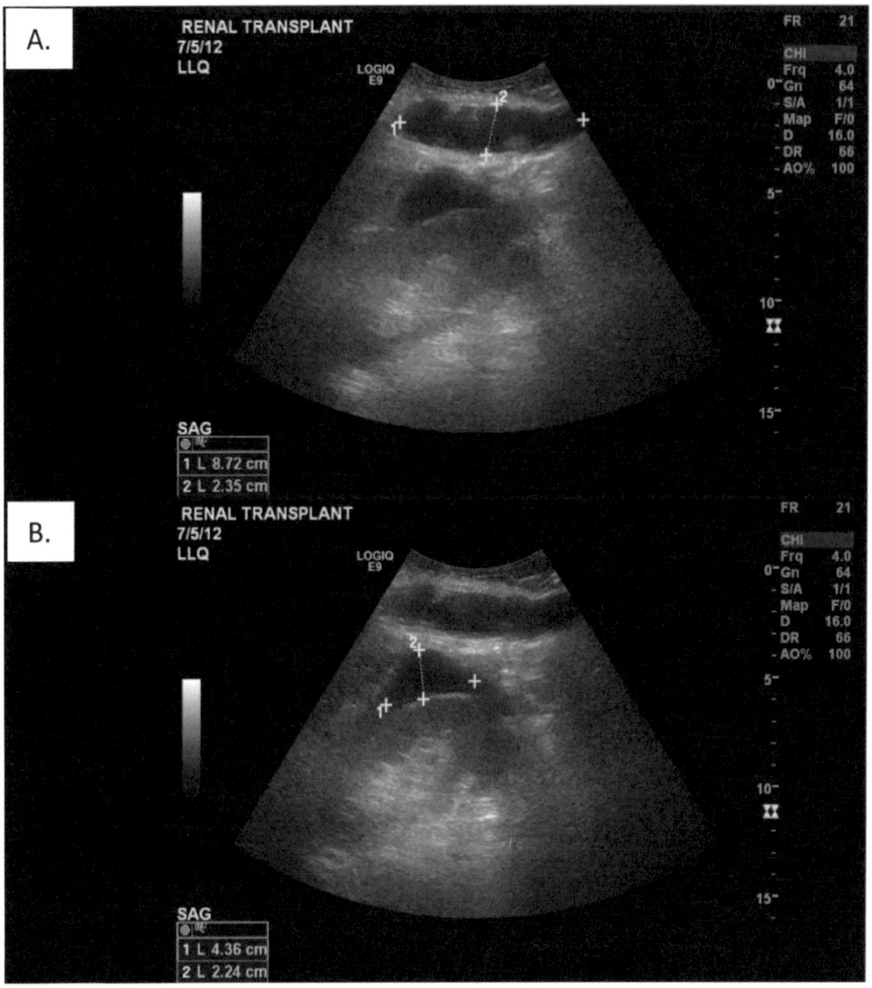

Figure 2. Panel A demonstrates an early postoperative hematoma (as outlined by plus signs) above the fascia in a transplant patient on systemic anticoagulation. Panel B illustrates a perinephric hematoma (as outlined by plus signs) in the same patient.

Patients requiring postoperative anticoagulation for prophylaxis of a vascular thrombotic event are at greatest risk of developing a hematoma [33,34]. The reported risk of a postoperative bleed on heparin requiring surgical exploration has been reported as high as 60% in patients on anticoagulation. Moreover, patients with a history of lupus and lupus anticoagulant are especially sensitive to heparin anticoagulation, leading to an increased risk of postoperative hemorrhage [35]. Percutaneous drainage of large hematomas is insufficient and operative exploration and evacuation should be undertaken to avoid vascular thrombosis and to remove clot as a potential nidus of infection.

5.1.4. Renal artery stenosis

Transplant renal artery stenosis is a late complication of kidney transplantation. The diagnosis is usually made with DUS, which demonstrates parvus tardus waveforms as well as elevated resistive indices. An MRA is necessary to confirm the diagnosis. Treatment includes interventional procedures involving balloon angioplasty and potentially stenting or surgical repair with cadaveric graft. This topic is discussed in detail in another chapter of this textbook.

5.2. Urinary

5.2.1. Ureteral obstruction

Pelvicaliceal dilation seen on DUS implies obstruction in the urinary flow. Placement of a foley catheter and examination of its patency can provide relief if the cause is from an enlarged prostate or dysfunctional bladder. Failure of the foley catheter to relieve obstruction necessitates immediate decompression via placement of a percutaneous nephrostomy tube. An antegrade pyelogram can be performed to visualize where the obstruction occurs (Figure 3). A decrease in the serum creatinine following decompression confirms the diagnosis. After 1-2 days of allowing the postoperative edema to subside, a nephrogram is performed to evaluate whether ureteral obstruction or stenosis remains. Early strictures usually require surgical repair, where as late strictures are more amenable to less invasive procedures, such as stent placement and angioplasty.

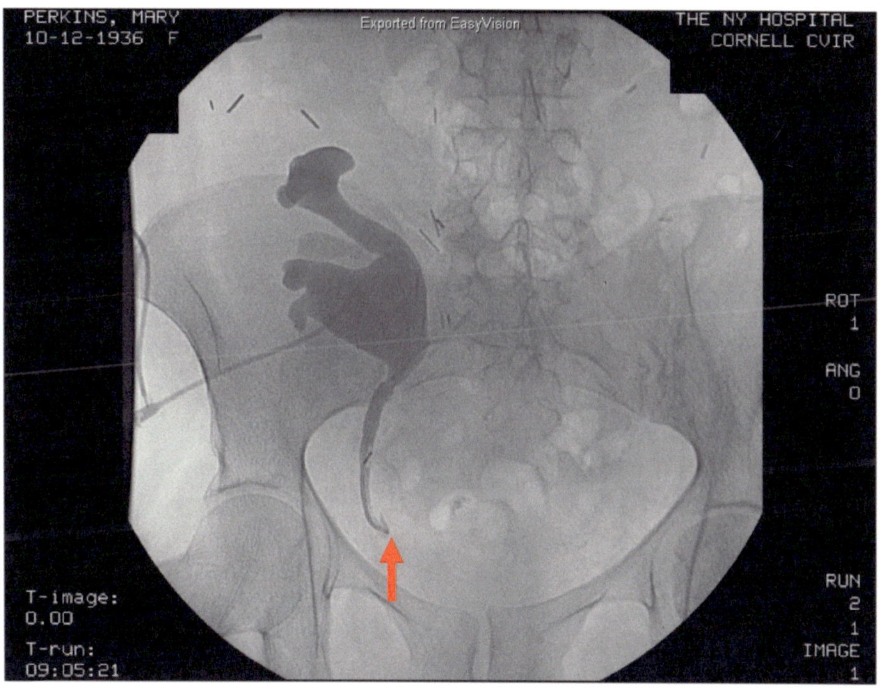

Figure 3. An antegrade pyelogram is shown demonstrating complete obstruction (red arrow) at the ureteroneocystostomy anastomosis of the transplanted kidney in the right lower quadrant.

Ureteral strictures in the early postoperative period are related to technical issues. Patients with ureteral stents will not present with obstruction in the early postoperative period. Rather they may present with this problem several weeks after stent removal. This complication is usually the result of a twist in the ureter or narrowing at the anastomosis due to distal ureteral ischemia [36]. Short segment strictures (< 2 cm) are usually amenable to percutaneous dilatation whereas longer strictures (>2 cm) and those involving the proximal or mid-ureter typically require surgical revision. The treatment options include excising the stricture and creating a new ureteroneocystostomy, if sufficient length is available on the transplant ureter. A psoas hitch or Boari flap can be performed to bring the bladder closer to the kidney to assist in this approach. Otherwise, a ureteroureterostomy using the ipsilateral native ureter or ureteropyelostomy may be required. A 6 French double-J stent can be left in place for 4 to 6 weeks. In cases where the ipsilateral native ureter is unavailable, the contralateral ureter can also be used. Graft survival is not significantly affected in patients undergoing correction or revision of urologic complications in the first year post-transplant [37].

5.2.2. Urine leak

Urine leak usually occurs in the first month after transplant and is due to a disruption in the ureteral-bladder anastomosis. Caliceal infarction from a partial thrombosis of the renal allograft can also present as a urine leak. The presenting symptoms include abdominal pain, increasing serum creatinine level and a decrease in urine output. Typically, a DUS or renal scan shows a fluid collection in the retroperitoneal space (Figure 4). Sampling of the fluid and analysis for creatinine can confirm the diagnosis of a urinoma.

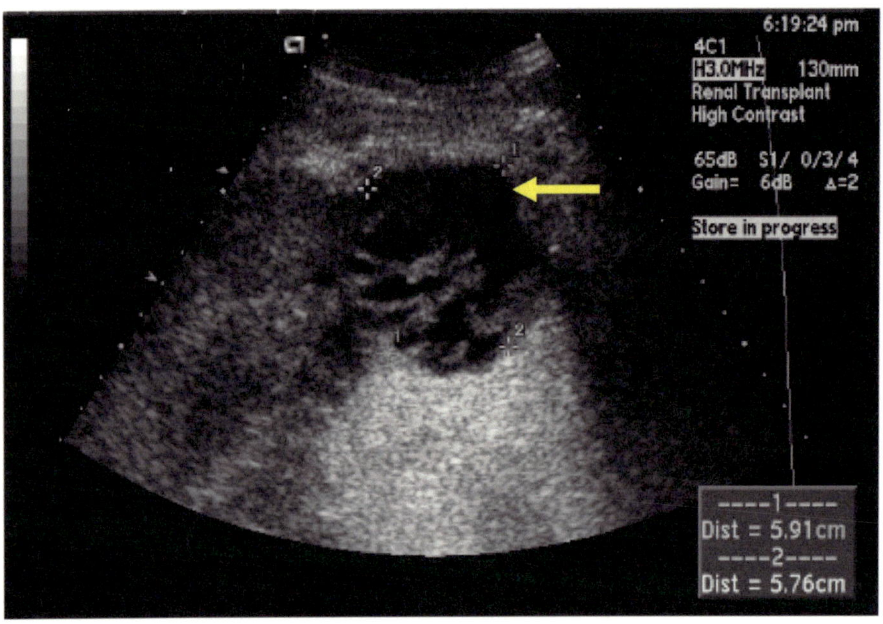

Figure 4. Urinoma (yellow arrow) located at the inferior pole of the transplanted kidney as a result of a urine leak.

Causes of urine leak include technical issues related to creation of the ureteroneocystostomy or ischemic necrosis of the distal ureter. Urgent surgical management of this condition is mandatory to decrease the risk of wound infection and improve potential for recovery of the allograft.

5.3. Lymphocele

A lymphocele is a collection of lymphatic fluid that develops in the postoperative field in a nonepithelialized cavity. These collections typically form around the divided lymphatics surrounding the recipient iliac vasculature. Most lymphoceles are asymptomatic and do not require any intervention; however, lymphoceles can cause compressive symptoms from mass effect on surrounding tissue and structures, or can become infected. Most lymphoceles occur between 2 weeks and 6 months post-transplant [38]. The peak incidence is about 6 weeks post-transplant. The source of the lymphocele is from disrupted lymphatic channels surrounding the iliac vasculature during implantation. Lymphocele formation can be prevented by meticulous dissection and ligation of all lymphatic trunks with a nonabsorbable suture. Some have even suggested that lymphocele formation can be avoided by anastomosing to the common iliac vasculature were less lymphatic tissue is present [39]. The use of mTOR inhibitors has been strongly and positively correlated with the development of lymphoceles in kidney transplantation [40].

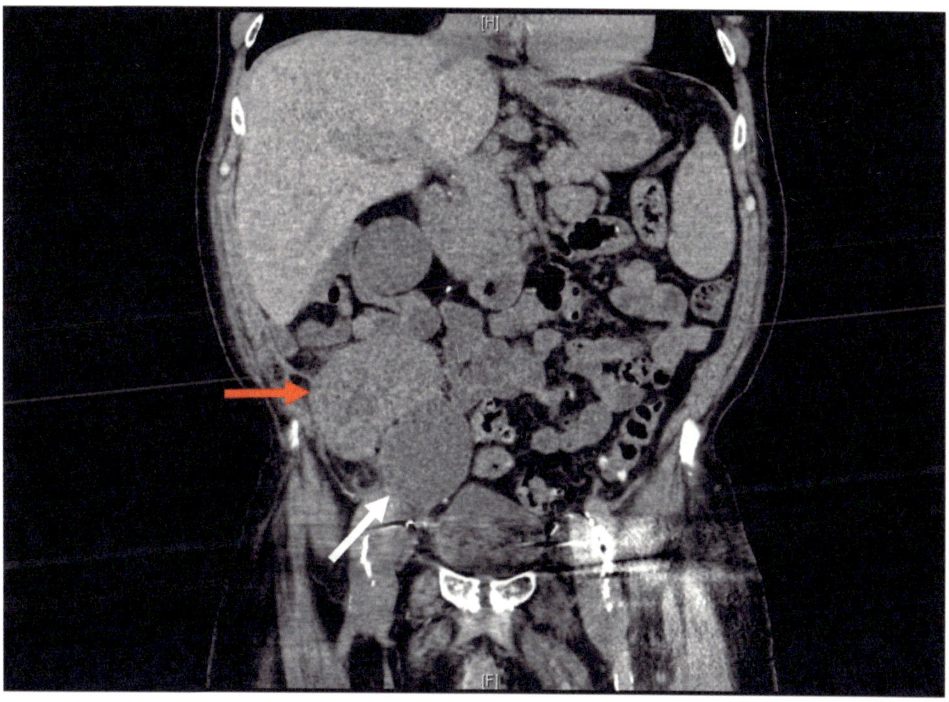

Figure 5. A lymphocele (white arrow) can be seen on CT scan compressing the right lower quadrant transplanted kidney (red arrow) causing hydronephrosis.

Lymphoceles are suggested by DUS or CT scan findings demonstrating a large fluid periallograft collection (Figure 5). The most common location is adjacent to the bladder and multiple collections may be present. Sending aspirated fluid for cytological and biochemical analysis for lymphocytes can confirm the diagnosis. Small, asymptomatic collections should be left alone, as spontaneous resolution is common. Larger collections and those that are causing obstructive symptoms can be initially managed by placement of a percutaneous drain. Recurrence is common and several aspirations may be necessary. Each aspiration carries a theoretical risk of infection. Sclerotherapy with povidone-iodine can be effective [41]. A possible complication of povidone-iodine is acute renal failure and this should be monitored during and after treatment [42]. Operative drainage of lymphoceles provides definitive therapy. The goal for drainage is to allow communication with the peritoneal cavity where it can be reabsorbed. This can be done via an open or the preferred laparoscopic approach [38]. The lymphocele is unroofed or fenestrated with a 5 cm opening to allow direct drainage into the peritoneal cavity.

6. Medical complications

6.1. Delayed graft function

Delayed graft function (DGF) is the most common cause of early graft dysfunction and is defined as the need for dialysis within the first week after transplant. DGF has been reported to affect approximately 20-25% of all deceased donor transplant recipients [43]. Recipients of marginal donors, including ECD and DCD, have rates of DGF as high as 70% in some studies [15, 44]. The use of pulsatile hypothermic machine perfusion has been shown in studies to reduce that risk, though the overall rate still remains higher than SCD allografts [44]. Various donor risk factors for DGF include age, cause of death, and ischemia reperfusion injury [45].

DGF is a well-documented risk factor for poor graft survival. In a 2011 study analyzing 40 years of deceased donor renal transplant recipients, the occurrence of DGF and acute rejection were the most significant predictors of renal allograft survival rates [26]. As previously discussed, marginal donors have the highest rates of DGF, while the rate of DGF in living donors is relatively uncommon. Additionally, patients undergoing retransplantation have higher rates of DGF than first time recipients of renal allografts. ECD allograft recipients may have a higher rate of acute rejection, which may be related to the higher rate of DGF in these allografts [46]. Prolonged cold ischemia has been a well-documented cause of DGF; however, recent data suggests that cold ischemia-induced DGF may play a limited role in long-term outcomes [47].

The use of DUS and biopsy can differentiate DGF from other causes of early graft dysfunction, such as acute rejection or surgical complications. A transplant biopsy is usually necessary to differentiate between other causal factors, such as acute rejection or recurrent disease. Radiographic studies in the proper clinical context can also aid in the diagnosis of DGF. Typically, transplants with DGF will demonstrate good renal perfusion and good parenchymal uptake of radionucleotide tracer with little or no renal excretion. Primary non-function should be considered in the differential at this time point.

6.2. Drug-induced nephrotoxicity

Calcineurin inhibitors (CNIs) have become the cornerstone of immunosuppression regimens. Early administration post-transplant has helped mitigate the risk of acute rejection in kidney transplantation. Most institutions have implemented the use of polyclonal antibody-depleting or monoclonal antibody induction therapy in conjunction with introduction of CNIs as early as postoperative day 1 or 2, as we do in our institution. CNIs can have a nephrotoxic effect on the allograft by decreasing renal blood flow in the afferent arteriole, leading to tubular injury [48]. Variable oral absorption of CNIs, especially cyclosporine, in the early postoperative period can lead to either overdosing or underdosing, causing either nephrotoxicity or acute rejection, respectively.

Differentiating calcineurin inhibitor toxicity from other causes of graft dysfunction is difficult based on clinical context. Percutaneous transplant biopsy can be used to diagnose other causes of graft dysfunction. Histologic findings are non-specific with tubular injury and tubular vacuolization being the most common early findings. Hyaline deposition and fibrosis can be found with chronic injury. Obtaining daily calcineurin inhibitor levels can prevent supratherapeutic dosing, predisposing patients to the nephrotoxic effects. Avoiding nephrotoxicity is important, as chronic nephrotoxicity has been shown to correlate with chronic transplant nephropathy, ultimately affecting long-term allograft survival [49].

6.3. Infectious complications

Infectious complications in the early postoperative period are typically related to the operation. The most common postoperative infections include surgical site infections, urinary tract infections, bacteremia from central venous catheters, and pneumonia [50]. Careful and meticulous surgical technique and attention to detail can help prevent most early infectious complications, such as surgical site infections, central venous catheter sepsis, and urinary tract infections from foley catheter placement. Encouraging early ambulation and the use of incentive spirometry decreases the incidence of atelectasis and the risk of postoperative pneumonia. Removing foley catheters and stents once they no longer serve an appreciable purpose can help prevent and eliminate urinary tract infections. Central venous catheters should be removed as early as possible to decrease the incidence of line sepsis.

Typically, opportunistic infections are relatively uncommon in the early postoperative period (<30 days). Cytomegalovirus (CMV) infection occurs, especially in seronegative recipients receiving allografts from seropositive donors. Institution of CMV prophylaxis with oral valganciclovir or high-dose oral acyclovir for a minimum of 3 months has significantly reduced the incidence and severity of CMV infection [51]. Once antiviral prophylaxis has been halted, CMV infection may still occur. Appropriate prophylaxis with trimethoprim/sulfamethoxazole has almost entirely eliminated early *Pneumocystis carinii* pneumonia. Prophylactic antifungal agents, such as nystatin or clotrimazole troches, have also been instituted to decrease the risk of oral *Candida* infections in the early postoperative period.

Prompt diagnosis and treatment of infectious complications leads to better outcomes. Aggressive treatment with intravenous antibacterial, antiviral or antifungal agents for severe infections improve outcomes. Infected intra-abdominal collections should be drained. Minimizing external instrumentation should be part of the fundamental strategy in preventing infectious complications.

6.4. Disease recurrence

The majority of causes of end-stage renal disease (ESRD) do not recur early in the post-transplant period. Disease processes such as diabetes mellitus and hypertension can cause recurrence of ESRD if poorly controlled over a long period of time. Two causes of ESRD, however, can recur immediately post-transplant: focal segmental glomerulosclerosis (FSGS) and thrombotic microangiopathy (TMA).

FSGS is a form of glomerulonephritis that can recur immediately post-transplant. Although the exact mechanism is unclear, a serum factor causes glomerular injury and early massive proteinuria [52,53]. The development of nephrotic range proteinuria can be suggestive of disease recurrence in a patient with a pretransplant diagnosis of FSGS. The diagnosis can be verified with electron microscopy demonstrating effacement of foot processes. Current treatment strategies include increasing calcineurin inhibitor dosing, steroids, and plasmapheresis, with the latter modality being the most effective [52]. If patients fail to respond over several weeks, then further treatments are not likely to be effective.

Thrombotic microangiopathy can also recur relatively quickly post-transplant. Causes of TMA include recurrent disease, endothelial damage from calcineurin inhibitor use, hypercoagulable disorders, or antibody-mediated rejection episodes [54]. Clinical manifestations include hemolysis and decreases in hemoglobin, platelet count, and haptoglobin. Additionally, microangiopathy will be present on peripheral blood smears. Patients will have increases in lactate dehydrogenase and serum creatinine, signifying allograft dysfunction. Transplant biopsy will show fibrin clot in arterioles. Treatment includes removing inciting factors, such as calcineurin inhibitors, as well as plasmapheresis [55]. Eculizumab, a humanized monoclonal antibody to complement component 5 (C5) to mediate complement-mediated injury, has emerged as a possible treatment option for TMA [56]. Blocking complement activation, especially the last step of the complement cascade, has important implications in TMA. Treatment of TMA posttransplant has been successfully reported [57], but still carries a poor prognosis.

7. Summary

Early management of the kidney transplant recipient is crucial for optimizing outcomes and avoiding early graft loss, or even death. Given the surgical and medical complexity of these patients, attention to detail and prompt diagnosis of complications is critical to achieving excellent outcomes. Clinical scenarios need to be recognized where early operative intervention is necessary to save the graft. However, whenever possible, prevention of complications provides the best outcomes.

Author details

Cheguevara Afaneh, Meredith J. Aull, Anthony Watkins, Sandip Kapur and Jim Kim
Department of Surgery, Division of Transplant Surgery, New York-Presbyterian Hospital- Weill Cornell Medical College, New York, NY, USA

8. References

[1] Almond, P.S.; Matas, A.; Gillingham, K., et al. (1993). Risk factors for chronic rejection in renal allograft recipients. *Transplantation*, Vol.55, No.4, (April 1993), pp. 752-6, ISSN 0041-1337.
[2] Aultman, D.F.; Sawaya, D.E.; Zibari, G.B., et al. (1999). Are all successful renal transplants really successful? *Am J Kidney Dis*, Vol.34, No.1, (July 1999), pp. 61-4, ISSN 0272-6386.
[3] Troppmann, C.; Gillingham, K.J.; Benedetti, E., et al. (1995). Delayed graft function, acute rejection, and outcome after cadaver renal transplantation: a multivariate analysis. *Transplantation*, Vol.59, No.7, (April 1995), pp. 962-8, ISSN 0041-1337.
[4] Nankivell, B.J.; Borrows, R.J.; Fung, C.L., et al. (2003). The natural history of chronic allograft nephropathy. *N Engl J Med*, Vol.349, No.24, (December 2003), pp. 2326-33, ISSN 0028-4793.
[5] Matsuoka, L.; Shah, T.; Aswad, S., et al. (2006). Pulsatile perfusion reduces the incidence of delayed graft function in expanded criteria donor kidney transplantation. *Am J Transplant*, Vol.6, No.6, (June 2006), pp. 1473-8, ISSN 1600-6135.
[6] Dawidson, I.J.; Sandor, Z.F.; Coorpender, L., et al. (1992). Intraoperative albumin administration affects the outcome of cadaver renal transplantation. *Transplantation*, Vol.53, No.4., (April 1992), pp. 774-82, ISSN 0041-1337.
[7] Buchler, M.; Hurault de Ligny, B.; Madec, C., et al. (2003). Induction therapy by anti-thymocyte globulin (rabbit) in renal transplantation: a 1-yr follow-up of safety and efficacy. *Clin Transplant*, Vol.17, No.6, (December 2003), pp. 539-45, ISSN 0902-0063.
[8] Dawidson, I.; Rooth, P.; Fry, W.R., et al. (1989). Prevention of acute cyclosporine-induced renal blood flow inhibition and improved immunosuppression with verapamil. *Transplantation*, Vol.48, No.4, (October 1989), pp. 575-80, ISSN 0041-1337.
[9] Dawidson, I.; Rooth, P.; Alway, C., et al. (1990). Verapamil prevents posttransplant delayed function and cyclosporine A nephrotoxicity. *Transplant Proc*, Vol.22, No.4, (August 1990), pp. 1379-80, ISSN 0041-1345.
[10] Cross, N.B.; Webster, A.C.; Masson, P.; O'connell, P.J.; Craig, J.C. (2009). Antihypertensives for kidney transplant recipients: systematic review and meta-analysis of randomized controlled trials. *Transplantation*, Vol.88, No.1, (July 2009), pp. 7-18, ISSN 0041-1337.
[11] Candan, S.; Pirat, A.; Varol, G.; Torgay, A.; Zeynelgolu, P.; Arslan, G. (2006). Respiratory problems in renal transplant recipients admitted to intensive care during long-term follow-up. *Transplant Proc*, Vol.38, No.5, (June 2006), pp. 1354-6, ISSN 0041-1345.
[12] Canet, E.; Osman, D.; Lambert, J., et al. (2011). Acute respiratory failure in kidney transplant recipients: a multicenter study. *Crit Care*, Vol.15, No.2, (March 2011), R91, ISSN 1364-8535.
[13] Sharifipour, F.; Resaeetalab, F.; Naghibi, M. (2009). Pulmonary fungal infection in kidney transplant recipients: an 8-year study. *Transplant Proc*, Vol.41, No.5, (June 2009), pp. 1654-6, ISSN 0041-1345.

[14] Green, H.; Paul, M.; Vidal, L.; Leibovici, L. (2007). Prophylaxis for pneumocystis pneumonia (PCP) in non-HIV immunocompromised patients. *Cochrane Database Syst Rev*, No.3, (July 2007), pp. CD005590, ISSN 1469-493X.

[15] Barba, J.; Zudaire, J.J.; Robles, J.E.; Rosell, D.; Berian, J.M.; Pascual, I. (2012). Complications of kidney transplantation with grafts from expanded criteria donors. *World J Urol*, (Jan 2012), Epub ahead of print, ISSN 1433-8726.

[16] Ledinh, H.; Weekers, L.; Bonvoisin, C., et al. (2012). Results of kidney transplantation from controlled donors after cardio-circulatory death: a single center experience. *Transplant Int*, Vol.25, No.2, (February 2012), pp. 201-9, ISSN 0934-0874.

[17] Stevens, R.B.; Skorupa, J.Y.; Rigley, T.H., et al. (2009). Increased primary non-function in transplanted deceased-donor kidneys flushed with histidine-tryptophan-ketoglutarate solution. *Am J Transplant*, Vol.9, No.5, (May 2009), pp. 1055-62, ISSN 1600-6135.

[18] Webber, A.; Hambleton, J.; Chami, A., et al. (2012). Mean arterial blood pressure while awaiting kidney transplantation is associated with the risk of primary nonfunction. *Transplantation*, Vol.93, No.1, (January 2012), pp. 54-60, ISSN 0041-1337.

[19] Woo, Y.M.; Jardine, A.G.; Clark, A.F., et al. (1999).Early graft function and patient survival following cadaveric renal transplantation. *Kidney Int*, Vol.55, No.2, (February 1999), pp. 692-9, ISSN 0085-2538.

[20] van der Vliet JA, Warlé MC, Cheung CLS, Teerenstra S, Hoitsma AJ. Influence of prolonged cold ischemia in renal transplantation. Clin Transplant 2011: 25: E612–E616

[21] Squifflet, J.P.; De Meyer, M.; Malaise, J.; Latinne, D.; Pirson, Y.; Alexandre, G.P. (2004). Lessons learned from ABO-incompatible living donor kidney transplantation: 20 years later. *Exp Clin Transplant*, Vol.2, No.1, (June 2004), pp. 208-13, ISSN 1304-0855.

[22] Leeser, D.B.; Aull, M.J.; Afaneh, C., et al. (2012). Living donor kidney paired donation transplantation: experience as a founding member center of the National Kidney Registry. *Clin Transplant*, Vol.26, No.3, (May/June 2012), pp. E213-22, ISSN 0902-0063.

[23] Jordan, S.C.; Vo, A.A.; Tyan, D.; Nast, C.C.; Toyoda, M. (2005). Current approaches to treatment of antibody-mediated rejection. *Pediatr Transplant*, Vol.9, No.3, (June 2005), pp. 408-15, ISSN 1399-3046.

[24] Racusen, L.C.; Solez, K.; Colvin, R.B., et al. (1999). The Banff 97 working classification of renal allograft pathology. *Kidney Int*, Vol.55, No.2, (February 1999), pp. 713-23, ISSN 0085-2538.

[25] Jamil, B.; Nicholls, K.; Becker, G.J.; Walker, R.G. (1999). Impact of acute rejection therapy on infections and malignancies in renal transplant recipients. *Transplantation*, Vol.68, No.10, (November 1999), pp. 1597-603, ISSN 0041-1337.

[26] Serur, D.; Saal, S.; Wang, J, et al. (2011). Deceased-donor kidney transplantation: improvement in long-term survival. *Nephrol Dial Transplant*, Vol.26, No.1, (January 2011), pp. 317-24, ISSN 0931-0509.

[27] Mohanka, R.; Basu, A.; Shapiro, A.; Kayler, L.K. (2008). Single versus en bloc kidney transplantation from pediatric donors less than or equal to 15 kg. *Transplantation*, Vol.86, No.2, (July 2008), pp. 264-8, ISSN 0041-1337.

[28] Singh, A.; Stablein, D.; Tejani, A. (1997). Risk factors for vascular thrombosis in pediatric renal transplantation: a special report of the North American Pediatric Renal Transplant Cooperative Study. *Transplantation*, Vol.63, No.9, (May 1997), pp. 1263-7, ISSN 0041-1337.

[29] Balachandran, V.P.; Aull, M.J.; Goris, M.; Figueiro, J.; Leeser, D.B.; Kapur, S. (2010). Successful transplantation of single kidneys from pediatric donors weighing less than or equal to 10 kg in standard weight adult recipients. *Transplantation*, Vol.90, No.5, (September 2010), pp. 518-22, ISSN 0041-1337.

[30] Benedetti, E.; Troppmann, C.; Gillingham, K., et al. (1995). Short- and long-term outcomes of kidney transplants with multiple renal arteries. *Ann Surg*, Vol.221, No.4, (April 1995), pp. 406-14, ISSN 1528-1140.

[31] Afaneh, C.; Ramasamy, R.; Leeser, D.B., et al. (2011a). Is right-sided laparoendoscopic single-site donor nephrectomy feasible? *Urology*, Vol.77, No.6, (June 2011), pp. 1365-1369, ISSN 0090-4295.

[32] Afaneh, C.; Aull, M.J.; Schubl, S., et al. (2011b). The evolution of laparoscopic right donor nephrectomy: Progression to single site surgery. *J Transplant Technol Res*, Vol.1, Issue.2, No.103, (November 2011), pp. 1-7, ISSN 2161-0991.

[33] Friedman, G.S.; Meier-Kriesche, H.U.; Kaplan, B., et al. Hypercoagulable states in renal transplant candidates: impact of anticoagulation upon incidence of renal allograft thrombosis. *Transplantation*, Vol.72, No.6, (September 2011), pp. 1073-8, ISSN 0041-1337.

[34] Kusyk, T.; Verran, D.; Stewart, G., et al. (2005). Increased risk of hemorrhagic complications in renal allograft recipients receiving systemic heparin early posttransplantation. *Transplant Proc*, Vol.73, No.2, (March 2005), pp. 1026-8, ISSN 0041-1345.

[35] Mathis, A.S. & Shah, N.K. (2004). Exaggerated response to heparin in post-operative renal transplant recipient with lupus anticoagulant undergoing plasmapheresis. *Transplantation*, Vol.77, No.6, (March 2004), pp. 957-8, ISSN 0041-1337.

[36] Ghasemian, S.M.; Guleria, A.S.; Khawand, N.Y.; Light, J.A. (1996). Diagnosis and management of urologic complications of renal transplantation. *Clin Transplant*, Vol.10, No.2, (April 1996), pp. 218-23, ISSN 0902-0063.

[37] van Roijen, J.H.; Kirkels, W.J.; Zietse, R.; Roodnat, J.I.; Weimar, W.; Ijzermans, J.N. (2001). Long-term graft survival after urological complications of 695 kidney transplantations. *J Urol*, Vol.165, No.6 pt 1, (June 2001), pp. 1884-7, ISSN 0022-5347.

[38] Bailey, S.H.; Mone, M.C.; Holman, J.M.; Nelson, E.W. (2003). Laparoscopic treatment of post renal transplant lymphoceles. *Surg Endosc*, Vol.17, No.12, (December 2003), pp. 1896-9, ISSN 1432-2218.

[39] Sansalone, C.V.; Aseni, P.; Minetti, E., et al. (2000). Is lymphocele in renal transplantation an avoidable complication? *Am J Surg*, Vol.179, No.3, (March 2000), pp. 182-5, ISSN 0002-9610.

[40] Pengel, L.H.; Liu, L.Q.; Morris, P.J. (2011). Do wound complications or lymphoceles occur more often in solid organ transplant recipients on mTOR inhibitors? A systematic review of randomized controlled trials. *Transplant Int*, Vol.24, No.12, (December 2011), pp. 1216-30, ISSN 0934-0874.

[41] Montalvo, B.M.; Yrizarry, J.M.; Casillas, V.J., et al. (1996). Percutaneous sclerotherapy of lymphoceles related to renal transplantation. *J Vasc Interv Radiol*, Vol.7, No.1, (January-February 1996), pp. 117-23, ISSN 1051-0443.

[42] Manfro, R.C.; Comerlato, L.; Berdichevski, R.H., et al. (2002). Nephrotoxic acute renal failure in a renal transplant patient with recurrent lymphocele treated with povidone-iodine irrigation. *Am J Kidney Dis*, Vol.40, No.3, (September 2002), pp. 655-7, ISSN 0272-6386.

[43] Cecka, J.M. (2003). The UNOS Renal Transplant Registry. In Cecka JM. Terasaki PI (eds): Clinical Transplants 2002. Los Angeles, UCLA Immunogenetics Center, 2003, pp. 1-20, ISSN 0890-9016.

[44] Jochmans, I.; Moers, C.; Smits, J.M., et al. (2010). Machine perfusion versus cold storage for the preservation of kidneys donated after cardiac death: a multicenter, randomized, controlled trial. *Ann Surg*, Vol.252, No.5, (November 2010), pp. 756-64, ISSN 1528-1140.

[45] Land, W. (1998). Postischemic reperfusion injury and kidney transplantation. *Transplant Proc*, Vol.30, No.8, (December 1998), pp. 4210-3, ISSN 0041-1345.

[46] Cecka, J.M. (2005). The UNOS Renal Transplant Registry. In Cecka JM. Terasaki PI (eds): Clinical Transplants 2004. Los Angeles, UCLA Immunogenetics Center, 2003, pp. 1-16, ISSN 0890-9016.

[47] Kayler, L.K.; Srinivas, T.R.; Schold, J.D. (2011). Influence of CIT-induced DGF on kidney transplant outcomes. *Am J Transplant*, Vol.11, No.12, (December 2011), pp. 2657-64, ISSN 1600-6135.

[48] Perico, N.; Ruggenenti, P.; Gaspari, F., et al. (1992). Daily renal hypoperfusion induced by cyclosporine in patients with renal transplantation. *Transplantation*, Vol.54, No.1, (July 1992), pp. 56-60, ISSN 0041-1337.

[49] Solez, K., Vincenti, F.; Filo, R.S. (1998). Histopathologic findings from 2-year protocol biopsies from a U.S. multicenter kidney transplant trial comparing tacrolimus versus cyclosporine: a report of the FK506 Kidney Transplant Study Group. *Transplantation*, Vol.66, No.12, (December 1998), pp. 1736-40, ISSN 0041-1337.

[50] Rubin, R.H. Infectious diseases in transplantation/pre- and post-transplantation. In Norman DJ, Suki, WN (eds): Primer on Transplantation. Thorofare, NJ, American Society of Transplant Physicians, 1998, pp. 141-152.

[51] Paya, C.; Humar, A.; Dominguez, E., et al. (2004). Efficacy and safety of valganciclovir vs. oral ganciclovir for prevention of cytomegalovirus disease in solid organ transplant recipients. *Am J Transplant*, Vol.4, No.4, (April 2004), pp. 611-20, ISSN 1600-6135.

[52] Artero, M.L.; Sharma, R.; Savin, V.J.; Vincentin, F. (1994). Plasmapheresis reduces proteinuria and serum capacity to injure glomeruli in patients with recurrent focal glomerulosclerosis. *Am J Kidney Dis*, Vol.23, No.4, (April 1994), pp. 574-81, ISSN 0272-6386.

[53] Savin, V.J.; Sharma, R.; Sharma, M., et al. (1996). Circulating factor associated with increased glomerular permeability to albumin in recurrent focal segmental glomerulosclerosis. *N Engl J Med*, Vol.334, No.14, (April 1996), pp. 878-83, ISSN 0028-4793.

[54] Chiurchiu, C.; Ruggenenti, P.; Remuzzi, G. (2002). Thrombotic microangiopathy in renal transplantation. *Ann Transplant*, Vol.7, No.1, (2002), pp. 28-33, ISSN 1425-9524.

[55] Kaplan, A.A. (2001). Therapeutic apheresis for renal disease. *Ther Apher*, Vol.5, No.2, (April 2001), pp.134-41, ISSN 1744-9979.

[56] Fehr, T. & Gaspert, A. (2012). Antibody-mediated kidney allograft rejection: therapeutic options and their experimental rationale. *Transpl Int*, Vol.25, No.6, (June 2012), pp. 623-32, ISSN 0934-0874.

[57] Wilson, C.H.; Brown, A.L.; White, S.A.; Goodship, T.H.; Sheerin, N.S.; Manas, D.M. (2011). Successful treatment of de novo posttransplant thrombotic microangiopathy with eculizumab. *Transplantation*, Vol.92, No.8, (October 2011), pp. e42-3, ISSN 0041-1337.

Section 2

Immunologic Considerations in Kidney Transplantation

Chapter 5

Immunologic Concepts in Kidney Transplantation

John R. Lee and Thangamani Muthukumar

Additional information is available at the end of the chapter

http://dx.doi.org/10.5772/53798

1. Introduction

On December 23, 1954, the first successful kidney transplantation was performed at the Peter Bent Brigham Hospital in Boston with the donor being an identical twin of the recipient [1]. This sentinel event marked one of the first in the history of modern medicine that a perfectly healthy individual underwent an invasive surgical procedure for the benefit of another. It also revealed that kidney donation and kidney transplantation were feasible and thus ushered the era of renal transplantation. Crossing immunological barriers between donor and recipient became the next major hurdle in the field. Over the past decades, advances in immunosuppression and crossmatch techniques have significantly improved the survival of renal transplants. Allograft survival has improved from 10% in the 1960's to over 90% in the modern era [2,3].

This chapter will introduce the basics of transplantation immunology with an emphasis on the HLA system and mechanisms for HLA typing. It will also provide an overview of different crossmatch techniques and also expound upon methods to determine sensitization to the donor. Lastly, it will introduce the basis for acute rejection, the diagnostic criteria that is currently employed, and noninvasive methods to diagnose acute rejection.

2. HLA system

The Human Leukocyte Antigen (HLA) is composed of proteins expressed on all nucleated cells encoded by a gene cluster called the major histocompatibility complex (MHC) and is the cornerstone of how mammals can differentiate between self and non-self. The work on MHC originated from Peter Gorer in the 1930's where he identified a set of four blood-group antigens [4]. Since these important findings, much research has been performed in investigating the MHC system and the equivalent H-2 system in mice. Understanding the

HLA system is critical to transplantation because differences in HLA between donor and recipient allow the immune system of a recipient to reject a donor's kidney. The HLA system is divided into two major classes of molecules: class I and class II.

2.1. HLA class I system

There are three major alleles of the HLA class I genes: HLA-A, HLA-B, and HLA-C. The HLA class I molecule is a membrane-bound glycoprotein that is expressed on the surface of all nucleated cells and presents peptides for recognition by the host immune cells. The structure of the HLA class I molecule can be divided into the following regions: a cytoplasmic tail, a transmembrane segment, and an extracellular alpha component that has three external domains: a1, a2, and a3. In order to be able to present antigen to lymphocytes for recognition, the HLA class I molecule must associate with B2-microglobulin. Between the a1 and a2 domains is a groove like structure that can bind peptides of 8 to 10 amino acids.

To understand the process of presentation in the HLA class I system, we will use an example of an intracellular bacteria that has invaded a nucleated cell of the host. Presentation of antigen by an HLA class I molecule requires an important step called loading of the antigen on the HLA class I molecule. Inside each cell is a protein-degrading machinery called the proteasome which constantly degrades proteins into amino acids. Following bacterial invasion, some of the bacterial proteins will be degraded by the cell's proteasome. The short peptide segments of the bacterial proteins are loaded onto the groove of the host HLA class I molecule. The HLA class I molecule is then brought to the surface of the cell and can now present the peptide to the host's circulating lymphocytes. If a lymphocyte recognizes the bacterial antigen in the groove of the host HLA class I molecule, it can become activated and can initiate a cascade of intracellular changes, resulting in the proliferation of lymphocytes that can specifically attack the infected cell. It is through the host HLA class I antigen processing and presentation that the immune system can eliminate cells infected with intracellular bacteria. If presented without the host HLA class I molecule, naked bacterial proteins are not recognized by the host immune system [4,5].

For transplantation, this process can be summarized in a similar way. Just as the proteasome processes proteins associated with intracellular bacteria, it also degrades all proteins in a foreign cell including the HLA class I molecules. As such, donor leukocytes that travel along the kidney at the time of transplantation undergo the fate of an intracellular bacteria. They present peptides of the donor HLA class I molecule to circulating host lymphocytes. Lymphocytes recognize the donor peptides and mount a response against the foreign HLA class I molecule.

2.2. HLA class II system

An important difference between HLA class I molecules and HLA class II molecules is that the HLA class II molecules are expressed in a limited number of cell lines such as dendritic cells, macrophages, and B lymphocytes. Certain other cells like vascular endothelial cells and various epithelial and mesenchymal cells can be induced to express class II molecules. There are 3 major alleles of the HLA class II genes: HLA-DP, HLA-DQ, and HLA-DR. The function of the HLA class II molecule is to present extracellular foreign antigens to the immune system.

The structure of the HLA class II molecule can be divided into the following regions: a cytoplasmic tail, a transmembrane segment, and an extracellular alpha component that has two external domains. Unlike the HLA class I molecule, the HLA class II molecule is composed of a dimer. Once a dimer is formed, the extracellular units of the dimer create a groove like structure that can bind peptides for presentation. This peptide binding groove is the place where foreign antigens can be presented to lymphocytes.

To understand the process of presentation in the HLA class II system, we will use an example of extracellular bacteria. A macrophage, which is one of the cell types that express HLA class II molecules, can endocytose an extracellular bacteria. The endocytosed bacteria fuse with lysosomes, which contain enzymes that will degrade peptides of the bacteria. Peptides from this degradation event are loaded onto the HLA class II molecules which are brought to the surface for display to the immune system. The HLA class II molecules present the peptides to the host lymphocytes resulting in various immune responses that culminate in the killing of the bacteria.

For transplantation, the immune response can be summarized in a similar way. Specialized recipient cells that express the HLA class II molecule routinely endocytose contents of their environment. As such, these specialized cells can endocytose the contents of donor cells which may include donor HLA class I or class II molecules. These peptides are subsequently loaded onto the HLA class II molecule and can now be presented to the recipient's circulating lymphocytes.

A major functional difference between the two classes of HLA is that the class I molecules present peptides derived from intracellular proteins to cytotoxic CD8 T cells, whereas class II molecules present peptides derived from extracellular proteins to CD4 T cells. After a kidney transplant, donor antigen presenting cells migrate to the draining lymph nodes of the recipient. The recipient CD4+T cells respond to donor class II HLA-peptide complex and the recipient CD8+T cells respond to donor class I HLA-peptide complex. This is called the direct pathway and is fundamentally different from the way the immune system responds to a foreign antigen. Contrary to MHC-restriction by which the T cells that respond to foreign peptides do so only when the foreign peptides are presented by antigen presenting cells expressing the same MHC as the responding T cells, T lymphocytes of the recipient respond and proliferative to donor derived non-self HLA molecules. In the indirect pathway, the sequence of events is similar to the host response towards an extracellular pathogen; recipient's antigen presenting cells internalize donor derived peptides and present as recipient HLA-donor peptide complex to the recipient lymphocyte [6].

2.3. HLA typing

Determining the HLA make up of an individual is called HLA typing. The HLA system is extremely diverse with hundreds of known alleles for each HLA class molecule. We have two alleles, one derived from each parent, for each HLA molecule. Alleles derived from each parent that are transmitted together is called a haplotype. Matching or mismatching between donor and receipient is reported based on haplotypes for living related transplants and on individual antigens for deceased donor transplants. Typically, there are three major HLA alleles that are routinely assessed: 2 alleles of HLA-A, 2 alleles of HLA-B, and 2 alleles of HLA-DR. It is important to remember that, immunologically, a 6-antigen matched deceased donation is not the same as a 2-haploidentical living-related donation. Similarly, due to differences in minor histocompatibility antigens, donation between 2-haploidentical siblings is not the same as donation between identical twins. In the following sections, we will review the methods for determining the composition of the HLA antigen system of an individual.

2.3.1. Serology based methods

Serology based typing was the first method used to identify the HLA of an individual. This technique is similar to blood group typing. It utilizes viable lymphocytes of the individual to be typed. The lymphocytes are mixed with antisera that contain antibodies to a wide spectrum of HLA. Although simple, there are several limitations with this method. The coverage of HLA antigen screening is not comprehensive as antisera for corresponding HLA have been largely developed in Caucasian population. Variability exists in the production of antisera resulting in differences among laboratories. Viable lymphocytes are necessary for serology typing. Given these limitations and the significant decrease in cost for DNA typing methods, serology based methods have been largely supplanted [7,8].

2.3.2. DNA typing methods

Currently, the major techniques in DNA typing include sequence-specific primers (SSPs), sequence-specific oligonucleotide probes (SSOPs), and sequencing-based typing (SBT). The SSP method takes advantage of the polymerase chain reaction (PCR) and the specificity of primers. A PCR will not undergo amplification unless the sequences of the primers are nearly perfect in binding. Primer sets have been designed in order to detect the variation in sequences for HLA typing. The SSP method can thus detect the HLA typing of an individual. Given the significant reduction in cost for PCR, the technique is inexpensive and can provide HLA typing in few hours. The SSOP method provides a complementary approach. The method utilizes 6 to 19 length nucleotide probes that will bind to DNA sequences specific to HLA alleles. The probes are labeled with a marker like digoxigenin that will allow for identification of HLA alleles.

Because of increasing number of HLA alleles being identified, higher resolution methods have been developed. Both the SSP and SSOP methods can only identify known HLA alleles. In contrast, SBT method does not require prior knowledge of the HLA alleles and can reveal new alleles. This method does provide the most comprehensive understanding of an HLA typing but is time consuming and expensive. Many centers utilize SSP method and SSOP method for routine identification of the typing of an individual [7,8,9].

2.4. HLA matching

It was recognized that allograft survival was superior in siblings who shared the same serologically typed HLA when compared to non-matched deceased donor transplants. Given advances in immunosuppressive therapy and improved crossmatching techniques, transplantation across HLA barriers is now routinely performed. In the early 1990s, it was shown that there was an increased rate of one-year graft survival and estimated half-life for matched grafts compared with mismatched grafts [10]. Long term graft survival rather than early rejection is affected by the degree of HLA mismatch. As per the 2010 annual report of the Scientific Registry of Transplant Recipients, the five-year allograft survival for deceased donor kidney transplants was 77% with zero HLA mismatch and 67% with six HLA mismatch (3). Two haplotype matched living transplants are estimated to have a half life of approximately 30 years while one haplotype matched living transplants have a half life of 18 years [11].

In addition to the major HLA described above, minor antigens may play a significant role in allograft survival. An important antigenic molecule that is well described is the MHC class I polypeptide-related sequence A encoded by the MICA gene. The MICA gene is located on human chromosome 6 but unlike class I molecule, does not associate with beta-2-microglobulin and thus does not present antigens like HLA class I molecules. However, it is highly polymorphic and over 50 antigens have been described. Transplant recipients who have antibodies to MICA have worse graft survival compared to those who do not [12,13,14].

3. Blood group matching

In order to transplant a kidney, the same rules of blood transfusion apply. Thus, ABO blood group matching is the fundamental first step. Rh matching, however, is not required as Rh proteins are predominantly expressed only on red blood cells. Aside from HLA matching, ABO incompatibility has been another successful barrier that has been crossed in renal transplantation. In Japan, over 1000 transplant patients have received ABO incompatible transplants with good allograft survival. One-year and 3-year graft survival rates in this cohort were 96% and 94%, respectively [15]. Desensitization protocols have been developed that include use of rituximab, splenectomy, or plasmapheresis to successfully achieve high rates of graft survival.

4. Complement Dependent Cytotoxicity (CDC) crossmatch test

The CDC crossmatch test was a landmark *in vitro* test that propelled transplantation into a new era. Developed by Paul Terasaki in the late 1960's, it is still used today and is a prerequisite for any renal transplantation. The CDC crossmatch test essentially screens for preformed antibodies in the recipient that may immediately react against the donor. In this test, T lymphocytes are isolated from the donor and mixed with serum from the recipient. When preformed antibodies from the recipient recognize the HLA class I molecule, these antibodies bind to them. Following the addition of complement, the cells undergo lysis. A dye that penetrates lysed cells is utilized to detect the strength of the cell death. In contrast, if no antibodies in the recipient's serum bind to the T-lymphocyes of the donor, complement will not be activated and there will be no cell death. No dye will be taken up by the cells and the test is considered a negative reaction. The result of the crossmatch test is reported as the percentage of dead cells relative to live cells as determined by microscopy. The reading is on a semi-quantitative scale with 0 representing no dead cells, 2, 4, and 6 representing increasing severity of cell death, and 8 representing complete lysis of cells. When there is greater than 20% cell lysis, the test is reported as positive and is generally considered a contraindication for transplantation [6].

The importance of the CDC crossmatch test in transplantation cannot be underscored. In Terasaki's initial series, 24 out of 30 transplants that tested positive for the CDC crossmatch test had immediate allograft failure while only 4 out of 17 transplants that tested negative had immediate allograft failure [16]. Since the development of this test, hyperacute rejection with immediate allograft failure has largely disappeared.

4.1. Significance of B lymphocyte CDC test

At the present time, a positive CDC crossmatch test utilizing T lymphocytes of the donor is considered an absolute contraindication for kidney transplantation. T cells do not constitutively express HLA class II molecules. Hence, the result of a positive T lymphocyte crossmatch test generally reflects antibodies to HLA class I only. A positive CDC crossmatch test using B lymphocytes of the donor has different implications. B lymphocytes express both HLA class I and HLA class II molecules. A CDC crossmatch test that is positive against donor B lymphocytes but negative against donor T lymphocytes can be interpreted to represent a HLA class II antibody that reacts against the donor or to represent low levels of HLA class I antibodies against the donor. The expression of HLA class II molecule is not universal like HLA class I molecule and is limited to macrophages, dendritic cells, and B lymphocytes. A positive B lymphocyte CDC crossmatch test is not an absolute contraindication to proceeding with the transplantation. However, it has been associated with reduced long term graft survival [17]. A positive T lymphocyte CDC crossmatch in the presence of a negative B lymphocyte CDC crossmatch could possibly be a technical error related to B lymphocyte viability and is usually repeated [18].

4.2. Advances in CDC testing

In order to enhance the sensitivity of the CDC crossmatch test, anti-human globulin (AHG) has been utilized [6]. Efficient complement activation in the CDC crossmatch test depends not only on the antibody binding to the donor cells but also the concentration of antibodies on the surface of the cells. It is possible to have a false negative T lymphocyte CDC crossmatch test if the concentration of antibodies binding to the T lymphocytes is below the threshold for complement activation. Addition of AHG will enhance the concentration of antibodies if specific binding of antibodies are already present and thus increase the sensitivity of the CDC crossmatch test.

As both IgG and IgM can fix complement, the CDC crossmatch test cannot distinguish IgG from IgM antibodies. IgM antibodies are usually autoantibodies. IgM antibody exists as a pentamer that is held by disulfide bonds. Such disulfide bonds can be broken down by the use of the reducing agents like 2-mercaptoethanol or dithiothreitol or by heating the serum to 63^{0}C for 10 minutes. As such, a CDC crossmatch test that is positive against B lymphocytes but negative when the same serum is treated with heat at 63°C likely indicates an IgM antibody. However, reducing agents or heat can also inactivate low levels of IgG antibodies. The significance of the presence of IgM antibodies is not well understood.

4.3. Caveats to CDC crossmatch testing

While the standard CDC crossmatch test with B lymphocytes and T lymphocytes has helped the transplant community to avoid hyperacute rejection, the test does have some limitations. Although lymphocytes express class I HLA and class II HLA molecules, they do not provide the full representation of all antigens against which antibodies from a recipient can react. Examples to consider are antibodies to MICA or anti-endothelial antibodies. MICA, as described previously, are HLA like molecules expressed on the surface of cells with many different allelic variations. Importantly, MICA is expressed on many cell lines like endothelial cells, dendritic cells, fibroblasts, and epithelial cells but not on lymphocytes. Thus, the standard CDC crossmatch tests with B lymphocytes and T lymphocytes are unable to detect donor specific antibodies against MICA. In a similar fashion, antibodies against donor endothelial cells may also be missed on the standard CDC crossmatch test as the targeted antigen may be present on the endothelial cells but not on the lymphocytes. A CDC test with endothelial cells has recently been developed and employed. In reports of hyperacute rejection despite a negative CDC crossmatch test, investigation with the endothelial cell CDC crossmatch test has revealed the presence of antibodies against donor endothelial cells [19]. While it is possible that non-HLA antibodies can cause a hyperacute rejection, this is likely a rare event.

5. Flow cytometry crossmatch test

Advances in the field of transplantation have led to the development of a more sensitive test called the flow cytometry crossmatch test. The flow cytometer utilizes laser-based technology to evaluate the status of single cells one at a time. In a flow crossmatch test, cells from the potential donor are isolated and are labeled using a fluorescent marker. A fluorescent labeled antibody against CD3 or CD19 is used as a marker to distinguish T from B lymphocytes. The donor cells are incubated with the recipient's serum to allow for potential antibodies to bind. If there are donor specific anti-HLA antibodies, the Fab portion of the antibody binds to the HLA antigens on the cell surface. Fluorescein-labeled goat anti-human antibody is then used as the reporter fluorescent dye to detect the binding of this alloantibody. This secondary antibody can detect either IgG or IgM antibodies. Thus, if there is a positive reaction between the recipient's serum and donor lymphocytes, the flow cytometer will be able to detect this interaction as it will recognize the fluorescent-labeled anti-CD3 or CD19 antibody and the fluorescent labeled antibody against the Fc portion of the donor specific antibody. If there is a negative reaction between the recipient's serum and donor lymphocyte, the flow cytometer will recognize the fluorescent labeled anti-CD3 or

CD19 antibody but not detect any fluorescent labeled antibody against the Fc portion of donor specific antibody [6].

The flow crossmatch test has many advantages and is now routinely used prior to renal transplantation. It is considered to be more sensitive than the CDC crossmatch test. Complement fixation or high-titer antibodies are not required to obtain a positive result. During the early years of transplantation, patients continued to experience hyperacute rejections despite a negative CDC crossmatch test. Studies using flow crossmatch tests found that many acute rejections were associated with a positive flow crossmatch [20]. More recent studies have also suggested that transplant recipients with negative flow cytometry crossmatch test have better renal survival compared with those with positive flow cytometry crossmatch [21,22].

It is important to note a few caveats in the interpretation of the flow crossmatch test. Flow cytometry results are reported as positive or negative based upon the median channel shift caused by the binding of a specific antibody. The number of channel shifts required to call a test positive or negative varies among laboratories and has not been standardized. Although modifications can be made to detect IgM antibodies, typically the standard flow crossmatch test only detects IgG that is bound to donor cells. A possible scenario is that the CDC crossmatch test is positive against T lymphocytes but negative against T lymphocytes when heated to 63°C, thus suggesting the presence of an IgM antibody. The flow crossmatch test will be negative as it cannot detect donor specific IgM antibody. Unlike the CDC crossmatch test, the flow crossmatch test is also not dependent on complement. A possible scenario is that the CDC crossmatch test is negative against T lymphocytes but the flow crossmatch test is positive against T lymphocytes. A possible interpretation of these results is that the antibodies that are binding to the donor T lymphocytes are non-complement fixing antibodies like IgG2.

5.1. Significance of a positive flow crossmatch test

The significance of a positive result in the presence of a negative CDC crossmatch is not entirely clear. In the absence of prior sensitization, a positive T or B lymphocyte flow crossmatch is not associated with increased risk of acute rejection. In patients who are sensitized prior to transplantation, the graft survival is inferior [18]. The outcome of a positive B lymphocyte flow crossmatch is less clear [23]. Some studies have not found that a positive B lymphocyte flow crossmatch influences graft function. These studies evaluated deceased donor transplantations and did not find a difference in the one year and three year graft survival [24]. Other studies have found that a positive B lymphocyte flow crossmatch test is associated with worse survival. One study evaluated 145 patients and found that patients with a positive B lymphocyte flow crossmatch had significantly poorer graft survival than those with a negative one (68% vs. 90% at 1 year) [25].

6. Panel Reactive Antibody test

Instead of utilizing donor T lymphocytes and B lymphocytes as used in the standard CDC, the panel reactive antibody (PRA) test utilizes a panel of lymphocytes from approximately

100 blood donors that represent the local population of potential donors. Percentage of PRA is the number of reactions within that panel. This test allows for characterizing the sensitization of a recipient. For example, if the serum of a recipient causes lysis of cells and hence a positive reaction in 80 out of 100 samples, the PRA is 80%. Theoretically, if a donor is available from that donor pool, the recipient would experience acute rejection 80% of the time (6). The PRA test, however, is not comprehensive. The panel of individuals does not represent all HLA class I and class II molecules. Moreover, the antigen specificity is not known. Despite these drawbacks, the PRA test has been extremely useful in providing information about the sensitization of a recipient.

Now, with refinement in technology, it is possible to determine the antigen specificity against which an individual produces antibody. These antigens against which an individual has antibodies are called unacceptable antigens. Currently, several centers do not perform routine PRA and instead calculate the PRA (CPRA). By knowing the frequency of unacceptable antigens in the national pool of donors, it is possible to calculate the likelihood that a recipient and a donor will be incompatible. Patients with CPRA that is greater than 80% receive additional points for the allocation of a kidney.

7. Solid phase assays for donor specific antibodies

Development of solid phase assays in the past decades has advanced the ability to identify antibodies in the blood to specific HLA. Two methods, one based on ELISA and one based on fluorescent microspheres (Luminex®), are currently being used to determine the presence of HLA class I and HLA class II antibodies.

In the ELISA method, specific purified HLA molecules are immobilized on a plastic surface. The serum of the patient of interest is then incubated on the plastic surface. If there are antibodies directed against a specific HLA, these antibody binds to the antigen. A second anti-human IgG directed against the Fc portion of antibody is now added to detect the serum antibodies that have bound to the HLA. An enzyme is usually attached to this second antibody. If the second antibody binds to the Fc portion of the specific anti-HLA antibody, addition of a substrate for the attached enzyme will generate a colored product that can be quantified.

In the fluorescent microsphere method, specific synthetic HLA molecules are immobilized on fluorescent microspheres. The Luminex® system consists of 100 fluorescently dyed 5.6 micron-sized polystyrene microspheres. These are internally dyed with red and infrared fluorophores. When excited with laser, each microsphere generates a unique spectral signature allowing for powerful multiplexing. The serum of the patient of interest is incubated with the microspheres coated with HLA molecules. A second fluorescent-labeled anti-human IgG directed against the Fc portion of the antibodies is then added to the system. A flow cytometer will detect the amount of fluorescent labeled anti-human IgG that is bound to a particular HLA molecule. The strength of the antibody titer is quantified as the mean fluorescence intensity (MFI). Currently, Luminex® based anti-HLA detection is available as a screen to determine the presence of anti-HLA antibodies (LABScreen PRA) as well as to detect the specificity of the antibodies (LABScreen single antigen) [26].

It is important to note some limitations with the solid phase assays. The chosen panel of HLA in solid phase assay usually represents the most prevalent HLA in the population and so can miss some of the less common HLA. The solid phase assay is also more of "in vitro" test as the HLA in the ELISA method and fluorescent microsphere method are not expressed on cells but are rather synthetically generated and placed on plastic plate or beads, respectively. As such, the solid phase assays will be able to detect HLA in secondary structure but may miss detection of antibodies to HLA in quaternary structure as might be detected on an assay like the CDC crossmatch test. Commonly used solid phase assays are currently designed to detect IgG antibodies and so an IgM antibody can be missed. Finally, the solid phase assays does not distinguish complement fixing from non-complement fixing antibodies. Despite these limitations, solid phase assays is the most robust test that is currently available to detect donor specific antibodies and have provided a wealth of information about a recipient's sensitization to a donor kidney.

7.1. Significance of donor specific antibodies

Due to sensitization from prior transplants, pregnancy, or transfusions, potential transplant recipients may have preformed donor specific antibody (DSA) against HLA. Several studies have examined the significance of having preformed antibodies and have found an association with worse graft survival and increased antibody mediated rejection. In one study that investigated DSA in over 400 transplant recipients, those with preformed anti-HLA DSA had inferior graft survival at 8 years as compared with those with no preformed DSA (93% vs. 61%) [27]. Another study investigated pre-transplant DSA in 334 patients and found a higher incidence of clinical/subclinical antibody mediated rejection in those with DSA (55% vs. 6%) [28]. The strength of the DSA as measured by MFI may also play a role in the development of antibody mediated rejection [27].

While many studies have found that the presence of pre-transplant anti-HLA DSA is a risk factor for inferior graft survival and increased AMR, not all anti-HLA DSA may be pathogenic. In one study, 30 out of the 67 patients who had anti-HLA DSA did not have a clinical/subclinical antibody mediated rejection [28]. Five-year death censored graft survival among this group was similar to the transplant patients without anti-HLA DSA. Clearly, further research is needed to elucidate the characteristics of anti-HLA DSA that are pathogenic.

Transplant recipients may not have anti HLA-DSA prior to the transplant but can develop them after transplantation. Similar to preexisting DSA, de novo anti-HLA DSA has been found to be a risk factor for graft failure. In an international cooperative study of transplant recipients who did not have anti-HLA antibodies prior to transplant, the one-year allograft survival after the detection of antibodies was worse among the post transplant recipients with de novo anti-HLA antibodies (9%) than among the post transplant recipients with no post transplant anti-HLA antibodies (3%) ($P<0.001$) [29].

7.2. Monitoring and treatment

Transplantation in the presence of preformed anti-HLA DSA is associated with increased risk of antibody mediated rejection and graft failure. Transplant centers have utilized desensitization protocols with agents like intravenous immunoglobulin or rituximab to reduce the antibody titers prior to transplant. Acceptable patient and graft survival have been reported [30]. Furthermore, transplanting highly sensitized patients after desensitization may be beneficial as compared to maintaining them on dialysis. One study that evaluated 211 HLA sensitized patients found a survival benefit of a desensitization protocol as compared with a matched control on dialysis awaiting a deceased donor transplant (81% vs. 31% survival at 8 years, $P<0.001$, respectively) [31]. It is not clear how patients who are sensitized and transplanted following desensitization should be monitored. One study found that an increase in DSA by one week after transplant following desensitization therapy was significantly associated with antibody mediated rejection [32].

8. Transplant rejection

Acute rejection continues to remain a significant problem after transplantation. Categorization of rejection is based on the Banff classification schema. In the early 1960's, hyperacute rejection was described in cadaveric kidney transplantations. Shortly after the vascular anastomosis, the allograft became cyanotic. On microscopic examination, the major findings included neutrophil and platelet margination in glomerular and peritubular capillaries, red blood cell stasis, acute tubular necrosis, and variable degree of cortical necrosis. Immunofluorescence studies demonstrated the presence of IgG in peritubular capillaries [33].

Many of these hyperacute rejections have largely disappeared following the development of the CDC crossmatch test. Currently, acute rejection is classified into two major categories: T cell mediated acute rejection (ACR) and acute antibody mediated rejection (AMR) (Table 1). The following sections will provide an overview of the evolution of the criteria for both major types of acute rejection.

8.1. Renal transplant biopsy adequacy

The gold standard for diagnosis of transplant rejection is a renal biopsy. Diagnosis of transplant rejection depends on the availability of an adequate specimen for evaluation. In 1991, the Banff schema defined an allograft biopsy specimen as adequate if it contained seven or more glomeruli [34]. Further revisions in 1997 required two cores of tissues, 10 or more total glomeruli, and the presence of at least two arteries [35]. The presence of seven glomeruli and one artery is the threshold for a minimal sample. The diagnosis of acute rejection thus depends on an adequate specimen as defined by the Banff criteria.

8.2. Acute T cell-mediated rejection

In the 1980's and 1990's it was observed that interstitial inflammation found in transplant kidney biopsies, in many cases, had a negligible effect on graft survival and thus was not pathognomonic for acute rejection [34]. Tubilitis, the infiltration of lymphocytes into the tubules of kidney, was associated with allograft dysfunction and became the hallmark of acute rejection. The Banff 1991 consensus defined acute rejection as the involvement of tubilitis (>4 mononuclear cells/tubular cross section) and/or intimal arteritis (the infiltration of lymphocytes in the arterial wall). Further revisions of the Banff criteria in 1997 provided a classification of acute T cell-mediated rejection that is currently used today [35]. Grade 1A rejection requires moderate to severe interstitial inflammation (>25% of parenchyma affected) (i2 or i3) and foci of moderate tubulitis (>4 mononuclear cells/tubular cross section) (t2). Grade 1B rejection requires moderate to severe interstitial inflammation (>25% of parenchyma affected) (i2 or i3) and severe tubulitis (>10 mononuclear cells/tubular cross section) (t3). Grade 2A rejection requires intimal arteritis (presence of lymphocytes within the intima) (v1). Grade 2B rejection requires severe arteritis (involving >25% of luminal area) (v2). Grade 3 rejection requires transmural arteritis and/or necrosis of medial smooth muscle cells (v3) (Table 1).

Banff 4: **Acute T Cell Mediated Rejection**	**Banff 2:** **Acute Antibody Mediated Rejection**
Grade IA:	**1. Morphological evidence of kidney injury**
>25% interstitial inflammation (i2,i3) AND foci of moderate tubilitis (t2)	A) Acute tubular necrosis or B) Neutrophils and/or mononuclear cells in peritubular capillaries and/or glomeruli, and/or capillary thrombosis or C) intimal arteritis/fibrinoid necrosis/intramural or transmural inflammation in arteries
Grade IB:	
>25% interstitial inflammation (i2,i3) AND foci of severe tubilitis (t3)	
Grade IIA:	**2. Immunopathological evidence of antibody action**
mild to moderate intimal arteritis (v1)	A) presence of C4d in peritubular capillaries or B) immunoglobulin and complement in arterial necrosis
Grade IIB:	**3. Serological evidence of circulating antibodies**
severe intimal arteritis involving >25% (v2) of luminal area	A) antibodies to donor HLA or B) antibodies to donor endothelial antigens
Grade III:	All 3 criteria are necessary to make a diagnosis of antibody mediated rejection; 2 out of 3 criteria makes a diagnosis of suspicious for antibody mediated rejection
transmural arteritis and/or arterial fibrinoid changes with accompanying lymphocyte infiltration (v3)	

I Scoring and V Scoring Definitions
I scoring: i0 (<10% parenchymal inflammation), i1 (10 to 25% parenchymal inflammation), i2 (25 to 50% parenchymal inflammation), i3 (>50% parenchymal inflammation)
T scoring: t0 (no mononuclear cells in tubules), t1 (foci of 1 - 4 mononuclear cells/tubular cross section), t2 (foci of 5-10 mononuclear cells/tubular cross section), t3 (foci of >10 mononuclear cells/tubular cross section)
V scoring: v0 (no arteritis), v1 (mild to moderate intimal arteritis in one arterial cross section), v2 (severe intimal arteritis with at least 25% luminal area lost), v3 (transmural arteritis and/or arterial fibrinoid change with lymphocytic infiltrate)

Table 1. Banff Classification of Acute Rejection (adapted from references 35.37.41)

8.3. Acute antibody mediated rejection

Feucht et al. reported the presence of complement-split products (C4d) in early biopsies of patients with high immunological risk [36]. The Banff 97 classification defined antibody mediated rejection as rejection demonstrated to be due, at least in part, to anti-donor antibody. Two forms, immediate and delayed, were recognized. With the description of staining for C4d as a marker for antibody mediated rejection, an update to the Banff 97 classification was reported in 2003 that defined AMR with three characteristics: i) evidence of morphological injury in the form of either a) acute tubular necrosis, b) neutrophils and/or macrophages in glomeruli or peritubular capillaries or thrombi in glomeruli, or c) intimal arteritis/fibrinoid necrosis/intramural inflammation; ii) immunological evidence of antibody as either a) presence of C4d in peritubular capillaries or b) immunoglobulins in arterial fibrinoid necrosis; and iii) serological evidence of circulating antibodies to donor HLA or other endothelial antigens. If 2 out of 3 characteristics are present, the renal biopsy is considered suspicious for antibody mediated rejection [35, 37] (Table 1).

8.4. Borderline changes

When there is tubulitis and interstitial inflammation but the definition of ACR is not met, the biopsy findings are categorized as borderline changes: 'suspicious' for acute cellular rejection. The criteria for this diagnosis includes: i) no intimal arteritis; ii) mild tubilitis (1 to 4 mononuclear cells/tubular cross section); iii) at least 'i1' inflammation (10-25% of parenchyma involved). The significance of borderline biopsies on renal outcomes is not clearly defined. One study of 100 kidney allograft biopsies categorized as borderline changes found a progressive increase in serum creatinine over time [38]. Nevertheless, management of a borderline diagnosis has not been clearly defined. More recently, a study that compared 40 borderline changes, 35 T-cell mediated rejection, and 116 nonrejection biopsies observed that most cases designated borderline by histopathology were found to be nonrejection by molecular phenotyping [39].

8.5. Other types of acute rejection

ACR and AMR are not mutually exclusive and frequently coexist. In a study of 87 patients with C4d positive AMR as defined by Banff criteria, 32 (37%) had evidence of concurrent ACR. The presence of concurrent ACR was an independent risk factor of allograft failure in kidney transplant recipients with C4d positive acute AMR [40]. It is important to emphasize that Banff criteria are not all-inclusive. Plasma-cell rich acute rejection is an entity where the interstitial inflammation and tubulitis are predominantly composed of plasma cells in addition to lymphocytes. Allergic interstitial nephritis closely resembles ACR and are all not always associated with eosinophil infiltrates. Thus, morphologically, it may be also be useful to categorize acute rejection as (i) interstitial rejection characterized predominantly by interstitial inflammation and tubulitis, (ii) vascular rejection characterized predominantly by intimal arteritis and (iii) capillary rejection characterized predominantly by glomerulitis and peritubular capillary inflammation usually in the presence of circulating DSA.

8.6. Chronic rejection

The Banff classification also defined three forms of chronic rejection: (i) chronic active T cell-mediated rejection characterized by arterial intimal fibrosis with mononuclear cell infiltration in fibrosis and formation of neo-intima, and (ii) chronic active antibody-mediated rejection characterized by C4d+, presence of circulating antidonor antibodies, and morphologic evidence of chronic tissue injury, such as glomerular double contours and/or peritubular capillary basement membrane multilayering and/or interstitial fibrosis/tubular atrophy and/or fibrous intimal thickening in arteries, and (iii) interstitial fibrosis and tubular atrophy without evidence of any specific etiology that may also include nonspecific vascular and glomerular sclerosis [41]. Morphological evidence of chronic active antibody mediated tissue injury but with negative C4d is being increasingly recognized.

9. Non-invasive molecular techniques for assessing acute rejection

The platforms for molecular based biomarker discovery and validation are: (i) Real-time polymerase chain reaction (RT-PCR), Microarray and RNA sequencing (detection of expression of single or multiple genes), (ii) Elisa and protein microarray (detection of single or multiple proteins), (iii) ELISPOT (detection of cytokine producing cells), (iv) Immuknow (detection of adenosine triphosphate [ATP] levels in activated T-lymphocytes), and (v) Luminex® (detection of cytokines or alloantibodies) [42].

Urinary cell and peripheral blood cell messenger RNA (mRNA) profiling of transplant recipients has been studied extensively as a tool for the noninvasive diagnosis and prognosis of kidney transplant rejection. This technique involves quantification of mRNA levels of mechanistically informative genes using RT-PCR assay from urinary cells or peripheral blood cells of kidney transplant recipients. As an example, measurement of granzyme B and perforin (m) mRNA activity in urinary cells has been reported to be a sensitive and specific marker for the detection of acute cellular rejection [43]. In a study of 83 kidney transplant recipients; 36 with acute rejection, 18 with chronic allograft nephropathy, and 29 with normal biopsy results, urinary cell mRNA levels of regulatory T-lymphocyte marker, FoxP3, quantified at the time of biopsy diagnosis predicted reversal of acute rejection with 90 percent sensitivity and 73 percent specificity. Urinary cell mRNA levels of FoxP3 also identified subjects at risk for graft failure within six months after the incident episode of acute rejection. Urinary cell mRNA levels of CD3 (marker of T lymphocytes), CD25 (marker of activated T-lymphocytes), and perforin did not predict rejection reversal or graft failure [44]. Recently, a large multi-center trial sponsored by the National Institutes of Health trial validated the utility of urinary cell mRNA levels in the diagnosis of ACR [45]. The role of urinary cell mRNA level as a noninvasive tool is not limited to the diagnosis of acute rejection. A recent study identified a urinary cell mRNA signature for the diagnosis of fibrosis in human kidney allografts [46].

The Cylex Immuknow assay is an FDA approved blood test for the detection of cell mediated immune response in populations undergoing immunosuppressive therapy for organ transplants. The test quantifies the amount of ATP produced by lymphocytes of the transplant recipient upon activation. Based on the ATP levels there are two cut-off values: $\leq$225 ng/ml represents a low immune cell response and $\geq$525 ng/ml represents a strong immune cell response. In between values represent moderate immune cell response. Some studies have found a relation between the Cylex Immuknow assay and acute rejection [47].

However, more recently, a study that evaluated 1330 ImmuKnow assay values in 583 renal transplant recipients at a single center from 2004 to 2009 failed to show an association between single time point ImmuKnow assay values and the subsequent development of an adverse event (acute rejection or opportunistic infections) in the subsequent 90 days [48].

In a recent study of 64 kidney transplant recipients with graft dysfunction, a panel of 21 cytokines secreted by peripheral blood mononuclear cells was assayed using the Luminex® platform. In the initial training cohort of 32 patients, IL-6 was the best predictor of acute rejection. In the validation cohort of 32 patients, IL-6 predicted acute rejection, using a training set derived cut-point, with 92% sensitivity and 63% specificity [49].

Rapid advancements in our understanding of the role of microRNAs in transplantation [50] and in molecular techniques such as RNA sequencing have opened up new avenues for biomarker discovery and has resulted in better insight on the mechanistic basis of allograft dysfunction. In the future, we anticipate personalized management of transplant recipients with a combination of traditional pathology and the 'omics' based approach (genomics, proteomics, and metabolomics).

Author details

John R. Lee and Thangamani Muthukumar
Division of Nephrology & Hypertension, Department of Transplantation Medicine,
NewYork-Presbyterian Hospital/Weill Cornell Medical College, New York, NY, USA

10. References

[1] Merrill JP, Murray JE, Harrison JH, Guild WR. Successful homotransplantation of the human kidney between identical twins. *JAMA* 1956; 160(4): 277-282. PMID: 13278189.
[2] Murray JE: Conference on human kidney transplant: proceedings. *Transplantation* 1964; 2: 147-165.
[3] Organ Procurement and Transplantation Network (OPTN) and Scientific Registry of Transplant Recipients (SRTR). OPTN / SRTR 2010 Annual Data Report. Rockville, MD: Department of Health and Human Services, Health Resources and Services Administration, Healthcare Systems Bureau, Division of Transplantation. 2011.
[4] Goldsby, R., Kindt, T., Osborne, B. *Kuby Immunology.* Fourth Edition. W.H. Freeman and Company. 2002.
[5] Sompayrac, L. *How the Immune System Works.* Third Edition. Blackwell Publishing. 2008.
[6] Danovitch, G. *Handbook of Kidney Transplantation.* Fifth Edition. Lippincott Williams & Wilkins. 2010.
[7] Middleton, D. HLA Typing from Serology to Sequencing Era. *Iran J Allergy Asthma Immunol* 2005; 4(2):53-66. PMID: 17301424.
[8] Dunn, PP. Human leucocyte antigen typing: techniques and technology, a critical appraisal. *Int J Immunogenet* 2011; 38(6): 463-473. PMID: 22059555.
[9] McClatchey, K. *Clinical Laboratory Medicine.* Second Edition. Lippincott Williams & Wilkins. 2002.

[10] Takemoto, S., Terasaki, PI, Cecka, JM, Cho, YW, Gjertson DW. Survival of nationally shared, HLA-matched kidney transplant from cadaveric donors. The UNOS Scientific Renal Transplant Registry. *N Engl J Med* 1992; 327(12): 834-839. PMID: 1508242.

[11] Jennette, J., Olson, J., Schwartz, M., Silva, F. *Heptinstall's Pathology of the Kidney.* Sixth Edition. Lippincott Williams & Wilkins. 2006.

[12] Zou, Y., Stastny, P., Susal, C., Dohler, B., Opeiz, G. Antibodies against MICA antigens and kidney-transplant rejection. *N Engl J Med* 2007; 357(13): 1293-1300. PMID: 17898098.

[13] Dragun, D., Philippe, A., Catar, R. Role of non-HLA antibodies in organ transplantation. *Curr Opin Organ Transplant* 17(4); 440-445, 2012. PMID: 22790079.

[14] Zou, Y., Stastny, P. Antibodies against major histocompatibility complex class I-related chain A in transplant recipients. *Chin Med J* 2011; 124(5): 764-770. PMID: 21518573.

[15] Takahashi, K. Recent findings in ABO-incompatible kidney transplantation: classification and therapeutic strategy for acute antibody-mediated rejection due to ABO-blood-group-related antigens during the critical period precding the establishment of accommodation. *Clin Exp Nephrol* 2007; 11(2): 128-141. PMID: 17593512.

[16] Patel, R., Terasaki, PI. Significance of the positive crossmatch test in kidney transplantation. *N Engl J Med* 1969; 280(14): 735-739. PMID: 4886455.

[17] Cho YW, Cecka JM. Crossmatch tests – an analysis of UNOS data from 1991-2000. *Clin Transpl* 2001 237-246. PMID: 12211787.

[18] Mulley WR, Kanellis J. Understanding crossmatch testing in organ transplantation: A case-based guide for the general nephrologist. *Nephrology (Carlton)* 2011; 16(2): 125-133. PMID: 21272123

[19] Grandtnerova B, Mackova N, Hovoricova B, Jahnova E. Hyperacute rejection of living related kidney grafts caused by endothelial cell-specific antibodies: case reports. *Transplant Proc* 2008; 40(7): 2422-2424. PMID: 18790254.

[20] Lazda VA, Pollak R, Mozes MF, Jonasson O. The relationship between flow cytometer crossmatch results and subsequent rejection episodes in cadaver renal allograft recipients. *Transplantation* 198; 45(30: 562-565, PMID: 3279580.

[21] Lazda VA. Identification of patients at risk for inferior renal allograft outcome by a strongly positive B cell flow cytometry crossmatch. *Transplantation* 1994; 57(6): 964-969. PMID: 8154041.

[22] Illham MA, Winkler S, Coates E, Rizzello A, Rees TJ, Asderakis A. Clinical significance of a positive flow crossmatch on the outcomes of cadaveric renal transplant. *Transplant Proc* 2008; 40(6): 1839-1843. PMID: 18675065.

[23] Delgado JC, Eckels DD. Positive B-cell only flow cytometric cromssatch: implications for renal transplantation. *Exp Mol Pathol* 2008; 85(1): 59 – 63. PMID: 18499103.

[24] Bryan CF, Wakefield M, Reese JC, Shield CF 3rd, Warady BA, Winklhofer FT, Murillo D. Renal graft survival is not influenced by a positive flow B-cell crossmatch. *Clin Transplant* 2007; 21(1): 72-79. PMID: 17302594.

[25] Bittencourt MC, Rebibou JM, Saint-Hillier Y, Chabod J, Dupont I, Chalopin JM, Herve P, Tiberghien P. Impaired renal graft survival after a positive B-cell flow-cytometry crossmatch. *Nephrol Dial Transplant* 1998; 13(8): 2059-2064. PMID: 9719165.

[26] Picascia A, Infante T, Napoli C. Luminex and antibody detection in kidney transplantation. *Clin Exp Nephrol* 2012; 16(3): 373-381. PMID: 22552384.

[27] Lefaucheur C, Loupy A, Hill GS, Andrad J, Nochy D, Antoine C, Gautreau C., Charron D, Glotz D, Suberbielle-Boissel C. Preexisting donor-specific HLA antibodies predict outcome in kidney transplantation. *J Am Soc Nephrol* 2010; 21(8): 1398-1406. PMID: 20634297.

[28] Amico P, Honger G, Mayr M, Steiger J, Hopfer H, Schaub S. Clinical relevance of pretransplant donor-specific HLA antibodies detected by single-antigen flow-beads. *Transplantation* 2009; 87(11): 1681-1688. PMID: 19502960.

[29] Terasaki PI, Ozawa M. Predicting kidney graft failure by HLA antibodies: a prospective trial. *Am J Transplant* 2004; 4(3): 438-443. PMID: 14961999.

[30] Vo AA, Peng A, Tovoda M, Kahwaji J, Cao K, Lai CH, Reinsmoen NL, Villicana R, Jordan SC. Use of intravenous immune globulin and rituximab for desensitization of highly HLA-sensitized patients awaiting kidney transplantation. *Transplantation* 2010; 89(9): 1095-1102. PMID: 20110854.

[31] Montgomery RA, Lonze BE, King KE, Kraus ES, Kucirka LM, Locke JE, Warren DS, Simpkins CE, Dagher NN, Singer AL, Zachary AA, SEgev DL. Desensitization in HLA-incompatible kidney recipients and survival. *N Engl J Med* 2011; 365(4): 318-326. PMID: 21793744.

[32] Mohamed MA, Muth B, Vidyasagar V, Foley D, Fernandez L, Hofmann RM, Mezrich J, Pirsch J, Odorico J, d'Allesandro T, Bellingham J, Torrealba J, Kaufman D. Post-transplant DSA monitoring may predict antibody-mediated rejection in sensitized kidney transplant recipients. *Clin Transplant* 2011; 389-394. PMID: 22755436.

[33] Racusen LC, Haas M. Antibody-mediated rejection in renal allografts: lessons from pathology. *Clin J Am Soc Nephrol* 2006; 1(3): 415-420. PMID: 17699240.

[34] Solez K, Axelsen RA, Benediktsson H, Burdick JF, Cohen AH, Colvin RB, Droz D, Dunnill MS, Halloran PF, et al. International standardization of criteria for the histological diagnosis of renal allograft rejection: the Banff working classificiation of kidney transplant pathology. *Kidney Int* 1993; 44(2): 411-422. PMID: 8377384

[35] Racusen LC, Solez K, Colvin RB, Bonsib SM, Castro MC, cavallo T, Croker BP, Demetris AJ, Drachenberg CB, Fogo AB, Furness P, Gaber LW, Gibson IW, Glotz D, Goldberg JC, Grande J, Halloran PF, Hansen HE, Hartley B, Hayry PJ, Hill CM, Hoffman EO, Hunsicker LG, Lindblad AS, Yamaguchi Y, et. al. The Banff 97 working classification of renal allograft pathology. *Kidney Int* 1999; 55(2): 713-723. PMID: 9987096.

[36] Feucht HE, Felber E, Gokel MJ, Hllebrand G, Nattermann U, Held E, Riethmuller G, Land W, Albert E. Vascular deposition of complement-split products in kidney allografts with cell mediated rejection. *Clin Exp Imunol* 1991; 86(3): 464-470. PMID: 1747954.

[37] Racusen LC, Colvin RB, Solez K, Mihatsch MJ, Halloran PF, Campbell PM, Cecka MJ, Cosyns JP, Demetris AJ, Fishbein MC, Fogo A, Furness P, Gibson IW, Glotz D, Hayry P, Hunsickern L, Kashgarian M, Kerman R, Magil AJ, Montgomery R, Morozumi K, Nickeleit V, Randhawa P, Regele H, Seron D, Seshan S, Sund S, Tripkov K. Antibody-mediated rejection criteria - an addition to the Banff 97 classification of renal allograft rejection. *Am J Transplant* 2003; 3(6): 708-714. PMID: 12780562.

[38] Matoza JR, Danguilan RA, Chicano S. Impact of Banff borderline acute rejection among renal allograft recipients. *Transplant Proc* 2008; 40(7): 2303-2306. PMID: 18790219.

[39] de Freitas DG, Sellarés J, Mengel M, Chang J, Hidalgo LG, Famulski KS, Sis B, Einecke G, Halloran PF. The nature of biopsies with "borderline rejection" and prospects for eliminating this category. *Am J Transplant* 2012; 12(1): 191-201. PMID: 21992503.

[40] Matignon M, Muthukumar T, Seshan SV, Suthanthiran M, Hartono C. Concurrent Acute Cellular Rejection is an Independent Risk Factor for Renal Allograft Failure in Patients C4d-Positive Antibody-Mediated Rejection. *Transplantation 2012; 94(6): 603-611.*

[41] Solez K, Colvin RB, Racusen LC, Sis B, Halloran PF, Birk PE, Campbell PM, Cascalho M, Collins AB, Demetris AJ, drachenberg CB, Gibson IW, Grimm PC, Haas M, Lerut E, Liapis H, Mannon RB, Marcus PB, Mengel M, Mihatsch MJ, Nankivell BJ, Nickeleit V, Pamadimitriou JC< Platt JL, Randhawa P, Roberts I, Salinas-Madriga L, Salomon DR, SEron D, Sheaff M, Weening JJ. Banff '05 Meeting Report: differential diagnosis of chronic allograft injury and elimination fo chronic allograft nephropathy ('CAN'). *Am J Transplant* 2007; 7(3): 518-526. PMID: 17352710.

[42] Hartono C, Muthukumar T, Suthanthiran M. Noninvasive diagnosis of acute rejection of renal allografts. *Curr Opin Organ Transplant* 2010; 15(1): 35-41. PMID: 19935064.

[43] Li B, Hartono C, Ding R, Sharma VK, Ramaswarmy R, Qian B, Serur D, Mouradian J, Schwartz JE, Suthanthiran M. Noninvasive diagnosis of renal-allograft rejection by measurement of messenger RNA for perforin and granzyme B in urine. *N Engl J Med 2001;* 44(13): 947-954. PMID: 11274620.

[44] Muthukumar T, Dadhania D, Ding R, Snopkowski C, Naqvi R, Lee JB, Hartono C, Li B, Sharma VK, Seshan SV, Kapur S, Hancock WW, Schwartz JE, Suthanthiran M. Messenger RNA for FOXP3 in the urine of renal-allograft recipients. *N Engl J Med* 2005; 353(22): 2342-2351. PMID: 16319383.

[45] Suthanthiran M, Ding R, Sharma V, Abecassis M, Dadhania D, Samstein B, Knechtle S, Hancock W, Schwartz J, Liu J, Bridges N, Shaked A. Validation of urinary cell biomolecular markers of acute cellular rejection: A report from CTOT-4 trial investigators. *Am J Transplant* 2010; 10 (suppl 4): 144.

[46] Anglicheau D, Muthukumar T, Hummel A, Ding R, Sharma VK, Dadhania D, Seshan SV, Schwartz JE, Suthanthiran M. Discovery and validation of a molecular signature for the noninvasive diagnosis of human renal allograft fibrosis. *Transplantation* 2012; 93(11): 1136-1146. PMID: 22592886

[47] Kowalski RJ, Zeevi A, Mannon RB, Britz JA, Carruth LM. Immunodiagnostics: evaluation of functional T-cell immunocompetence in whole blood independent of circulating cell numbers. *J. Immunotoxicol* 2007; 4(3): 225-232. PMID: 18958732.

[48] Huskey J, Gralla J, Wiseman AC. Single time point immune function assay (Immuknow) testing does not aid in the prediction of future opportunistic infections or acute rejection. *Clin J Am Soc Nephrol* 2011; 6(2): 423-429. PMID: 21088287.

[49] De Serres SA, Mfarrej BG, Grafals M, Riella LV, Magee CN, Yeung MY, Dyer C, Ahmad U, Chandraker A, Najafian N. Derivation and validation of a cytokine-based assay to screen for acute rejection in renal transplant recipients. *Clin J Am Soc Nephrol* 2012; 7(6): 1018-1025. PMID: 22498498.

[50] Anglicheau D, Muthukumar T, Suthanthiran M. MicroRNAs: small RNAs with big effects. *Transplantation* 2010; 90(2): 105-112. PMID: 20574417.

Chapter 6

Transplanting Against Histocompatibility Barriers

Dinesh Kannabhiran, Michelle L. Lubetzky and Darshana Dadhania

Additional information is available at the end of the chapter

http://dx.doi.org/10.5772/54346

1. Introduction

Currently there are over 90,000 patients awaiting a kidney transplant in the United States. Despite the large number of wait-listed patients, just over 16,000 were transplanted in 2009 [1]. Mean waiting times for transplantation can range from 2 years to over 5 years depending on a variety of factors including blood type, sensitization status and deceased donor availability in the region. Despite the availability of a willing living donor, a patient may be forced to remain on the deceased donor waiting list because of ABO incompatibility (ABOi) and/or the presence of a positive crossmatch due to donor specific anti-HLA antibodies. Those with blood O and B tend to have the longest wait times (median waiting time for O:1852 days; A:1208 days; B:1937 days; AB: 855 days) and may also have difficulty finding a compatible living donor [2]. Sensitized patients are those with high levels of anti-HLA (Human Leukocyte Antigen) antibodies in their blood. These antibodies form as a result of exposure to foreign HLA during pregnancy, transfusions and exposure to previous organ transplants. Approximately 16% of patients on the waiting list are re-transplants. Patients who are sensitized (Panel Reactive Antibody, PRA 10% or greater) make up roughly 25% of the current waiting list, 16% of which have a PRA >80% [1]. In some cases, a highly sensitized patient can wait up to 10 years before being transplanted. These wait times a negative impact on patients as the morbidity and mortality of dialysis patients are higher compared to kidney transplant recipients[3]. In 2010 over 5,000 patients died while waiting to receive a kidney transplant [1]. Given the increased mortality associated with dialysis, renal transplantation remains the preferred treatment for patients with end stage renal disease [4].

Historically, ABO compatibility has been a requirement for renal transplantation due to high rates of rejection seen in ABO incompatible transplants. In blood group compatible transplants, a negative T cell CDC (complement dependent cytotoxicity) crossmatch with a donor is required for kidney transplantation. It is not only difficult to find a compatible donor for the highly sensitized patients, but also difficult to achieve good long-term graft survival due to higher rates of acute and chronic rejection. In the last two decades, technology for assessment of histocompatibility barriers (ABO and anti-HLA antibodies) have advanced significantly. These new assays (advanced flow cytometry crossmatches, ELISA crossmatches, solid phase anti-HLA antibody assays) have improved our ability to determine the risk of acute rejection in the presence of these types of histocompatibility barriers. Complementary to these innovations, there have been great advancements in therapeutic options to remove and decrease production of anti-AB and anti-HLA antibodies for treatment of acute and chronic antibody mediated rejection and for reducing the risk of acute rejection episodes by providing treatments to modulate the immune response prior to transplantation. In this section, we will review the data on kidney transplantation in the ABO incompatible and crossmatch incompatible recipient-donor pairs.

2. Current therapies used for preparing patients for transplantation using donors with ABO and crossmatch incompatibility

In order to effectively reduce the immune response, a multi-faceted approach must be used for removal of antibodies prior to proceeding with an ABO or crossmatch incompatible transplant. For crossmatch incompatible patients, treatment protocols have been referred to as "desensitization" protocols. We will refer to these protocols as immunomodulatory or pre-transplant conditioning protocols since one is not actually changing the "sensitized" status of the patient. Figure 1 provides the basic mechanisms that are addressed to modulate the immune system of a potential recipient of an ABO or crossmatch incompatible organ. Splenectomy and cytotoxic therapies such as rituximab and bortezomib decrease the size of B and plasma cell clones. Physical removal of circulating antibodies is accomplished by procedures such as plasmapheresis or double filtration or immunoadsorption. Other additional immunosuppressive medications as well as IVIG via Fc receptor signaling impair the ability of cells to make antibodies. IVIG may also directly inhibit the function of circulating antibodies. A brief overview of the mechanisms is provided below and an in-depth review of immunosuppressive medications used in kidney transplantation is provided in Chapter 9.

2.1. Plasmapheresis (PP) and Immunoadsorption (IA)

Physical removal of antibodies can be accomplished by several different procedures such as conventional plasmapheresis, double-filtration plasmapheresis, semi-selective and antigen-specific immunoadsorption. Treatment with these procedures leads to serial reduction in antibody titer. However, without additional therapies to prevent production of these antibodies, the antibody titers rebound and return to baseline values once the treatments have stopped.

Plasmapheresis is the most commonly used method in the United States. It is a procedure in which the blood passes through a medical device that separates plasma from cellular components of blood allowing for physical removal of plasma prior to returning the blood back to the patient. Patient's plasma volume that is removed is replaced with a replacement solution such as colloid solution (e.g. albumin and/or plasma) or a combination of crystalloid/colloid solution [5]. In Japan, double filtration plasmapheresis has been used. In this procedure, plasma is removed as for plasmapheresis and then passed through a second filter (plasma separator), whose smaller pore size traps only larger molecules like immunoglobulins. Thus, lower molecular weight plasma components can be passed back into the patient and less replacement fluid is needed. Although these procedures are not 100% efficient, sequential therapies allow for treatment of higher plasma volumes and greater reduction in antibody titers. These procedures are very effective for removal of antibodies against A and B blood group antigens and are associated with approximately 20% reduction in titer with each treatment. Common adverse reactions include hypocalcemia and pruritis seen in 5% of all patients [6].

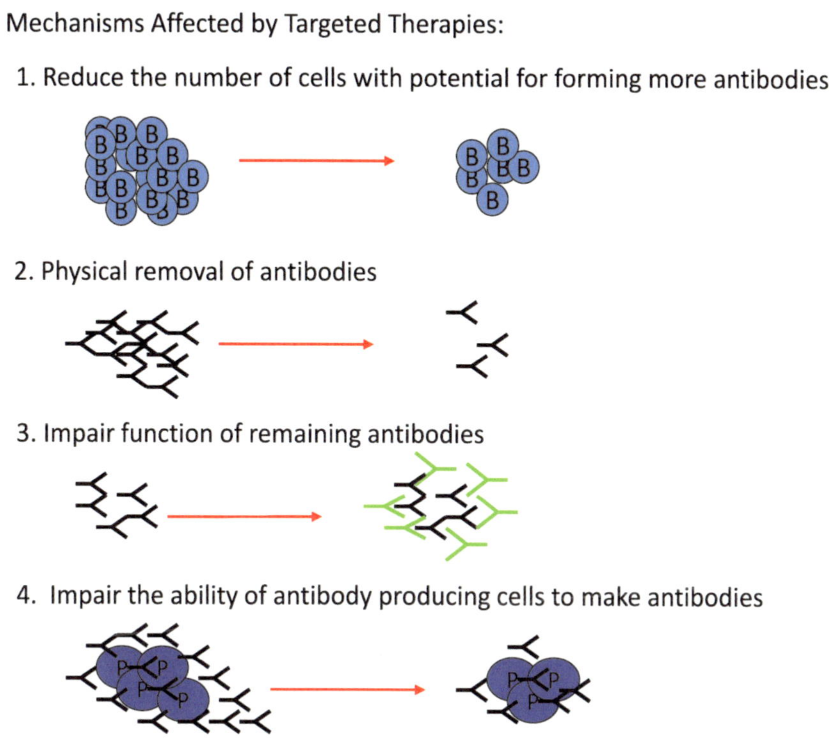

Figure 1. Immune Modulation of ABO or Crossmatch Incompatible Recipients

Immunoadsorption is a procedure in which plasma of the patient, after separation from blood, passes thru a column containing an active component that binds or removes immunoglobulins specifically [5]. A newer column for Immunoadsorption was created by Glycorex Transplantation AB (Lund, Sweden). This Glycosorb® ABO column has a matrix of sepharose beads coated with blood group A or B carbohydrate antigens that removes isohemagglutinins against the corresponding blood group. The Glycosorb® columns effectively remove anti-A or anti-B antibodies with approximately a 30% reduction in A/B

IgM and approximately a 20% A/B IgG levels after a single treatment. Importantly, titers of other antibodies, particularly those against Pneumococcus, Hemophilus, Diphtheria and tetanus seem largely unchanged [2, 7].

2.2. Splenectomy

Since the 1980s, splenectomy was performed in all successful ABOi kidney transplants to reduce the risk of rejection. The benefit for splenectomy was based on a small case series demonstrating a reversal of AMR (antibody mediated rejection) with splenectomy [8]. Since then, splenectomy had been a part of immunosuppressive regimen in most of the ABOi protocols and some early crossmatch incompatible protocols. The rationale was to physically remove the source of antibody producing cells and thus prevent rebound in antibody titer after plasmapheresis. In the past few years with the availability of new drugs such as rituximab, splenectomy is no longer a requirement for transplantation with incompatible donors.

2.3. Anti-CD20 antibody as surrogate for splenectomy

Rituximab, a monoclonal anti-CD20 antibody, was initially used for the treatment for Non Hodgkins lymphoma in 1997. Since then, it has been used in patients with immune complex mediated renal diseases and in kidney transplant recipients for treatment of rejection. It is a chimeric monoclonal antibody with human constant region and murine variable region that targets human CD20 molecule. CD20 is expressed on naive and mature activated B cells as well as some memory B cells. B cell depletion occurs via antibody dependent cytotoxicity and can be rapid, over 3-4 days and sustained, lasing for almost up to a year [9].

Tyden et al. [10] were first to demonstrate successful ABOi kidney transplantation in 4 patients with the use of single dose rituximab (375mg/m^2) in lieu of splenectomy. Since then, rituximab has been included in many immunosuppressive protocols for facilitating incompatible transplantation. The optimal dose of rituximab remains unknown. Toki [9] et al. studied the effect of B cell depletion with increasing doses of rituximab (10, 15, 35, 150, 300 mg/m^2) in 5 patients. All but one dosage of rituximab (10 mg/m^2) was able to completely eliminate B cells from circulation in 30 days. However, depletion of circulating B cells may not correlate with depletion of B cells within the lymph nodes and/or spleen.

2.4. Proteasome inhibition to target plasma cells

Plasma cells produce antibodies within one week after antigen exposure in large volumes- approximately several thousand antibodies per second. The excess protein synthesis leads to increased number of misfolded protein accumulating in the endoplasmic reticulum and these proteins are naturally degraded by proteasomes. Degradation of these proteins via the ubiquitin-proteasome dependent pathways is important for maintaining cellular homeostasis. Bortezomib, the first drug of its kind, inhibits ubiquitin-proteasome pathway by binding to the 26S proteasome and promotes G2-M cell cycle arrest and cell apoptosis. Because of the potential for reducing antibody producing plasma cells, bortezomib has been utilized with increased frequency for treatment of antibody mediated rejection and is being studied in conditioning regimens for recipients with incompatible donors [11, 12].

2.5. Intravenous immunoglobulin (IVIG)

IVIG is a commercial preparation of immune globulin which predominantly consists of intact IgG molecules and trace IgA obtained from pooled plasma from approximately 3000 to 10,000 healthy blood donors. These natural antibodies that are formed in the absence of immunization or foreign antigen exposure are thought to be essential in immunoregulatory effects. IVIG exerts its effect on immune systems through multiple mechanisms which include neutralization of circulating anti-HLA antibodies through anti-idiotypic antibodies, inhibition of complement activation, enhancing clearance of anti-HLA antibodies, negative signaling through Fcγ receptors, and selective down-regulation of antibody production. Two commonly used preparations are the pooled IVIG and the cytomegalovirus hyperimmune globulin (CMVIG). In the early 1990s there were both in vitro and in vivo studies that demonstrated high doses of IVIG could decrease PRA and increase rates of transplantation in highly sensitized individuals. IVIG is commonly administered following plasmapheresis to treat antibody mediated rejection and has been used in immunomodulatory therapies for ABOi and crossmatch incompatible transplants [13].

2.6. Other immunosuppressive therapies

Concurrent with these therapies, many protocols designed to precondition patients for incompatible transplants utilize standard maintenance immunosuppressive medications such as tacrolimus, mycophenolate mofetil and prednisone. The intention is to suppress the immune system and impair the ability of the immune cells to make more antibodies.

3. Renal transplantation with ABO incompatible donors

3.1. Patient assessment: ABO blood grouping

Blood group of an individual is defined by cell surface molecules that are present on all nucleated cells and platelets. Of the 30 blood group systems, the major blood group system is the ABO system, discovered by Karl Landsteiner in 1901. The blood group antigens consist of carbohydrates moieties attached to a glycosphingolipid and glycoprotein backbone. The major blood groups are A, B, AB and O and are defined by the type of molecules that are present on cell surface (A or B). Individuals develop naturally acquired antibodies against the molecules that are not present on their own cells. The antigenic stimulus for the development of these naturally occurring antibodies is believed to come from exposure to gut bacteria that express similar antigens.

These naturally occurring antibodies against A/B antigens are termed isohemagglutinins because of their ability to agglutinate cells (RBCs) that express the target molecules. This ability to cause agglutination in vivo results in acute thrombosis and inflammation when a recipient receives an ABO incompatible organ without any therapy to modulate the immune response and reduce the number of circulating antibodies directed against the ABO group [14, 15]. In organ transplantation, ABO compatibility is the first step in determining the suitability of a donor for a particular recipient. Group A individuals express the A antigen on cell surface and produce antibodies against the non-expressed B antigen (anti B antibodies). Group B individuals express the B antigen on cell surface and produce anti A antibodies. Group AB individuals express both A and B antigens on cell surface and therefore do not produce either anti-A or anti-B antibodies. They are referred to as the "universal recipients" and can receive an organ from any individual. Individuals with blood group O express neither A or B antigen on cell surface and therefore produce antibodies against both A and B antigens. Given the lack of cell surface expression of A and B antigens, these individuals are considered "universal donors." However because they express antibodies against both A and B antigens, they can only receive a donor from blood group O individuals.

Blood group A has two major subtypes, A1 and A2. A2 is expressed in approximately 20% of the US population and these individuals have lower cell surface expression of the blood group antigen compared to individuals with blood type A1. In addition, antibodies directed against the A antigen do not cause efficient agglutination of RBC from individuals with blood type A2. Given the lower cell surface expression of A2 antigen and less robust binding of anti- A to the A2 molecules resulting in less agglutination, donors with A2 subtype are considered to be less immunogenic. In fact, A2 donor kidneys have been transplanted to B recipients without the use of treatment protocols for immune modulation prior to transplantation [8], however, most patients do require some form of immunomodulatory therapy prior to transplantation [16]. The long-term outcomes were similar to that of ABO compatible transplantation [17].

3.1.1. Isohemagglutinin measurement

In addition to ABO grouping, the strength of the anti-A and anti-B titers need to be determined prior to initiating therapy for an ABOi kidney transplant. The presence of anti-A and anti-B causes hyperacute rejection within days to weeks in the setting of ABOi transplantation. These antibodies can be removed by plasmapheresis or immunoadsorption. Different centers use different goals for isohemagglutinin titers ranging from <1/8 to <1/32. Antibodies are measured using serial dilutions of a patient's sample, which are incubated for a period of time at 37°C with RBC aliquots with the appropriate blood group antigen. The sample is then checked for macroscopic agglutination of red blood cells (for IgM) or undergoes additional incubation with antihuman globulin to detect IgG agglutination [2]. The reagents for these tests are not standardized and therefore inter-laboratory variation does occur (up to 32-fold for IgM and 256-fold for IgG). ELISA and flow cytometry methods may be more accurate and reproducible [18].

3.2. Brief history of kidney transplantation with ABO incompatible donors

In 1954, Hume et al. [19] reported the first ABOi renal transplantation where the patient lost the graft on the 5th post-operative day. Though Starzl et al. [20] in 1964 reported 3 successful kidney transplants across the ABO barrier, over the next 2 decades several case reports of unsuccessful attempts at kidney transplant across ABO antigens were published. Cooke et al. [21] reported a graft survival rate of 4% at 1 year in ABOi transplants. Therefore, ABO incompatibility generally was considered an absolute contraindication to kidney transplantation.

In 1981, Slapak et al. first reported the use of plasmapheresis (PP) as a tool to remove the anti-A and anti-B when a patient with blood group O inadvertently received a kidney from a donor with blood group A. Acute antibody mediated rejection was reversed with PP and the patient had normal renal function 20 months after transplantation. Six years later, Alexandre et al. [22] reported the successful outcome of ABOi transplantation in 26 patients with splenectomy and PP. The overall outcome of ABO incompatible transplants has improved over the years with the introduction of PP and more potent immunosuppressive therapies including the use of poly and monoclonal antibody therapies. As a result, splenectomy is no longer a required procedure for ABO incompatible kidney transplants. Today, ABO incompatible transplants are routinely performed in Japan where approximately 20% of living donor recipients receive a kidney from an ABO incompatible donor. The option of receiving an ABO incompatible transplant is being utilized more frequently in other countries as well.

3.3. Modulation of the immune response in recipients with ABO incompatible donors

A review of the major immunosuppressive protocols that have been studied to facilitate ABO incompatible transplants is summarized in Table 1. Most studies utilized some form of antibody removal via PP, double-filtration or immunoadsorption and the target anti-A/B titer was between 1:8 and 1:32. In the '80s and '90s, splenectomy was commonly performed in recipients of ABO incompatible transplants. In 2004, Squifflet et al. found that the outcome of splenectomized ABOi living related transplant recipients was similar to the outcome of ABO compatible living related transplant recipients maintained on cyclosporine based immunosuppression [23].

Overall, rejection rates were relatively high (29.3%- 58%), in patients who underwent splenectomy as part of the treatment protocol (Table 1- #1-3) [24-26]. With the introduction of rituximab, splenectomy was no longer required for successful transplantation with ABO incompatible donors and rituximab has been referred to as "medical splenectomy". Gloor et al. found that the incidence of antibody mediated rejection in the splenectomy group was 30 % compared to 18% in the rituximab group (p=0.68) [24]. Patient and graft survival were similar. Genberg et al. found that the combination of immunoadsorption and rituximab improved outcomes similar to that of ABO compatible living donor kidney transplants (graft survival was 86.7% in both the groups) [7].

More recently, Montgomery et al. [25] found that a conditioning regimen using PP and IVIG alone may be effective in successful ABOi transplantation. The group transplanted 28 ABOi patients who had received plasmapheresis and CMVIG alone without B cell ablative therapy and followed them for 2 years. The incidence of humoral rejection was 17.8% which was similar to those patients who had splenectomy (n=17) or rituximab (n=15) in addition to PP and CMVIG [25]. In Japan where ABOi transplants are very common, acute rejection rates have decreased to less than 10%. In a series of 74 patients who received rituximab and PP for immunomodulation, the incidence of humoral rejection was only 6.7%. Patient survival was 100% and the graft survival was 97% [27].

Overall the goal of the pre-transplant conditioning regimen is to reduce the anti-A and/or anti-B titers to a low level. The acceptable titer for transplantation varies significantly among the centers, ranging from 1:32 to <1:8. Generally patients receive additional PP treatment in the early post-transplant period. The anti-A and anti-B titers are followed routinely post-transplant and a rise in the titer may be used as an indication to reinitiate PP and/or a biopsy procedure. For long term immunosuppression, these patients are usually maintained on triple drug therapy (calcineurin inhibitors, antimetabolites and steroids). Acute rejection episodes are treated as per center protocols.

3.4. Clinical outcomes of recipients with ABO incompatible donors

The major goal of conditioning regimens for recipients of ABOi donors is to reduce the anti-A and/or anti-B titers to a level that allows for transplantation without hyperacute rejection and early graft loss. We reviewed some of the protocols that have led to successful transplantation using ABOi donors. However, these patients are still at risk for acute rejection episodes and acute rejection rates can be as high as 30% in some series. Acute antibody mediated rejection (AMR) has also been shown to affect graft survival in ABOi kidney transplants. Toki [28] et al. showed that the graft survival is much lower when patients have AMR compared to patients who do not experience AMR (5 year survival- 84% vs. 95%). Presence of AMR also correlates with the development of transplant glomerulopathy at 1 year (64% vs. 3%). Since any episode of AMR has a profound effect on the graft outcomes despite treatment, optimizing the evaluation and management of recipients with ABOi transplants is important to mitigate the risk of rejection episodes (Figure 2).

Most centers utilize some form of monitoring protocol that includes anti-A/anti-B titers as well as protocol biopsies. However, recent data does not indicate that titers are predictive of early acute rejection and/or poor allograft outcomes. In a study by Shimmura et al. pre-transplant anti-A/anti-B titers were not found to correlate with graft survival in the patients with anti A/B IgG titers [29]. However, the presence of donor specific anti-HLA antibodies did appear to have a more significant association with poor allograft outcomes than anti-blood group antibodies [28]. In another study, the authors found that the median anti-A/anti-B titer in those who had antibody mediated rejection was 16 (range 8-256). However, the positive predictive value of a high anti-A/B titers for AMR was poor (33.3%) [30]. Other studies have found that the absence of mycophenolate mofetil in the conditioning regimens was also associated with an increased risk of rejection [2, 28-30].

Acute antibody-mediated rejection requires morphologic evidence of acute tissue injury, circulating donor-specific alloantibodies, and immunological evidence of antibody-mediated process (particularly C4d positive staining). C4d is a degradation product of the classic complement pathway. A unique feature of C4d is that it binds covalently to the endothelial and collagen basement membranes, thereby avoiding removal and raising the possibility of serving as an immunologic footprint of complement activation and antibody activity. Presence of C4d correlates with the presence of donor specific anti HLA antibodies and also poor graft survival. But the significance of C4d deposition is not clear. C4d deposition has been seen in up to 80% of protocol biopsies in ABOi transplantation without any sign of graft dysfunction. Platt et al. suggested that perhaps the binding of anti-donor antibodies and complement to the graft induces accommodation. So, the presence of C4d alone does not signify endothelial damage or rejection [31].

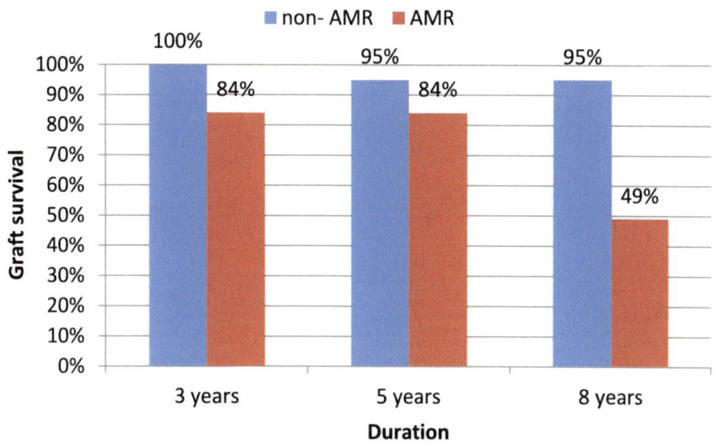

Difference in Graft Survival between AMR vs. Non-AMR at 5 years was significant, P=0.009
AMR – antibody mediated rejection; Data adapted from Toki et al., AM J Transplant, 2008

Figure 2. Graft survival rate influenced by antibody mediated rejection in recipients of ABOi kidney transplants.

Despite the acute rejection complication, long term outcomes for recipients of ABOi transplants are good and similar to the outcomes seen in ABO compatible transplantation. Results from Japan, where the largest number of ABOi transplants have been performed, are also promising. Ichimaru et al. [32] published a review of 1,012 ABOi transplants performed from 1989-2006 at 92 institutions. The 1-year, 3- year, 5- year and 10- year patient survival rates were 95%, 93%, 91% and 87% and the corresponding graft survival rates were 90%, 86%, 80% and 63%, respectively (Figure 3). Graft survival was significantly better in patients aged 15 or younger and in patients transplanted after 2001.

Futagawa and Terasaki [33] published an analysis of registry data of UNOS examining ABOI kidney recipients compared to ABO compatible transplantation. There was no significant difference in allograft survival at 1 and 5 years after transplantation (66.9 versus 66.7 %). These results were also validated in other studies (Figure 3). Genberg et al. [7] analyzed the protocol on 60 consecutive ABOi kidney transplants that included immunoadsorption (used primarily in Europe) instead of plasmapheresis. At 5- year follow-up, graft survival was 97% for the ABOi group vs. 95% for the ABO compatible recipients. Patient survival was identical (98%).

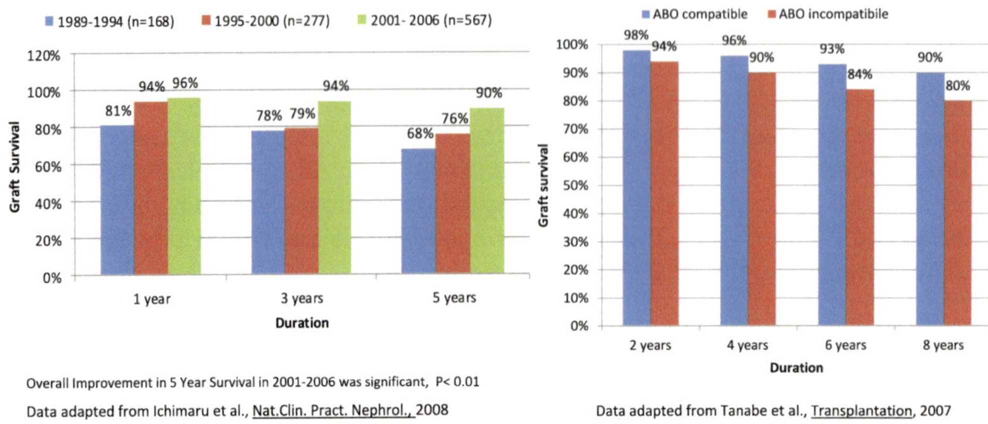

a) b)

Figure 3. a) Trends in graft survival rates of ABOi kidney transplant recipients from 1989-2006 b) Comparison of graft survival rates in ABOi and ABO compatible kidney transplant recipients

3.5. Accommodation

After a successful ABOi transplantation, many allografts exhibit signs of "accommodation" which is defined as the absence of allograft injury in the presence of alloantibodies. Many of the recipients of ABOi kidney transplants demonstrate C4d deposition in protocol biopsies without any signs of acute or chronic rejection [34]. Haas and colleagues found that in ABOi graft recipients, individuals with diffuse C4d deposition without other signs of graft dysfunction did better than those without significant C4d deposition. Several experimental models have attempted to elucidate the mechanism of these findings. One explanation is that the binding of anti-A/B to the endothelium leads to upregulation of protective genes such as CD55 and CD59 which inhibit complement mediated cell injury and protects the graft acutely [35, 36]. It is postulated that reduction in cell surface expression of A /B antigens in the graft and development of endothelial chimerism may protect the graft long-term [37-39].

3.6. Future of transplantation with ABO incompatible donors

Using blood group frequencies in the US population, 30–35% of potential living donors will be blood group incompatible. Other than continuing on renal replacement therapy and waiting for a deceased donor transplant, the options for patients with ABOi donors are kidney paired donation or ABO incompatible transplantation. Not all recipient-donor pairs find a suitable donor exchange option quickly. Similar to waiting for a donor on the deceased donor list, blood type O recipients have an increased wait time on the kidney paired donation registry. This topic is covered in more detail in Chapter 9.

Research to facilitate ABOi transplants and reduce acute rejection rates in these individuals would be of value. Experimental therapies are being investigated to reduce the antibody target on the endothelium. This is achieved either through the use of enzymes that cleave the carbohydrate antigen or by blocking antibody preventing isohemagglutinin binding. Kobayashi and others have shown that recombinant ABase infusion (an enzyme which removes A/B antigen from cell surface) in baboons leads to significant reduction in expression of blood group antigens on its kidneys. Hasegawa isolated a novel antibody (K7508) which targets blood group A antigen. They showed that group A red cells coated with the blocking antibody (K7508) were not recognized by other anti-A antibodies, indicating that antigen A was masked by K7508. Both these options reduce antibody-antigen binding in recipients of ABOi transplants and may improve our management of ABOi recipient-donor pairs [40, 41].

4. Renal transplantation with crossmatch incompatible donors

4.1. Patient assessment: Histocompatibility testing

The predominant method of evaluating a patient's sensitization is using the panel reactive antibody (PRA). Historically, this was done using a complement dependent cytotoxicity (CDC) assay. In this assay, the patient's serum is incubated with a panel of donor lymphocytes in the presence of rabbit complement which results in lymphocyte death in the presence of patient's antibodies binding to the cell surface and activating complement cascade. The percentage of lymphocytes giving a positive reaction (cell death) over the total number tested is the PRA of the patient. Sensitized patients who have been exposed to Class I and Class II HLA (human leukocyte antigens) via transfusions, pregnancies and previous transplants are likely to have PRA because they harbor many anti-HLA antibodies that react with larger pool of the donor leukocyte panel [42]. In this assay, it was difficult to determine the exact target of the anti-HLA antibodies since each lymphocytes of the donor would express more than one Class I and II HLA molecules. More recently, with the advent of solid phase assays (where HLA antigens are immobilized in a tray well or on a bead) using ELISA, flow-Cytometry, and Luminex technologies, we can be more precise about the specificity of the anti-HLA antibody when assessing the sensitization of a given patient [43]. We can also calculate the PRA (cPRA) based on the frequency of the HLA antigens in a larger pool of donors and perform a "virtual crossmatch" in which we try to predict the possibility of a positive crossmatch based on the semiquantitative strength of the anti-HLA antibodies present in the donor's serum and the HLA typing of the potential donor. These solid phase anti-HLA antibody assays allow each center to minimize the number of positive crossmatches for their recipients and assess relative risk of immunological complications early post-transplantation [44].

Prior to any kidney transplant, a prospective sensitive CDC (complement dependent cytotoxicity) crossmatch is required. The standard crossmatch at most centers is the AHG-CDC (anti-human immunoglobulin enhanced CDC) crossmatch). A positive donor T cell AHG-CDC is a contraindication to transplantation. In this crossmatch, the donor cells are mixed with the patient's serum and incubated with rabbit complement to evaluate if the recipient antibodies are able to elicit donor cell death. The strength of the reaction is graded and any significant cell death above and beyond the negative control well is considered positive. If there is a positive reaction, it suggests that the patient is sensitized against the donor and is at high risk of hyperacute or accelerated rejection episode. The flow cytometry crossmatch is also utilized to identify any donor specific antibodies and it is considered to be a more sensitive crossmatch than the standard AHG-CDC crossmatch. The flow crossmatch is performed by incubating an individual's sera with donor lymphocytes (T & B) that are stained with a fluorochrome-conjugated anti-IgG. The fluorescence of the bound antibody is then detected using a laser and compared to a negative control. The difference in the signal between the donor crossmatch and the negative control is calculated and reported as a mean channel shift (MCS). The CDC crossmatch identifies complement activating antibodies but does not distinguish anti-HLA from non anti-HLA antibodies. Similarly the standard flow cytometry crossmatch detects both anti-HLA and non anti-HLA antibodies but does not distinguish between complement activating antibodies and non-complement activating antibodies. Both of these tests are used to assess donor-reactivity [45]. The association between positive flow cytometry crossmatch and acute rejection rates and graft survival is still being debated. Only one prospective blinded study has been performed and it showed that a positive flow cytometry crossmatch did not affect graft outcomes [46]. However, there are multiple other studies demonstrating increased acute rejection risk associated with a positive flow cytometry crossmatch. At some centers a positive flow cytometry crossmatch is considered a contraindication to transplantation while at other centers may utilize condition therapies or modify induction therapies to avoid early acute rejection episodes [47, 48].

To distinguish between anti-HLA and non anti-HLA antibodies, a series of solid phase antibody detection systems have been developed [49]. In these assays, the HLA antigens eluted from cell lines are immobilized on an artificial surface and patient's serum is incubated with the bound HLA antigens. If the patient has an anti-HLA antibody, it will bind to the antigen. The bound antibodies are detected using some type of fluorescence signal. Different platforms are used for solid phase antibody screening including ELISA, standard flow cytometer and the multiplexing assays on the Luminex® platform. At this time a solid phase antibody screening is required to list unacceptable antigen on the UNOS waiting list.

When performing histocompatibility testing, most centers are reporting DSA (donor specific antibodies) as part of the assessment. Although the term DSA can refer to any type of antibody directed against the donor, it commonly refers to the anti-HLA antibodies detected against the donor using solid phase antibody screening. The most commonly used platform, Luminex® platform, is able to provide the relative strength of the antibody in terms of MFI values (mean fluorescence intensity). However, it is not considered an absolute quantitative assay and the assay is not standardized across laboratories.. Therefore, MFI values obtained at one center cannot be compared directly to the MFI values obtained at another center. However, the relative strength (low, medium, strong) should be comparable [50].

Solid phase antibody assays are routinely used to report DSA and identify patients at risk for AMR (antibody mediated rejection) post-transplantation. Akalin and colleagues found in their treatment protocols that AMR was observed only in patients with strong DSAs (MFI >6000 on Luminex® platform) [51]. Similarly Mayo clinic also found that the development of AMR was more likely in patients with strong DSAs and higher MCS on flow cytometry crossmatch [52]. Lefaucher et al. showed that patients with DSA MFI >6000 were 100 times more likely to develop AMR [53].

A prospective CDC crossmatch is performed on all patients. A positive donor CDC T cell crossmatch is considerted to be a contraindication to transplantation in routine practice. However, other techniques are routinely used to measure the sensitization status of the patient, determine whether the antibody is directed against HLA or non-HLA, and assess risk for early acute rejection episodes [54]. These techniques also aid in measuring the response to immunomodulation treatment protocols and understanding when transplantation can safely be performed while minimizing the risk of acute rejection. New technology is continuously emerging and new assays to look at complement binding antibodies, IgG subtypes and endothelial antibodies are currently being studied [55-57].

4.2. History of kidney transplantation with crossmatch incompatible donors

In 1969, Patel and Terasaki were the first to demonstrate that the presence of pre-formed antibodies significantly affects transplant outcomes and that the crossmatch could help define who could be safely transplanted. Their pivotal paper showed that when transplanted with a positive crossmatch, 80% of patients would go on to lose their grafts, however with a negative crossmatch, only 4% of patients lost their grafts [58]. Since then our techniques for measuring antibodies and assessing sensitization have become quite sophisticated. Additionally, multiple studies have demonstrated that the presence of preformed antibodies predisposes patients to hyper-acute rejection as well as acute and chronic AMR. We now understand that simply the presence of preformed antibodies leads to decreased graft survival even in the absence of clinical signs of AMR [53].

Because of the shortage of available organs and the high percentage of sensitized patients on the wait-list for transplantation, many centers began looking into methods for immunomodulation to improve the rates of transplantation and outcomes in highly sensitized individuals since the early 90s. These early studies as well as many recent protocols involve the use of low or high dose IVIG and PP. The mechanism of action of these therapies was described earlier. More recently newer protocols have begun using rituximab, anti-CD20 antibody, bortezomib, the protease inhibitor and eculizumab, the anti-C5, terminal complement inhibitor.

4.3. Modulation of the immune response in recipients with crossmatch incompatible donors

Immunomodulation therapy can be given prior to transplantation to facilitate transplantation or at the time of transplantation to reduce acute rejection related complications. Because the earliest forms of immunomodulation focused on obtaining a negative CDC crossmatch to allow transplantation of sensitized patients, only individuals with living donors were enrolled to determine if the treatment protocols utilizing PP and IVIG were successful in obtaining a negative crossmatch. With more experience, some centers have begun to treat patients who are on the waiting list for a transplant and suggested that PRA levels and time to transplantation can be decreased. Since 2000, there have been many studies describing protocols used for conditioning prior to transplantation [Table 2] as well as protocols administered peri-transplantation [Table 3] to reduce the risk of acute rejection in sensitized patients. We have divided data into two tables. Table 2 describes the protocols from 8 studies that predominantly focused on pre-transplant conditioning therapies to lower antibodies to a level that results in a negative crossmatch (some transplants occurred with persistent weakly positive crossmatches). The goal of these therapies was to reduce anti-HLA antibodies and allow for successful transplantation. If immunomodulation was unsuccessful, patients did not proceed to transplant. Three of the studies focused on use of high dose IVIG for immunomodulation [59-61]. In these studies rejection rates were 31-59% and patient and graft survival was 96-100% and 75-100% respectively. Four of the studies included rituximab as a part of their pre-transplant conditioning regimens [62-65]. Despite the addition of rituximab, AMR rates remained high, 37-50% and patient and graft survival were similar to the IVIG alone groups 86-100% and 79-94% respectively. Of these trials, only one was a randomized control trial and focused on treatment of patients awaiting a deceased donor transplant. Jordan et al published their data on the use of IVIG versus placebo. They found that transplantation rates improved and time to transplantation decreased significantly with the use of high dose IVIG. Additionally they demonstrated significant reductions in PRA after the use of IVIG ($p<0.03$).

It is unclear whether high dose IVIG is an improved therapy over PP and low dose IVIG. The study in Table 2 by Stegall et al. compared PP/IVIG with IVIG alone using anti-thymocyte globulin (ATG) induction [66]. In their study they looked at transplantation outcomes in 3 treatment groups. The first group received high dose IVIG, the second received PP, low dose IVIG and rituximab, and the third received PP, low dose IVIG, rituximab with close post-transplant monitoring. All groups received anti-thymocyte globulin induction. In the first group only 5/13 (38%) had pre transplant tyhomglobulin a negative crossmatch while 84% in group 2 and 88% in group 3 ultimately had a negative crossmatch. AMR rates in the first group were quite high (80%), and significantly lower in group 2 (37%) and group 3 (29%). Additionally they noted that at baseline, patients with higher AHG titers were less likely to achieve a negative crossmatch at the time of transplant. Among the small number of patients that went on to receive a transplant with a persistently positive crossmatch, 70% developed AMR and 50% went on to lose their grafts.

Table 3 describes protocols that were used to reduce the risk of acute rejection episodes and graft loss in sensitized patients who had an acceptable crossmatch to proceed with transplantation. These patients did not have contraindications to transplantation but were sensitized and deemed to be at high risk for early acute rejection episodes based on the presence of donor specific antibodies. These patients were treated either prior to transplantation or at the time of transplantation (Table 3) [61-63, 65, 67-77]. In these studies, AMR rates were lower and improved in some studies compared to historical controls. It is difficult, however, to compare one center's results to another's as there are no standardized methods to compare the strength of the antibodies in one group to another group at a different center. Acute rejection rates do appear to be lower compared to the studies in Table 2, a result attributable to the fact that this group's antibody titers were not high enough to cause a positive CDC crossmatch. Patient and graft survival ranged from 87-100% and 78-100% respectively.

The lowest rejection rates from Table 3 are seen in the data published by Mount Sinai using the addition of PP to IVIG/ATG pre-transplant conditioning protocols based on the intensity of DSA [51]. They studied a group of patients with CDC T cell negative crossmatch but T and/or B cell positive flow crossmatch. In their initial protocol patients were given low dose IVIG (300mg/kg) and ATG. However, they found with the initial 15 patients, 3 developed AMR so they increased their IVIG dosing to 2gm/kg. This still resulted in an AMR rate of 66% in patients with strong DSA and they altered their protocol to add PP in patients with strong DSA. They also noted that in the group of patients with weak DSA, there were no episodes of rejection. Once augmenting the protocol with PP, the AMR rate in the patients with strong DSA decreased to 7%. This study suggested that it was important to achieve MFI<6000 (at their center) to minimize the risk of acute rejection. Our center compared 33 flow XM positive patients treated with rituximab and IVIG prior to transplantation (living) or at the time of transplantation (deceased) to 16 flow crossmatch positive patients who had only received IVIG [78]. In our study cohort, use of rituximab was associated with a significant lower acute rejection rate at one year (16% vs. 45%; P=0.03). Despite these promising data, the majority of studies [Table 3] have much higher rates of AMR, significantly higher than the rejection rate of 13% reported across all transplants in the tacrolimus/MMF era of immunosupression [79].

Not all studies have reported success when using IVIG and rituximab for immunomodulation. Recently Marfu et al. examined the use of IVIG (2g/kg) and rituximab (1 dose 375mg/m2) for immunomodulation of patients on the deceased donor waiting list [80]. They found that in patients with cPRA >50%, treatment with IVIG and rituximab did not increase rates of transplantation. Compared to the Cedars Sinai group, their subjects had higher cPRA values. Post conditioning therapy, there was no improvement in cPRA values, nor was there a significant reductions in DSAs. They also performed whole blood genome analysis on their desensitized patient and demonstrated reductions in some B cell transcripts. In particular they found that specific genes previously shown to be associated with tolerance were down-regulated in their patients treated with IVIG/rituximab [81]. It is unclear what effect these changes in B cell transcripts resulting from IVIG and rituximab therapy will have on long term graft survival.

Although there has been some success with IVIG, PP and rituximab based protocols, the rates of AMR are still quite high and the success of decreasing PRA on patients waiting to receive a transplant is marginal at best. Newer therapies are currently being evaluated to improve these results.

4.4. Clinical outcomes of recipients with crossmatch incompatible donors

While the initial studies on immunomodulation quoted AMR rates as high as 100%, more recent studies that incorporates the use of stronger induction therapy, as well as use of the strength of DSA to guide PP and higher dose IVIG, suggest lower AMR rates. Short term graft survival ranges from 78-96%. To date only a few studies have looked at long term graft outcomes. Haririan et al. looked at living donor transplantation against a positive crossmatch and compared outcomes to negative cross-match living donor controls [69]. They found that 1 and 5 year allograft survival rates were 90% and 69% in the positive crossmatch group as compared to 98% and 81% in controls. More recently Johns Hopkins published their outcomes data comparing desensitized patients (using IVIG and PP) with two groups, a dialysis only group and a dialysis or transplantation group [82]. They found that patients who underwent immunomodulation had a survival of 90.6% at 1 year, 85.7% at 3 years and 80.6% at 8 years as compared with 91.1%, 67.2% and 30.5% in the dialysis only group and 93.1%, 77% and 49.1% in the dialysis or transplantation group respectively ($P<0.001$). While this group included only patients with live donors, there clearly remains a survival benefit to undergoing transplantation despite the need for immunomodulation. This survival benefit remained even in the group that was unable to obtain a negative crossmatch prior to transplantation. This data demonstrates a benefit to transplantation if a living donor is available over remaining on the wait list. However, it is unclear whether this can be extrapolated to those who received therapy prior to a deceased donor transplant.

Additionally there continues to be convincing evidence that the presence of DSA leads to poor graft outcomes, including increased incidence of chronic AMR and transplant glomerulopathy [83]. While there are no consensus guidelines as to the follow up of the sensitized patient post transplantation, it is clear that they should be followed more closely for monitoring of both acute and chronic AMR. In many centers this includes protocol biopsies and frequent monitoring of DSA. Any increase in serum creatinine or development of proteinuria should prompt repeat measurement of DSA and renal biopsy. Follow up should also include monitoring for sequalae of over-immunosuppression such as the development of BK viremia at regular intervals. At our center we currently monitor for DSA and BKV at 1 and 12 months in the highly sensitized patient.

Many studies have been done examining the use of protocol biopsies in transplanted patients, including those at high risk. The ability to detect and treat subclinical rejection at an early stage may have long term benefits on allograft survival [84, 85]. Persistent donor specific antibodies has been linked to the development of transplant glomerulopathy [86, 87]. Stegall and colleagues evaluated the incidence of transplant glomerulopathy in a large cohort of patients with protocol and diagnostic biopsies and found an incidence of 49% in well function renal allograft. The risk factors for transplant glomerulopathy included anti-HLA antibodies and history of prior acute rejection episode [88].The implementation of protocol biopsies has been shown to increase detection of subclinical rejection and Rush et al. found that treatment of subclinical rejection reduced rates of early and late rejection as well as improved graft survival at 2 years. Therefore it would be reasonable to perform protocol biopsies in a patient who undergoes immunomodulation and is at high risk for development of AMR and transplant glomerulopathy.

4.5. Future of crossmatch incompatible donors

While conditioning regimens for immunomodulation have shown some success in increasing transplantation rates in highly sensitized individuals, the rates of acute and chronic rejection remain high. Additionally, graft outcomes in patients with DSA are known to be worse than patients who are not sensitized to their donors [89, 90]. With the emergence of kidney paired donation programs (KPD), new options are now available for those patients who have a living donor but are highly sensitized. Given the growth and pool of donors in the current KPD programs, finding a compatible donor without the need for immunomodulation (prior to transplantation) is a more viable option. Segev et al. analyzed the benefits of a national KPD optimization scheme and found that highly sensitized patients would increase their rate of transplantation 6-fold (from 2.3% to 14.1%) [91]. Some highly sensitized patients may require immunomodulatory therapy even with the donors from the KPD program. However, data from more sensitive crossmatch techniques and solid phase antibody testing can be used to determine which donor would be associated with the the lowest relative risk of rejection for the recipient. Clearly this ability to assess relative risk with different donors will increase options for sensitized patients and allow us to optimize the donor selection process. Decision for whether or not to undergo pre-transplant conditioning therapy versus wait for a kidney to become available through KPD should be considered on a case by case basis.

Other novel therapies are currently being explored for immunomodulation. Bortezomib is a proteasome inhibitor that is FDA approved for the treatment of multiple myeloma. Its application in the field of transplantation is relatively new and based upon both in vitro and in vivo evidence of its activity against plasma cells. This agent is now being used to attempt reduction of DSA in sensitized patients [92, 93]. While many centers have incorporated this agent into treatment of AMR [94-96], its use for immunomodulation is limited to case reports. There have been 2 case reports that examined the use of bortezomib as a desensitizing agent pre-transplant. In the first, it was reported that one patient achieved a decrease in PRA from 57% to 31% and was able to be transplanted successfully [97]. In the other study, 2 patients received treatment with bortezomib and dexamethasone, and the effects were more modest, reduction of PRA from 87% to 80% and 37% to 13% [98]. Additionally at the 2010 American Transplant Congress, data was presented on the use of bortezomib in 6 patients for immunomodulation prior to transplantation. Compared to those treated with PP, 50% (3/6) received a transplant in the bortezomib group, while only 11% (1/9) in PP alone group [99]. There have also been small studies showing early treatment with bortezomib post-transplant can provide some modest reduction in DSAs that are detected during the early post-transplant period [100]. Whether bortezomib will become a meaningful agent for immunomodulation prior to transplantation remains to be determined.

Eculizumab is the newest agent to be considered for therapy of AMR and immunomodulation. It is a humanized monoclonal antibody against complement protein C5. It binds to C5 protein inhibiting its cleavage to C5a and C5b and preventing formation of the terminal complement complex C5b-9. It is FDA approved for paroxysmal nocturnal hemoglobinuria and for the prevention of atypical hemolytic uremic syndrome post-transplant [101]. More recently its use as an agent to prevent and treat AMR is being studied. An abstract presented at the 2010 American Transplant Congress from the Mayo Clinic showed that in 16 sensitized living donor transplant recipients treated with eculizumab, at the time of transplant, the AMR rate was as low as 6.25% [102]. Despite the reduced rates of AMR, 6 patients developed signs of chronic antibody mediated rejection. Again, this is a promising new agent whose role in the treatment of the sensitized patient is still being assessed.

5. Summary - Transplantation with incompatible donors

We have come a long way since the earliest studies in transplanting both the ABOi donor and the highly sensitized patient. Using blood group frequencies in the US population, 30–35% of potential living donors will be blood group incompatible. Other than continuing on renal replacement therapy and waiting for deceased donor transplant, the options for patients with ABOi donors are kidney paired donation (KPD) programs and ABO incompatible transplantation. Similar to compatible transplants, the waiting time for recipients with blood group O and B are longer in KPD programs (unless the donor is blood group O, universal donor). The mortality rate on dialysis while awaiting a transplant is very high (5-7 deaths per patient year) and therefore, for some individuals ABOi transplantation is not only a viable but a better option [2].

For the highly sensitized patient, sophisticated techniques to evaluate the level of sensitization and solid phase antibody screening tools can help to identify which antigens are unacceptable and likely to cause a positive crossmatch. With this information we can select recipient-donor combinations that would be amenable to immunomodulation and allow for successful transplantation with good long-term outcomes. For patients who have a living donor, KPD programs can be used to increase opportunities for the recipient and optimize chances for successful transplantation.

Conditioning therapies for immunomodulation do not come without a cost. AMR, chronic rejection and transplant glomerulopathy are frequent complications in recipients of incompatible donors. Patients must be monitored frequently for any signs of rejection as well as the infectious complications associated with high dose immunosuppressive therapies. The use of protocol biopsies should be considered and maintenance immunosuppression should be individualized. With the advent of non-invasive techniques for evaluating allograft function and the use of urinary biomarkers to detect early signs of graft dysfunction, monitoring of the highly sensitized patient will continue to evolve.

5.1. Economic considerations

The USRDS reports the annual cost of maintaining a patient on dialysis is $70,000$/year and the cost of an uncomplicated transplant is $25,000 but improves to $17,000/year when the graft is functioning well. Schwartz et al. performed a resource utilization study on 40 ABOi transplants and compared them with match ABO compatible transplants. The graft survival was similar in both the groups but, as expected, there was an increased rate of rejection in incompatible group. The average cost of an ABO-incompatible living donor kidney transplant is approximately $38,000 more than that of conventional ABO-compatible living donor kidney transplant. The major areas contributing the high cost were nursing (due to increased length of stay), plasmapheresis treatments and pharmacy (rituximab dosing). However, this was much more cost effective when compared to long term maintenance hemodialysis [103]. The high costs of induction therapy, PP, and other immunomodulatory agents can significantly increase the cost of transplantation and must be considered when evaluating the cost-effectiveness of immunomodulation. A functioning graft over time will be more cost effective than remaining on hemodialysis but this needs to be further explored in the current era with expensive novel therapeutic options.

5.2. Recommendations and alternatives

Overall, if given the option, it would be best for a recipient to have an ABO and crossmatch compatible donor where additional therapies for immunomodulation are not required and the risk of acute and chronic rejection are lower. If a patient has an incompatible living donor, encouraging them to enroll in the KPD program can maximize their chances for a compatible donor. However, if the patient is not able to find a compatible donor within a reasonable time, histocompatibility data should be evaluated to identify options for transplantation with an incompatible donor given the benefits of transplantation over continuing dialysis therapy. Post transplantation, patients should be monitored closely for acute and chronic rejection using protocol biopsies as well as infectious complications. This type of approach is being utilized by many centers and we feel this approach will lead to the best outcome for a patient with an ABOi or crossmatch incompatible donor [104, 105].

Author details

Dinesh Kannabhiran, Michelle L. Lubetzky and Darshana Dadhania

Department of Transplantation Medicine and Extracorporeal Therapy, Division of Nephrology and Hypertension, Department of Medicine, NewYork-Presbyterian Hospital- Weill Cornell Medical College, New York, NY, USA

Acknowledgement

The authors gratefully acknowledge the expert assistance of Dr. Melissa Cushing for her review of the testing protocols for ABO grouping and antibody titers and the assistance of Sue Pino for her careful review of the manuscript.

Appendix

Renal Transplantation In ABO incompatible Kidney Transplant Recipients								
Study	**n**	**Follow up Months**	**Conditioning regimen[a]**	**Target Anti-A/B Titer**	**Induction**	**Maintenance[b]**	**AR (%)**	**Survival (%)**
Takahashi et al. AJT 2004 Japan[26]	441	108 (9yrs)	ImmunoAd (n=51)→ DF-PP[a,c] (n=390) + Splenectomy (n=433)	8-16 fold ↓	Varied by center	Anti-metabolite + Tacrolimus (36%) or cyclosporine (64%)	58 (overall)	3yr: P-87 3yr: G-71 9yr: P-84 3yr: G-59
Gloor et al. Txp. 2005 USA[24]	34	24	Group1(g1)n-23: PP with IVIG (0.1g/kg)[a] + MMF+ splenectomy Group2(g2)n-11: PP with IVIG (0.1 g/kg)[a] + MMF+ rituximab(375 mg/m^2)x1	≤1:8	rATG	MMF Tacrolimus	AMR g1- 30 g2- 18	P-96 / 91 G-87 / 82
Montgomery et al. Txp. 2009 USA[25]	57	42 (median)	Group1(g1)n-14: PP with CMVIg (0.1 g/kg)[a] + splenectomy Group2(g2)n-15: PP with CMVIg (0.1 g/kg)[a] + rituximab (375 mg/m^2)x1 Group3(g3)n-28: PP with CMVIg (0.1 g/kg)[a] (all 3 groups also received tacrolimus / MMF)	≤1:16	daclizumab	MMF Tacrolimus	AMR/ACR g1-36/ 14 g2-27/ 14 g3-29/ 14	(3 groups) 3yr: P-96 3yr: G-93
Genberg et al. Txp. 2008 Sweden[7]	15	36 (median)	rituximab (375 mg/m^2)x1+ Ag-ImmunoAd[a] + MMF/Tacrolimus/steroids IVIG (0.5 g/kg) x1	<1:8	None	MMF Tacrolimus	AMR- 0 ACR- 7	P-100 G-87
Wilpert et al. NDT 2010 Germany[106]	40	39 (median)	rituximab (375 mg/m^2)x1+ Ag-ImmunoAd[a] + MMF/tacrolimus/steroids IVIG (0.5 g/kg) x1	<1:4	basiliximab	MMF Tacrolimus	AMR- 5 ACR- 28	P-98 G-100
Fuchinoue et al. Txp. 2011 Japan[107]	113	60	All – PP or DF-PP[a] + Group1(g1)n-63: splenectomy Group2 (g2)n-50: rituximab (dose varied)	<1:16	basiliximab	MMF Tacrolimus or cyclosporine	AMR/ACR g1: 16 /10 g2: 4 /4	P:100/100 G-90/100
Shirakawa et al. Clinical Txp. 2011 Japan[27]	74	>22	All- DF-PP[a] + MMF/tacrolimus/steroids+ rituximab Group1(g1)n-24: 0.5g vs. Group2(g2)n-24: 0.2g	<1:32	basiliximab	MMF Tacrolimus	AMR/ACR g1: 8 /16 g2: 6 /14	P-100/100 G-96/98

DF- Double filtration; Ag- Antigen specific; ImmunoAd- immunoadsorption; PP- Plasmapheresis; IVIG- Intravenous Immunoglobulin; MMF- Mycophenolate mofetil; rATG- rabbit anti-thymocyte globulin; CTX- cyclophosphamide; AR- Acute rejection (clinical & subclinical where reported) AMR-antibody mediated rejection; ACR- Acute cellular rejection; P- patient, G- graft;
[a]Number of treatments pre and post-transplant varied based on baseline titers; [b]Everyone received steroids; [c]Pre- transplant treatment only

Table 1. Conditioning Regimens for Facilitating Renal Transplantation In Blood Type Incompatible Kidney Transplant Recipients

Crossmatch Incompatible Kidney Transplant Recipients								
Study	**n**	**Follow Up Months**	**Conditioning regimen and Goal of Therapy**	**% Transplanted (txp/treated)**	**Induction**	**Maintenance[a]**	**AR (%)**	**Survival (%)**
Schweitzer et al. Txp. 2000 USA[1]	11 LD	13	PP / IVIG (0.5g/kg) (# varied) MMF / Tacrolimus/steroids Goal: Neg. CDC XM	73% (11/15)	OKT3	MMF + tacrolimus	36	P- 100 G- 100
Jordan et al. Txp. 2003 USA[2]	42 (26 LD, 15 DD)	>24	LD- IVIG 2gm/kg x 1 DD – IVIG 2g/kg x 4 (monthly) Goal: Neg. CDC XM	LD-92% (24/26) DD-93% (14/15)	daclizumab	MMF + tacrolimus	31	P-98 G- 89
Jordan et al. JASN 2004[3] USA	DD RTC[b] 48 IVIG vs. 50placebo	30	IVIG 2gm/kg x 4 vs. Placebo x 4 (monthly) Goal: Neg. CDC XM	IVIG-35% (17/48) Placebo -20% (10/50)	Varied by center	Varied by center	IVIG 53 placebo 10	P-100 G-75 vs. 62
Gloor et al. AJT 2003 USA[4]	14 LD	15	PP/IVIG (0.1mg/kg) x 4 rituximab(375mg/m^2) x1 Goal: Neg. CDC XM	reviewed only those transplanted	rATG splenectomy	MMF + tacrolimus	43	P-86 G-79
Stegall et al. AJT 2006 USA[5]	61 LD (3 groups)	12	<u>Group1:</u> IVIG 2g/kg x1 <u>Group2:</u> PP/IVIG (0.1mg/kg) + rituximab (375mg/m^2) <u>Group3:</u> PP/IVIG (0.1mg/kg) + rituximab (375mg/m^2) + monitoring post-txp therapy	Group 1: 36%(5/13) Group 2: 84%(27/32) Group 3: 88% (14/16)	rATG	MMF + tacrolimus	Group 1: 80 Group 2: 37 Group 3: 29	P-93 G-82
Magee et al. Txp. 2008 USA[6]	29 LD	22	PP / IVIG (10g) (# varied) Tacrolimus. / MMF Goal:Neg. CDC T-cell XM	97% (28/29) 15 w/ weak Pos XM (3-Tcell XM, 12-Bcell XM)	rituximab (n=21) rATG OR basiliximab	MMF + tacrolimus	39	P-96 G- 89
Thielke et al. Txp. 2009 USA[7]	51 LD	23	PP/IVIG (0.1g/kg)x3-4 rituximab(375mg/m^2) x 1-2 Goal: Neg. T cell Flow XM	89% (51/57) 2 with Pos.Flow XM	rATG	MMF + tacrolimus	43	P-95 G- 93
Vo et al. NEJM 2008 USA[8]	16 (10 LD, 6DD)	12	IVIG 2gm/kg x2 monthly rituximab 1g x2 Goal[c]: Neg. CDC Tcell XM at 1:2 dilution & Flow Tcell XM -MCS<250	80% (16/20)	alemtuzumab	MMF + tacrolimus	50	P-100 G-94
Vo et al, Txp. 2010 USA[9]	76 (31 LD, 45 DD)	24	IVIG 2gm/kg (day 1 &30) Rituximab 1g (day 15) Goal[c]: Neg. CDC T cell XM at 1:2 dilution & Flow Tcell XM- MCS<250	reported only those transplanted	alemtuzumab or daclizumab or rATG	MMF + tacrolimus	37	P-95 G-84

Txp-Transplantation; LD- Living donor; DD-Deceased Donor; Neg.-negative; Pos.- positive; PP-plasmapheresis; IVIG- Intravenous Immunoglobulin; OKT3-Muromonamab CD3; MMF- Mycophenolate mofetil; rATG- rabbit anti thymocyte globulin; PRA-panel reactive antibodies; AR-acute rejection; P- patient; G- graft; [a]Everyone received prednisone [b]Only RTC (randomized controlled trial); [c]These criteria for transplantation were not standard protocol but were specific for sensitized patients treated with the protocol.

Table 2. Conditioning Regimens for Facilitating Renal Transplantation and Prevention of Rejection In Crossmatch Incompatible Kidney Transplant Recipients

Prevention of Rejection in Sensitized Kidney Transplant Recipients								
Study	**n**	**Follow Up Months**	**Conditioning regimen[a]**	**% Transplanted (txp/treated)**	**Induction**	**Maintenance[b]**	**AR (%)**	**Survival (%)**
Montgomery et al. Txp. 2000 USA[10]	4 LD	6 (approx.)	PP / IVIG (0.1g/kg) (# varied)	all	daclizuma b	MMF + tacrolimus	100	P-100 G-100
Glotz et al. AJT 2002 France[11]	13 (11 DD, 2LD)	>12	IVIG (2gm/kg) q monthly x 3 Goal: 50%↓ in PRA	87% (11/13)	rATG	MMF + tacrolimus	8	P-87 G-87
Akalin et al. CJASN 2008 USA[12]	21 LD 14 DD	18 (median)	Group1:LR- IVIG 2g/kg (peri-transplant divided doses) Group2: HR- above IVIG+ PP pre/post (# varied)	all	rATG	MMF + tacrolimus	Group 1: 29 Group 2: 7	P-100/ 93 G-89/ 86
Anglicheau et al. AJT 2007 France[13]	38 DD	>12	IVIG 2gm/kg on POD 0/ 21/ 42/63	all	rATG or basilixima b	MMF + tacrolimus or cyclosporin	26	P-97 G-95
Lefaucher et al. AJT 2007 France[14]	32 (16LD, 16 DD)	30 (mean)	Pre: IVIG 2gm/kg x3 (monthly) (pre or peri-transplant)	all	rATG	MMF + tacrolimus	41	P-95 G-78
Mai et al. Txp. 2009 USA[15]	20 (5 LD, 15 DD)	36	IVIG 500mg/kg x 3 (peri-transplant)	all	rATG	MMF + tacrolimus	50	P-94 G-89
Bachler et al. AJT 2010 Switzerland[16]	37 (11 LD, 26 DD)	>12	IVIG 2gm/kg total at time of induction	all	rATG	MMF + tacrolimus	38	P-95 G-92

PP- Plasmapheresis; LD- Living donor; DD-Deceased Donor; IVIG- Intravenous Immunoglobulin; OKT3- murineAnti-CD3; MMF- Mycophenolate mofetil; rATG- rabbit anti-thymocyte globulin; AR-acute rejection; P- patient; G- graft; LR-low risk; HR – high risk;
[a]Patients were sensitized but they did not have a contraindication to transplantation; [b]Everyone received prednisone

Table 3. Conditioning Regimens for Prevention of Rejection in Sensitized Kidney Transplant Recipients

6. References

[1] Network, O.P.a.T. *www.optn.org/data.* 2012 [cited 2012.

[2] Crew, R.J. and L.E. Ratner, *ABO-incompatible kidney transplantation: current practice and the decade ahead.* Curr Opin Organ Transplant, 2010. 15(4): p. 526-30.

[3] Port, F.K., et al., *Comparison of survival probabilities for dialysis patients vs cadaveric renal transplant recipients.* JAMA, 1993. 270(11): p. 1339-43.

[4] Russell, J.D., et al., *The quality of life in renal transplantation--a prospective study.* Transplantation, 1992. 54(4): p. 656-60.

[5] Szczepiorkowski, Z.M., et al., *Guidelines on the use of therapeutic apheresis in clinical practice--evidence-based approach from the Apheresis Applications Committee of the American Society for Apheresis.* J Clin Apher, 2010. 25(3): p. 83-177.

[6] Tobian, A.A., et al., *Therapeutic plasma exchange reduces ABO titers to permit ABO-incompatible renal transplantation.* Transfusion, 2009. 49(6): p. 1248-54.

[7] Genberg, H., et al., *ABO-incompatible kidney transplantation using antigen-specific immunoadsorption and rituximab: a 3-year follow-up.* Transplantation, 2008. 85(12): p. 1745-54.

[8] Gloor, J.M. and M.D. Stegall, *ABO incompatible kidney transplantation.* Curr Opin Nephrol Hypertens, 2007. 16(6): p. 529-34.

[9] Toki, D., et al., *Impact of low-dose rituximab on splenic B cells in ABO-incompatible renal transplant recipients.* Transpl Int, 2009. 22(4): p. 447-54.

[10] Tyden, G., G. Kumlien, and I. Fehrman, *Successful ABO-incompatible kidney transplantations without splenectomy using antigen-specific immunoadsorption and rituximab.* Transplantation, 2003. 76(4): p. 730-1.

[11] Everly, M.J. and P.I. Terasaki, *The state of therapy for removal of alloantibody producing plasma cells in transplantation.* Semin Immunol, 2012. 24(2): p. 143-7.

[12] Woodle, E.S., et al., *Proteasome inhibitor therapy for antibody-mediated rejection.* Pediatr Transplant, 2011. 15(6): p. 548-56.

[13] Kazatchkine, M.D. and S.V. Kaveri, *Immunomodulation of autoimmune and inflammatory diseases with intravenous immune globulin.* N Engl J Med, 2001. 345(10): p. 747-55.

[14] Kahwaji, J., A.A. Vo, and S.C. Jordan, *ABO blood group incompatibility: a diminishing barrier to successful kidney transplantation?* Expert Rev Clin Immunol, 2010. 6(6): p. 893-900.

[15] Stegall, M.D., P.G. Dean, and J. Gloor, *Mechanisms of alloantibody production in sensitized renal allograft recipients.* Am J Transplant, 2009. 9(5): p. 998-1005.

[16] Norman, D.J., et al., *Use of A(2) kidneys for B and O kidney transplant recipients: report of a series of patients transplanted at a single center spanning a decade.* Transplant Proc, 2001. 33(7-8): p. 3327-30.

[17] Nelson, P.W., et al., *Ten-year experience in transplantation of A2 kidneys into B and O recipients.* Transplantation, 1998. 65(2): p. 256-60.

[18] Kobayashi, T. and K. Saito, *A series of surveys on assay for anti-A/B antibody by Japanese ABO-incompatible Transplantation Committee.* Xenotransplantation, 2006. 13(2): p. 136-40.

[19] Hume, D.M., et al., *Experiences with renal homotransplantation in the human: report of nine cases.* J Clin Invest, 1955. 34(2): p. 327-82.

[20] Starzl, T.E., et al., *Renal Homografts in Patients with Major Donor-Recipient Blood Group Incompatibilities.* Surgery, 1964. 55: p. 195-200.

[21] Cook, D.J., B. Graver, and P.I. Terasaki, *ABO incompatibility in cadaver donor kidney allografts.* Transplant Proc, 1987. 19(6): p. 4549-52.

[22] Alexandre, G.P., et al., *Present experiences in a series of 26 ABO-incompatible living donor renal allografts.* Transplant Proc, 1987. 19(6): p. 4538-42.

[23] Squifflet, J.P., et al., *Lessons learned from ABO-incompatible living donor kidney transplantation: 20 years later.* Exp Clin Transplant, 2004. 2(1): p. 208-13.

[24] Gloor, J.M., et al., *A Comparison of splenectomy versus intensive posttransplant antidonor blood group antibody monitoring without splenectomy in ABO-incompatible kidney transplantation.* Transplantation, 2005. 80(11): p. 1572-7.

[25] Montgomery, R.A., et al., *ABO incompatible renal transplantation: a paradigm ready for broad implementation.* Transplantation, 2009. 87(8): p. 1246-55.

[26] Takahashi, K., et al., *Excellent long-term outcome of ABO-incompatible living donor kidney transplantation in Japan.* Am J Transplant, 2004. 4(7): p. 1089-96.

[27] Shirakawa, H., et al., *The low dose of rituximab in ABO-incompatible kidney transplantation without a splenectomy: a single-center experience.* Clin Transplant, 2011. 25(6): p. 878-84.

[28] Toki, D., et al., *Acute antibody-mediated rejection in living ABO-incompatible kidney transplantation: long-term impact and risk factors.* Am J Transplant, 2009. 9(3): p. 567-77.

[29] Shimmura, H., et al., *Lack of correlation between results of ABO-incompatible living kidney transplantation and anti-ABO blood type antibody titers under our current immunosuppression.* Transplantation, 2005. 80(7): p. 985-8.

[30] Tobian, A.A., et al., *ABO antibody titer and risk of antibody-mediated rejection in ABO-incompatible renal transplantation.* Am J Transplant, 2010. 10(5): p. 1247-53.

[31] Haas, M., et al., *C4d and C3d staining in biopsies of ABO- and HLA-incompatible renal allografts: correlation with histologic findings.* Am J Transplant, 2006. 6(8): p. 1829-40.

[32] Ichimaru, N. and S. Takahara, *Japan's experience with living-donor kidney transplantation across ABO barriers.* Nat Clin Pract Nephrol, 2008. 4(12): p. 682-92.

[33] Futagawa, Y. and P.I. Terasaki, *ABO incompatible kidney transplantation - an analysis of UNOS Registry data.* Clin Transplant, 2006. 20(1): p. 122-6.

[34] Haas, M., et al., *C4d deposition without rejection correlates with reduced early scarring in ABO-incompatible renal allografts.* J Am Soc Nephrol, 2009. 20(1): p. 197-204.

[35] Iwasaki, K., et al., *Comparative study on signal transduction in endothelial cells after anti-a/b and human leukocyte antigen antibody reaction: implication of accommodation.* Transplantation. 93(4): p. 390-7.

[36] Chen Song, S., et al., *Complement inhibition enables renal allograft accommodation and long-term engraftment in presensitized nonhuman primates.* Am J Transplant. 11(10): p. 2057-66.

[37] Varga, Z., et al., *Tubular and endothelial chimerism in renal allografts using fluorescence and chromogenic in situ hybridization (FISH, CISH) technology.* Pathol Int. 62(4): p. 254-63.

[38] Dehoux, J.P. and P. Gianello, *Accommodation and antibodies.* Transpl Immunol, 2009. 21(2): p. 106-10.

[39] Tanabe, T., et al., *Decrease of blood type antigenicity over the long-term after ABO-incompatible kidney transplantation.* Transpl Immunol. 25(1): p. 1-6.

[40] Kobayashi, T., et al., *Removal of blood group A/B antigen in organs by ex vivo and in vivo administration of endo-beta-galactosidase (ABase) for ABO-incompatible transplantation.* Transpl Immunol, 2009. 20(3): p. 132-8.

[41] Hasegawa, Y., et al., *Neutralization of blood group A-antigen by a novel anti-A antibody: overcoming ABO-incompatible solid-organ transplantation.* Transplantation, 2008. 85(3): p. 378-85.

[42] Barama, A., et al., *Effect of recipient sensitization (peak PRA) on graft outcome in haploidentical living related kidney transplants.* Clin Transplant, 2000. 14(3): p. 212-7.

[43] Bray, R.A., et al., *Evolution of HLA antibody detection: technology emulating biology.* Immunol Res, 2004. 29(1-3): p. 41-54.

[44] Cecka, J.M., *Calculated PRA (CPRA): the new measure of sensitization for transplant candidates.* Am J Transplant. 10(1): p. 26-9.

[45] Gebel, H.M., R.A. Bray, and P. Nickerson, *Pre-transplant assessment of donor-reactive, HLA-specific antibodies in renal transplantation: contraindication vs. risk.* Am J Transplant, 2003. 3(12): p. 1488-500.

[46] Wen, R., et al., *Biomarkers in transplantation: Prospective, blinded measurement of predictive value for the flow cytometry crossmatch after negative antiglobulin crossmatch in kidney transplantation.* Kidney Int, 2006. 70(8): p. 1474-81.

[47] O'Rourke, R.W., et al., *Flow cytometry crossmatching as a predictor of acute rejection in sensitized recipients of cadaveric renal transplants.* Clin Transplant, 2000. 14(2): p. 167-73.

[48] Akalin, E., et al., *Intravenous immunoglobulin and thymoglobulin facilitate kidney transplantation in complement-dependent cytotoxicity B-cell and flow cytometry T- or B-cell crossmatch-positive patients.* Transplantation, 2003. 76(10): p. 1444-7.

[49] Tait, B.D., *Solid phase assays for HLA antibody detection in clinical transplantation.* Curr Opin Immunol, 2009. 21(5): p. 573-7.

[50] Cecka, J.M., *Current methodologies for detecting sensitization to HLA antigens.* Curr Opin Organ Transplant. 16(4): p. 398-403.

[51] Akalin, E., et al., *Addition of plasmapheresis decreases the incidence of acute antibody-mediated rejection in sensitized patients with strong donor-specific antibodies.* Clin J Am Soc Nephrol, 2008. 3(4): p. 1160-7.

[52] Gloor, J.M., et al., *Baseline donor-specific antibody levels and outcomes in positive crossmatch kidney transplantation.* Am J Transplant, 2010. 10(3): p. 582-9.

[53] Lefaucheur, C., et al., *Preexisting donor-specific HLA antibodies predict outcome in kidney transplantation.* J Am Soc Nephrol, 2010. 21(8): p. 1398-406.

[54] Salvalaggio, P.R., et al., *Crossmatch testing in kidney transplantation: patterns of practice and associations with rejection and graft survival.* Saudi J Kidney Dis Transpl, 2009. 20(4): p. 577-89.

[55] Tait, B.D., et al., *Review article: Luminex technology for HLA antibody detection in organ transplantation.* Nephrology (Carlton), 2009. 14(2): p. 247-54.

[56] Xavier, P., et al., *XM-ONE detection of endothelium cell antibodies identifies a subgroup of HLA-antibody negative patients undergoing acute rejection.* Transplant Proc. 43(1): p. 91-4.

[57] Lobashevsky, A., et al., *Subtypes of immunoglobulin (Ig)-G antibodies against donor class II HLA and cross-match results in three kidney transplant candidates.* Transpl Immunol. 23(1-2): p. 81-5.

[58] Patel, R. and P.I. Terasaki, *Significance of the positive crossmatch test in kidney transplantation.* N Engl J Med, 1969. 280(14): p. 735-9.

[59] Jordan, S.C., et al., *Evaluation of intravenous immunoglobulin as an agent to lower allosensitization and improve transplantation in highly sensitized adult patients with end-stage renal disease: report of the NIH IG02 trial.* J Am Soc Nephrol, 2004. 15(12): p. 3256-62.

[60] Jordan, S.C., et al., *Intravenous immune globulin treatment inhibits crossmatch positivity and allows for successful transplantation of incompatible organs in living-donor and cadaver recipients.* Transplantation, 2003. 76(4): p. 631-6.

[61] Magee, C.C., et al., *Renal transplantation in patients with positive lymphocytotoxicity crossmatches: one center's experience.* Transplantation, 2008. 86(1): p. 96-103.

[62] Thielke, J.J., et al., *Living donor kidney transplantation across positive crossmatch: the University of Illinois at Chicago experience.* Transplantation, 2009. 87(2): p. 268-73.

[63] Gloor, J.M., et al., *Overcoming a positive crossmatch in living-donor kidney transplantation.* Am J Transplant, 2003. 3(8): p. 1017-23.

[64] Vo, A.A., et al., *Rituximab and intravenous immune globulin for desensitization during renal transplantation.* N Engl J Med, 2008. 359(3): p. 242-51.

[65] Vo, A.A., et al., *Use of intravenous immune globulin and rituximab for desensitization of highly HLA-sensitized patients awaiting kidney transplantation.* Transplantation, 2010. 89(9): p. 1095-102.

[66] Stegall, M.D., et al., *A comparison of plasmapheresis versus high-dose IVIG desensitization in renal allograft recipients with high levels of donor specific alloantibody.* Am J Transplant, 2006. 6(2): p. 346-51.

[67] Schweitzer, E.J., et al., *A high panel-reactive antibody rescue protocol for cross-match-positive live donor kidney transplants.* Transplantation, 2000. 70(10): p. 1531-6.

[68] Montgomery, R.A. and A.A. Zachary, *Transplanting patients with a positive donor-specific crossmatch: a single center's perspective.* Pediatr Transplant, 2004. 8(6): p. 535-42.

[69] Haririan, A., et al., *Positive cross-match living donor kidney transplantation: longer-term outcomes.* Am J Transplant, 2009. 9(3): p. 536-42.

[70] Glotz, D., et al., *Desensitization and subsequent kidney transplantation of patients using intravenous immunoglobulins (IVIg).* Am J Transplant, 2002. 2(8): p. 758-60.

[71] Jordan, S.C., et al., *Posttransplant therapy using high-dose human immunoglobulin (intravenous gammaglobulin) to control acute humoral rejection in renal and cardiac allograft recipients and potential mechanism of action.* Transplantation, 1998. 66(6): p. 800-5.

[72] Akalin, E. and J.S. Bromberg, *Intravenous immunoglobulin induction treatment in flow cytometry cross-match-positive kidney transplant recipients.* Hum Immunol, 2005. 66(4): p. 359-63.

[73] Anglicheau, D., et al., *Posttransplant prophylactic intravenous immunoglobulin in kidney transplant patients at high immunological risk: a pilot study.* Am J Transplant, 2007. 7(5): p. 1185-92.

[74] Lefaucheur, C., et al., *Determinants of poor graft outcome in patients with antibody-mediated acute rejection.* Am J Transplant, 2007. 7(4): p. 832-41.

[75] Bachler, K., et al., *Efficacy of induction therapy with ATG and intravenous immunoglobulins in patients with low-level donor-specific HLA-antibodies.* Am J Transplant, 2010. 10(5): p. 1254-62.

[76] Mai, M.L., et al., *Excellent renal allograft survival in donor-specific antibody positive transplant patients-role of intravenous immunoglobulin and rabbit antithymocyte globulin.* Transplantation, 2009. 87(2): p. 227-32.

[77] Vo, A.A., et al., *Analysis of subcutaneous (SQ) alemtuzumab induction therapy in highly sensitized patients desensitized with IVIG and rituximab.* Am J Transplant, 2008. 8(1): p. 144-9.

[78] Dadhania, D.S., V. Wang, K. Friedlander, R. Menon, A. Serur, D. Aull, M. Kapur, S. Fotino, M. Suthanthiran, M., *Rituximab Therapy Decreases Acute Rejection Rates Among Sensitized Renal Allograft Recipients.* Transplantation, 2008. 86(2S): p. 151.

[79] Meier-Kriesche, H.U., et al., *Immunosuppression: evolution in practice and trends, 1994-2004.* Am J Transplant, 2006. 6(5 Pt 2): p. 1111-31.
[80] Marfu K. Ling M, B.Y., Calder B, Ye B, Hayde N, Greenstein S, Chapochnick-Friedman J, Glicklich D, de Boccardo G, Kinkhabwala M, Akalin E, *Lack of effect in desensitization with intravenous immunoglobulin and rituximab in highly-sensitized patients.* Transplantation, 2012. In Press.
[81] Newell, K.A., et al., *Identification of a B cell signature associated with renal transplant tolerance in humans.* J Clin Invest, 2010. 120(6): p. 1836-47.
[82] Montgomery, R.A., et al., *Desensitization in HLA-incompatible kidney recipients and survival.* N Engl J Med, 2011. 365(4): p. 318-26.
[83] Gloor, J., et al., *The spectrum of antibody-mediated renal allograft injury: implications for treatment.* Am J Transplant, 2008. 8(7): p. 1367-73.
[84] Rush, D., *Protocol transplant biopsies: an underutilized tool in kidney transplantation.* Clin J Am Soc Nephrol, 2006. 1(1): p. 138-43.
[85] Wilkinson, A., *Protocol transplant biopsies: are they really needed?* Clin J Am Soc Nephrol, 2006. 1(1): p. 130-7.
[86] Issa, N., et al., *Transplant glomerulopathy: risk and prognosis related to anti-human leukocyte antigen class II antibody levels.* Transplantation, 2008. 86(5): p. 681-5.
[87] Wavamunno, M.D., et al., *Transplant glomerulopathy: ultrastructural abnormalities occur early in longitudinal analysis of protocol biopsies.* Am J Transplant, 2007. 7(12): p. 2757-68.
[88] Gloor, J.M., et al., *Transplant glomerulopathy: subclinical incidence and association with alloantibody.* Am J Transplant, 2007. 7(9): p. 2124-32.
[89] Terasaki, P.I. and M. Ozawa, *Predictive value of HLA antibodies and serum creatinine in chronic rejection: results of a 2-year prospective trial.* Transplantation, 2005. 80(9): p. 1194-7.
[90] Terasaki, P.I., M. Ozawa, and R. Castro, *Four-year follow-up of a prospective trial of HLA and MICA antibodies on kidney graft survival.* Am J Transplant, 2007. 7(2): p. 408-15.
[91] Segev, D.L., et al., *Kidney paired donation and optimizing the use of live donor organs.* JAMA, 2005. 293(15): p. 1883-90.
[92] Everly, J.J., et al., *Proteasome inhibition for antibody-mediated rejection.* Curr Opin Organ Transplant, 2009. 14(6): p. 662-6.
[93] Trivedi, H.L., et al., *Abrogation of anti-HLA antibodies via proteasome inhibition.* Transplantation, 2009. 87(10): p. 1555-61.
[94] Everly, M.J., et al., *Protective immunity remains intact after antibody removal by means of proteasome inhibition.* Transplantation, 2010. 90(12): p. 1493-8.
[95] Walsh, R.C., et al., *Early and late acute antibody-mediated rejection differ immunologically and in response to proteasome inhibition.* Transplantation, 2011. 91(11): p. 1218-26.
[96] Walsh, R.C., et al., *Proteasome inhibitor-based primary therapy for antibody-mediated renal allograft rejection.* Transplantation, 2010. 89(3): p. 277-84.
[97] Raghavan, R., et al., *Bortezomib in kidney transplant desensitization: a case report.* Clin Transpl, 2009: p. 339-42.
[98] Wahrmann, M., et al., *Effect of the proteasome inhibitor bortezomib on humoral immunity in two presensitized renal transplant candidates.* Transplantation, 2010. 89(11): p. 1385-90.

[99] Raghavaiah SR, D.T., Burns JM, Gloor JM, Gandi MJ, Winters JL, Groettum CM, Dean PG, Stegall MD, *Depletion of alloantibody-secreting plasma cells by proteasome inhibition improves desensitizaiton [Abstract].* American Journal of Transplantation, 2010. 10(supl4): p. 44.

[100] Idica, A., et al., *Elimination of post-transplant donor-specific HLA antibodies with bortezomib.* Clin Transpl, 2008: p. 229-39.

[101] Risitano, A.M., et al., *Complement fraction 3 binding on erythrocytes as additional mechanism of disease in paroxysmal nocturnal hemoglobinuria patients treated by eculizumab.* Blood, 2009. 113(17): p. 4094-100.

[102] Stegall, M.D., Diwan T, Cornell DL, Burns J, Patrick DG, Gloor MJ, *Terminal completment inhibition deceases early acute humoral rejection in sensitized renal transplant recipients.* Am J Transplant, 2010. 10(suppl4): p. 39.

[103] Schwartz, J., et al., *Complications, resource utilization, and cost of ABO-incompatible living donor kidney transplantation.* Transplantation, 2006. 82(2): p. 155-63.

[104] Montgomery, R.A., *Renal transplantation across HLA and ABO antibody barriers: integrating paired donation into desensitization protocols.* Am J Transplant. 10(3): p. 449-57.

[105] Doxiadis, II, *Compatibility and kidney transplantation: the way to go.* Front Immunol. 3: p. 111.

[106] Wilpert, J., et al., *Long-term outcome of ABO-incompatible living donor kidney transplantation based on antigen-specific desensitization. An observational comparative analysis.* Nephrol Dial Transplant, 2010. 25(11): p. 3778-86.

[107] Fuchinoue, S., et al., *The 5-year outcome of ABO-incompatible kidney transplantation with rituximab induction.* Transplantation. 91(8): p. 853-7.

[108] Montgomery, R.A., et al., *Plasmapheresis and intravenous immune globulin provides effective rescue therapy for refractory humoral rejection and allows kidneys to be successfully transplanted into cross-match-positive recipients.* Transplantation, 2000. 70(6): p. 887-895.

Chapter 7

Modern Immunosuppression Regimens in Kidney Transplantation

Cheguevara Afaneh, Meredith J. Aull and Sandip Kapur

Additional information is available at the end of the chapter

http://dx.doi.org/10.5772/54092

1. Introduction

1.1. Historical Background of Induction Therapy

The initial results of kidney transplantation were significantly affected by a high rate of acute rejection as well as significant perioperative morbidity. Historically, the armamentarium of the transplant physician consisted of glucocorticoids and azathioprine. Significant improvements in the science and understanding of kidney transplantation immunology have lead to the development of induction therapy agents. Early induction therapy agents possessed little specificity and delivered a broad spectrum of effects; however, their potent ability to prevent early acute rejection episodes led to their widespread use [1].

The extensive use of these formulations exposed their flaws. The cross-reactivity with hematopoietic cells revealed dose-limiting side effects including thrombocytopenia, anemia, and neutropenia [2, 3]. Moreover, the lack of standardized preparation led to variations in dosing. In addition, these formulations had significant antigenic properties as a result of using horse or rabbit based formulations, which lead to significant side effects, such as serum sickness, cytokine release syndrome, or even anaphylaxis [4-6].

The development of specific, monoclonal antibodies by Kohler and Milstein circumvented many of the drawbacks of polyclonal formulations, including lack of specificity and variability in preparation [7]. Muromonab, or OKT3, was the first monoclonal antibody prepared from mouse specific for cluster of differentiation 3 (CD3) [8]. OKT3 was effective at specifically depleting T cells from the circulation, and became widely used as a valuable tool to combat acute rejection episodes [9, 10]. Nevertheless, these monoclonal formulations still maintained some of the similar side effect profile of the polyclonal formulations, including an antigenic response to the protein or cytokine release syndrome, which lead to limited dosing in some patients [11].

The 1980's marked an important era in transplantation with new advances in genetic engineering. Monoclonal antibodies became more sophisticated, targeting specific T cell populations and allowing blockade of T cell activation, such as the interleukin 2 receptor (IL-2R) or CD25 [12]. Moreover, the ability to avoid antigenic proteins by encoding genetic sequences of DNA binding sites of animal proteins onto human antibodies led to the development of chimeric monoclonal antibodies [13-15]. Using these techniques, soluble fusion proteins can be formed by merging nonantibody receptors with the Fc portion of antibodies.

1.2. Antibodies

Understanding the structure and function of antibodies is critical to understanding the efficacy of antibody induction therapy. Antibodies are composed of two identical heavy chains (either μ, γ, α, ε, or δ) and two identical light chains (either κ or λ). The heavy and light chain portions create two identical antigen binding sites (Fab fragment) which are held together by the common region, termed the Fc portion [16]. The type of heavy chain differentiates the immunoglobulin type as IgM, IgG, IgA, IgE, and IgD. In clinical transplantation, the IgG molecule is typically utilized, as it's readily produced and structurally feasible to manipulate (Fig. 1).

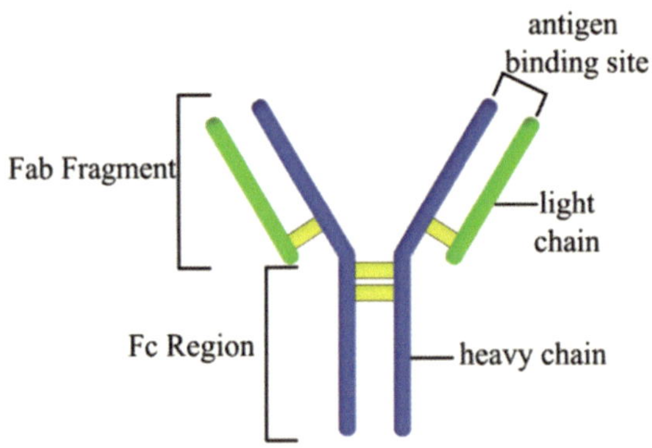

Figure 1. Basic antibody structure. Depicted is a standard IgG molecule. The heavy chains are colored in blue, while the light chains are colored in green. The yellow lines signify the disulfide bonds.

Antibodies are present on the surface of B cells. Upon secretion into the serum, antibodies are able to neutralize circulating antigens. Antibodies maintain their effector functions irrespective of species. Antibodies are capable of various functions, including mimicking activating ligands of receptors and serving as receptor inhibitors by blocking the ligand binding site [17, 18]. In some instances, antibody binding can lead to both activation and inhibition by inducing surface molecule internalization, whereby the molecule is removed from the surface of the cell [19]. This results in a negligible net effect. A major limitation of antibody use is the inability to directly bind intracellular molecules.

Antibodies have the ability to deplete target cells through two basic mechanisms. First, antibodies can activate the complement system resulting in complement-mediated lysis of target cells. Second, certain cells with Fc region receptors have the ability to phagocytose cells covered with antibodies through a mechanism termed antibody-dependent cellular cytotoxicity (ADCC) (Fig.2). The efficacy with which this occurs depends upon the Fab fragment and the Fc region [20]. It is important to note that cells which have significantly matured, or memory cells, are somewhat resistant to antibody-dependent depletion mechanisms, possibly due to increased expression of anti-apoptotic or complement regulatory genes [21].

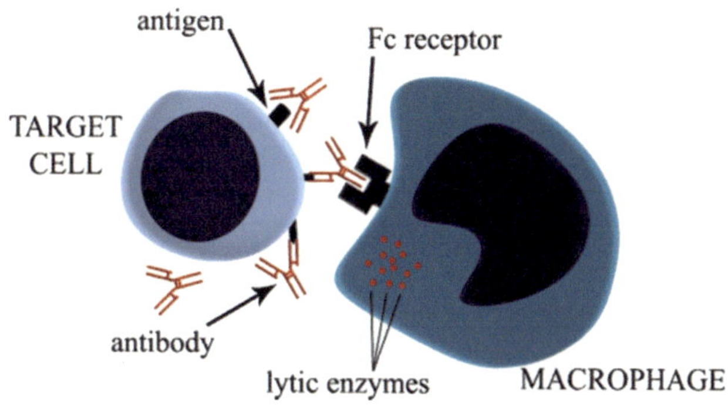

Figure 2. Antibody-dependent cellular cytotoxicity (ADCC). The Fc receptor on the macrophage is used to bind the constant Fc portion of antibodies to facilitate engulfment of cells coated with antibodies.

1.3. Classifying induction therapy agents

Induction therapy agents can be classified into two groups: depleting agents and non-depleting agents (Table 1). This distinction is based on the ability to target specific antigens or cells, leading to a decrease in the total expression or cell count. Most depleting agents are relatively potent with potential for toxicity with prolonged administration, while non-depleting agents are generally well-tolerated. In addition, the use of induction therapy agents has decreased the rates of acute rejection in the first 6 months compared to no induction therapy [22]. Although these short-term benefits appear promising, long-term outcomes, including patient and graft survival rates, have not been shown to be altered by the use of induction therapy, possibly the effect of long-term maintenance immunosuppressive therapy or even patient co-morbidities.

The overall success of a kidney transplant is contingent on both surgical technique and potent immunosuppressive medications. Although induction therapy has not affected surgical morbidity, the rate of allograft thrombosis has been shown to be reduced in children with the use of induction agents [23, 24]. However, not all medications used are FDA-approved for induction therapy. Additionally, these medications are not without risks, including infectious complications and the development of post-transplant lymphoproliferative disorder (PTLD), which has been well-described with the use of OKT3 and maintenance immunosuppression [25, 26]. Because of the effects of depleting agents on T cells, appropriate infectious prophylaxis should be instituted for all transplant recipients.

In 1995 induction therapy was used in less than half of all kidney transplants in the United States, while 10 years later, approximately 70% of all kidney transplant recipients received

Agent	Clonality	Targets	Dosing	Halflife	Duration of effects	Cytokine Release Syndrome?
rATG[1]	Polyclonal	Various immune targets, especially T cells	Multiple doses (POD[2]#0-4)	29.8-37.7 days	Months to years	Yes
Basiliximab	Monoclonal	CD25 (predominantly activated T cells)	2 doses (POD[2]#0 & 4)	7.2 days	Weeks	No
Daclizumab	Monoclonal	CD25 (predominantly activated T cells)	Multiple doses (POD[2]#0, then every 2 weeks)	20 days	Weeks	No
Alemtuzumab	Monoclonal	CD52 (naïve T cells, some B cells, and monocytes)	Typically 1 dose (POD[2]#0)	12 days	Months to years	Yes (less than rATG[1])

[1]rabbit Antithymocyte globulin, [2]post operative day

Table 1. Pharmacological Comparison of Induction Therapy

induction therapy [27]. Given the availability of various potent, specific induction agents in modern transplantation, the clinical dilemma lies in selecting the most appropriate agent for a given patient, taking into account co-morbidities, donor quality, immunological status, and planned immunosuppression maintenance therapy.

2. Induction therapy agents

2.1. Depleting agents

2.1.1. Rabbit Antithymocyte globulin (rATG)

2.1.1.1. Mechanism of Action

Rabbit antithymocyte globulin (rATG) is a polyclonal heterologous antibody produced from immunizing rabbits with human thymocytes, which serve as the immunogens (Fig. 3) [28]. The rabbit serum is then gathered and purified to remove antibodies with potentially detrimental effects and only the IgG isotypes are collected. Despite these purification techniques, it is possible that the majority of antibodies in these formulations serve no therapeutic purpose [29, 30]. When administered to humans, the rATG antibody formulations bind all antigens that the rabbits were exposed to during the immunization process.

rATG binds multiple T cell surface antigens and receptors involved in antigen recognition, adhesion and costimulation, including CD2, CD3, CD4, CD5, CD8, CD28, CD45, and CD40L. In addition, rATG may also bind non-T cell molecules such as CD16, CD20, CD56, and the major histocompatibility molecules (class I and II) [28-30]. The depleting effect of rATG occurs within 24 hours of administration and can persist with a prolonged serum half-life of several weeks [31, 32]. The effects of lymphocyte depletion are persists for years following administration, as evidenced by selectively low $CD4^+$ T cell counts [33, 34].

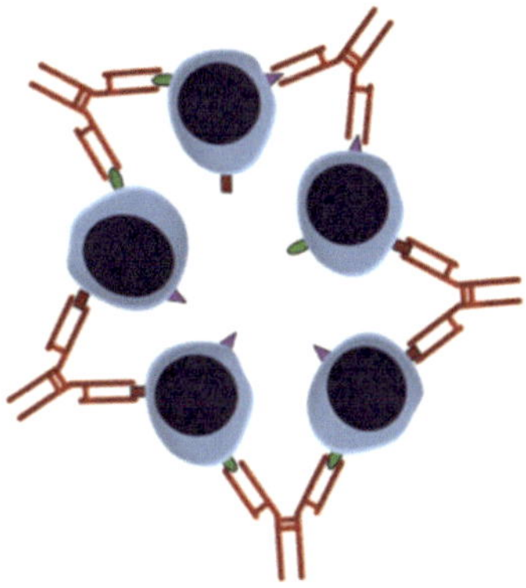

Figure 3. Polyclonal antibodies. Polyclonal antibodies are non-specific and bind multiple antigens as shown in the figure.

2.1.1.2. Clinical applications

rATG has been approved for use as an induction agent and for the treatment of acute rejection in Europe since 1984 [35]. However, in the United States, it is only indicated for the treatment of acute rejection. Nevertheless, it is routinely administered as induction therapy in many centers in the United States. Although early studies demonstrated an increased infectious risk and post-transplant malignancy when administered in conjunction with cyclosporine [36], improvements in infectious prophylaxis and lower doses have significantly alleviated these risks.

rATG administration improves early outcomes in kidney transplantation. Although the exact mechanism leading to this is unclear, rATG may minimize ischemia-reperfusion injury and potentially prevent the development of delayed graft function, which has been associated with poorer outcomes [37]. rATG has been used in patients at higher risk of developing delayed graft function, including recipients of donation after cardiac death donors, and recipients of extended criteria donors [38-40]. It is also administered in patients at higher immunologic risk, such as retransplants. Finally, it may help minimize the need for maintenance immunosuppression therapy facilitating early corticosteroid withdrawal [40, 41].

2.1.1.3. Adverse effects

Patients treated with rATG may experience a variety of side effects. It has been associated with a syndrome called cytokine release syndrome (Fig. 4), which is common to many polyclonal antibody formulations. Patients may experience mild flu-like symptoms, such as fever, chills, nausea, urticaria, rash, and headache [32]. This occurs as a result of increased production of tumor necrosis factor-α, IL-1, and IL-6 [28, 32, 42]. Premedication with corticosteroids, antipyretics, and antihistamines can prevent or treat these flu-like symptoms. In some cases, patients may develop more severe shock-like reactions, such as dyspnea, severe hypotension, pulmonary edema, or even anaphylaxis. Although patients frequently experience the mild flu-like symptoms and not the more severe reactions, recipient co-morbid conditions, such as cardiac or pulmonary disease, should be considered when selecting rATG as an induction agent. Serum sickness has also been associated with rATG administration in up to 7-10% of patients [43, 44].

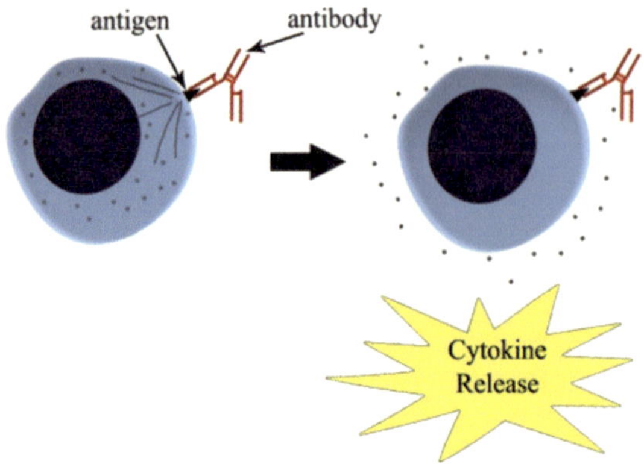

Figure 4. Antibody activation and cytokine release. Antibodies can bind antigens resulting in activation of the cell and cytokine release as illustrated in the figure.

Hematological adverse events may occur, including leucopenia and thrombocytopenia. It is important to monitor white blood cell, lymphocyte, and platelet counts daily. Effectively, these adverse events may lead to an increase in infectious complications, including cytomegalovirus (CMV), herpes simplex virus, Epstein-Barr virus (EBV), and varicella [45, 46].

2.1.2. *Alemtuzumab*

2.1.2.1. Mechanism of action

Alemtuzumab, or Campath-1H, is a monoclonal antibody to rat antihuman CD52 (Fig. 5). It is an IgG1 humanized molecule [47]. CD52 is present in high abundance on most lymphocytes, including T cell, B cells, and monocytes, but not hematopoietic precursors [48]. It effectively depletes T cells, and some B cells and monocytes in the circulation as well as the allograft [49].

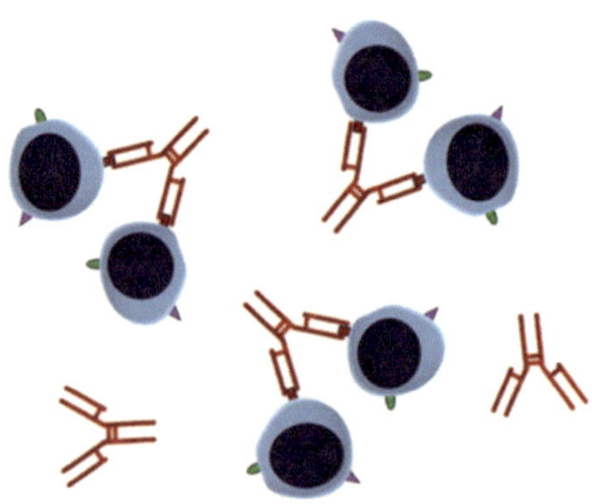

Figure 5. Monoclonal antibodies. Monoclonal antibodies are specific and bind a single antigen as shown in the figure.

2.1.2.2. Clinical applications

Alemtuzumab has not been approved for use as an induction agent; however, this is a common off-label use. At this time, it is only approved to treat lymphogenous malignancies.

As an off-label induction agent, it's been used with various immunosuppression regimens, including steroid-sparing regimens. Effectively, it depletes lymphocytes at the time of transplantation and last for several months to a year before the immune system is reconstituted [50]. Alemtuzumab is given at a dose of 30 mg or 0.3 mg/kg through a peripheral line over 3 hours. Sometimes 2 doses are given, although T cells are expectedly removed within 1 hour of initial administration [21, 49].

Alemtuzumab depletes all T cell subsets, but has a predilection for more naïve T cells [21]. Memory T cell subsets may not be depleted with this therapy, but these cell types are especially susceptible to calcineurin inhibitors. Because of the prompt and intense depletion, alemtuzumab is especially appealing to use in patients with delayed graft function, as calcineurin inhibitor therapy can be withheld to avoid concomitant calcineurin-induced renal insults.

Early studies of alemtuzumab demonstrated its efficacy as a treatment therapy for acute rejection; however, it was associated with significant infectious morbidity and mortality [47]. Patients were significantly over-immunosuppressed, especially on a triple maintenance therapy. More recent literature has been small studies or anecdotal data [51-53]. Because its efficacy is greatest against naïve T cells, its use in sensitized patients may-be limited.

In a recent study, alemtuzumab was prospectively compared to basiliximab and rATG as an induction agent in patients on a steroid-sparing immunosuppressive regimen [54]. Alemtuzumab demonstrated lower short-term rates of acute rejection compared to basiliximab in patients at low-risk of developing acute rejection. At 3-years, however, the rates of acute rejection were no different between alemtuzumab and rATG. Patients receiving alemtuzumab did not experience an increased incidence of adverse events.

2.1.2.3. Adverse effects

Similar to rATG, alemtuzumab has been associated with cytokine release syndrome, but to a lesser extent. With adequate premedication with methylprednisolone, acetaminophen, and diphenhydramine, the cytokine release is blunted. Rash is one of the most common manifestations, while anaphylaxis and hypotension have been reported. It has been linked to the development of autoimmune thyroiditis in patients treated with alemtuzumab for multiple sclerosis [55]. This has also been reported in a renal transplant recipient treated with alemtuzumab [56].

2.2. Non-depleting agents

2.2.1. Basiliximab

2.2.1.1. Mechanism of action

Basiliximab is a chimeric mouse-human monoclonal IgG1 antibody to CD25, the α-subunit of the IL-2 receptor. Basiliximab inhibition of IL-2 binding occurs through steric hindrance (Fig. 6). Effectively, basiliximab causes prevention of early T cell activation, as opposed to T cell depletion [50].

2.2.1.2. Clinical applications

Basiliximab targets naïve T cells, limiting its role to induction therapy. The first dose is administered on the day of transplant with the final dose administered on postoperative day 4 (20 mg per dose) via a peripheral line. Its use has been associated with decreased rates of acute cellular rejection compared to no formal induction agent on either triple or double drug immunosuppression regimens [57, 58]. Additional studies comparing basiliximab induction to polyclonal antibody depleting induction agents in the setting of triple maintenance immunosuppression regimens have shown similar outcomes with respect to acute rejection rates and delayed graft function [59, 60]. Basiliximab induction therapy has been successfully used in steroid avoidance immunosuppression regimens [61]. In the setting of monotherapy or calcineurin inhibitor free regimens; however, basiliximab has not been shown to be effective in preventing early immunologic events [62, 63]. In cases of excellent human leukocyte antigen (HLA)-matching (i.e. 2-haplotype matches), it's been used as an effective induction agent with steroid avoidance immunosuppressive regimens [61]. Given the relatively mild side effect profile, basiliximab is well-tolerated in all patients, even those with significant cardiac or pulmonary co-morbidities.

2.2.1.3. Adverse effects

The side effect profile of basiliximab is relatively mild [57, 58]. Because of the lack of T cell activation or stimulation, cytokine release syndrome does not occur. The most serious adverse event is hypersensitivity, which is rare (<1%) [50]. There is no increased risk of infectious complications or PTLD compared to no induction therapy [64].

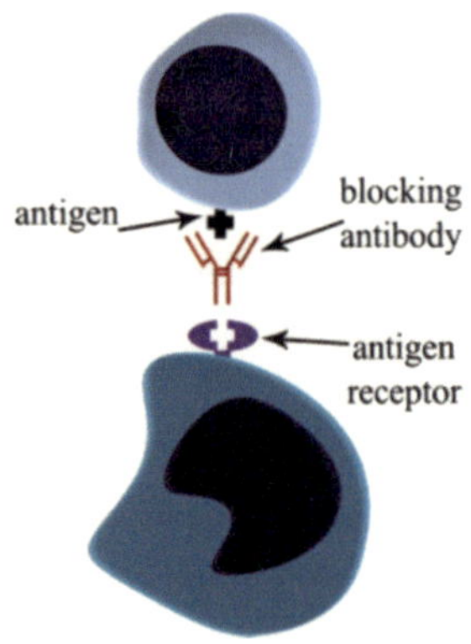

Figure 6. Antibody blockade. In this figure the antibody functions by blocking the antigen from binding to the receptor.

2.2.2. Daclizumab

2.2.2.1. Mechanism of Action

Daclizumab, like basiliximab, is a CD25 antagonist; however, it is a humanized IgG1 antibody. The CD25 molecule was the first humanized monoclonal antibody to be successfully targeted in the field of transplantation [65]. The mechanism of action of daclizumab essentially duplicates that of basiliximab.

2.2.2.2. *Clinical applications*

Daclizumab has been shown to decrease the incidence of acute cellular rejection when administered as an induction agent [66, 67]. Given the favorable side effect profile, it is well tolerated, irrespective of co-morbid conditions. The main disadvantage of daclizumab, as compared to basiliximab, is that it is more costly and requires repeated administrations [50]. Given the low demand for the medication, it has been discontinued by the manufacturer.

2.2.2.3. *Adverse effects*

The generally favorable side effect profile resembles that of basiliximab. Cytokine release is not typically associated with this agent [66, 67]. Like basiliximab, the risk of infectious complications or PTLD is not significantly increased with use [64].

3. Desensitizing agents

3.1. Rituximab

3.1.1. *Mechanism*

Rituximab is a monoclonal chimeric antibody to the CD20 molecule. CD20 is a glycoprotein on the cell surface of circulating, mature B cells. Rituximab effectively depletes CD20+ cells from the circulation by inducing apoptosis [68]. These cells are precursors to antibody-producing plasma cells, and their role in transplantation is only partially characterized. They may play a role in acute rejection, as B cells can act as antigen presenting cells.

3.1.2. *Applications*

Rituximab is approved for use in various lymphomas, leukemias, PTLD, and rheumatoid arthritis [50, 69]. Peripheral veins can be used for administration and dosing is dependent on the indication. A recent study examining the role of rituximab as an induction agent found no benefit compared to placebo [70]. However, it does play a role as a desensitizing agent in patients with preformed donor specific antibodies (DSA), in conjunction with total plasmapheresis and/or intravenous immunoglobulin (IVIG) [71, 72].

Additionally, it has been used to aid in transplanting across blood group barriers in donor recipient pairs and in patients with positive crossmatches following antibody elimination.

Rituximab is increasingly being used to treat episodes of vascular rejection and antibody mediated rejections [73, 74]. Finally, rituximab is a proven and effective agent in the treatment of PTLD [75]. Administration does not replace immunosuppression reduction or chemotherapy, but rather supplements the other modalities.

3.1.3. *Adverse effects*

Rituximab is generally well-tolerated with minimal side effects. Anaphylaxis remains a theoretical concern, as is the case with most agents. Reports on infectious complications related to rituximab have been variable [76-78]. In some instances there was no difference in bacterial, viral, or fungal infections in kidney transplant recipients treated with rituximab, however, this remains controversial.

3.2. Bortezomib

3.2.1. Mechanism

Bortezomib is a proteasomal inhibitor that causes apoptosis of plasma cells. It binds the 26S subunit of the proteasome [79]. Proteasome inhibition ultimately leads to apoptosis during mitosis. Bortezomib selectively causes apoptosis in CD138+ plasma cells [80]. Additionally, Bortezomib may block T cell cycling and decrease the number of circulating B cells by reducing bone marrow levels of IL-6 [81].

3.2.2 .Applications

Bortezomib has not been approved for use in kidney transplantation; however, it has been used in sensitized patients [80]. Bortezomib has been successfully used to decrease DSA levels, which may play a role in acute antibody-mediated rejection (AMR) Induction Therapy in Renal Transplant Recipients [82]. Furthermore, in vivo data has demonstrated a decrease in the percentage of bone marrow plasma cells, antibody production, and allospecificities of plasma cells in bone marrow aspirates of patients treated with bortezomib i in the setting of AMR [80].

3.2.3. Adverse events

Bortezomib has been associated with various side effects. Although gastrointestinal side effects are the most common, peripheral neuropathy has also been reported, especially in patients with a pre-existing history of neuropathy [79]. Moreover, myelosuppression and shingles has been reported.

3.3. Intravenous Immunoglobulin (IVIG)

3.3.1. Mechanism

Intravenous immunoglobulin, or IVIG, is pooled polyclonal antibodies from different human donors. These are high-dose human IgG fractions with a wide range of specificities. These are non-T cell specific formulations and have no specific cell targets [83]. It is able to bind activated complement components or even inhibit complement activation [84]. IVIG may also modulate the alloimmune response by binding to the Fc receptor of antigen-presenting cells, effectively quelling the alloimmune response [85].

3.3.2. Applications

Despite the inability to deplete T cells, IVIG is an effective treatment of acute cellular rejection. Early studies showed that IVIG was as effective as OKT3 in reversing steroid resistant acute rejection episodes [86]. In the setting of antibody-mediated rejection, IVIG has been shown to be beneficial when used in conjunction with plasmapheresis and/or rituximab [87-88]. As a desensitization agent alone, no study has demonstrated a clear benefit [88, 89]. Definitive reduction of antibody was not shown and a survival advantage was not evident.

3.3.3. Adverse effects

The side-effect profile of IVIG increases with dosing. High-dose IVIG is associated with more infusion-related complications, such as headache, thrombotic incidents, hemolysis, bronchospasms, osmotic nephropathy, or even aseptic meningitis [83, 90]. Sucrose-based and high osmolality products have a higher risk of developing osmotic nephropathy as opposed to other preparation. Nevertheless, it is typically well-tolerated, especially at lower doses and most patients report only headache.

4. Maintenance immunosuppression regimens

4.1. Historical background

The initial transplant armamentarium consisted only of azathioprine and steroids for maintenance immunosuppression in renal transplantation until the 1980's, when the first calcineurin inhibitor, cyclosporine became available. Over the next 20 years, azathioprine had been largely replaced by mycophenolate (MMF), an antiproliferative agent. Standard therapy in most modern immunosuppression regimens now consists of a calcineurin inhibitor, mycophenolate, with or without steroid maintenance.

Minimizing global immunosuppression in the modern era of transplantation has become an important goal. The use of induction therapy has allowed for steroid avoidance immunosuppression regimens. The goal of steroid avoidance immunosuppression is to decrease the negative cardiovascular profile associated with long-term administration of steroids. Specifically, steroid-free regimens should decrease the negative effects on blood pressure control as well serum glucose and lipid metabolism [91]. Moreover, the leading cause of death in kidney transplant patients is cardiovascular events [92].

4.2. Steroid maintenance versus withdrawal

Advocates of steroid-maintenance regimens suggest that steroids may allow for lower doses of calcineurin inhibitors, such as cyclosporine or tacrolimus. Moreover, steroids may decrease the incidence of nephrotoxicity perioperatively. However, there has been insufficient data to support either conclusion [93].

The effectiveness of steroid-withdrawal and cyclosporine-based therapy has been clearly associated with timing. Early studies of cyclosporine-based regimens demonstrated that cessation of steroids prior to the 6 month period post-transplantation increased the risk of acute rejection [94]. Furthermore, a meta-analysis of seven randomized-controlled trials of steroid avoidance and/or withdrawal demonstrated an increased risk of acute rejection with steroid avoidance or early withdrawal (most steroids were withdrawn in the first 3 months post-transplant) [95]. However, patient and graft survival were not adversely affected in the meta-analysis.

The ability to withdrawal steroids appears to be better with tacrolimus-based immunosuppression regimens. An early report by Shapiro et al. demonstrated that patients receiving tacrolimus and steroid-sparing immunosuppression had excellent early and intermediate-term patient and graft survival compared to kidney transplant recipients receiving standard steroid-maintenance immunosuppression [96]. Later, various randomized-controlled trials were undertaken to assess the initial outcomes. A meta-analysis of six randomized, controlled-trials comparing a calcineurin inhibitor-based immunosuppression regimen with MMF demonstrated a slightly increased risk of acute rejection once steroids were discontinued; however, this did not affect the incidence of graft failure [97]. Shortly thereafter, a randomized trial from Europe assigned low immunologic risk patients to receive either triple immunosuppression with tacrolimus, MMF, and steroids, a tacrolimus-based steroid withdrawal regimen, or a tacrolimus-based steroid-maintenance regimen without MMF [98]. At 6 months, the incidence of acute rejection was not different between the groups. Furthermore, the steroid withdrawal group benefited from an improved lipid profile. Kumar et al. reported on a series of 300 kidney transplant recipients receiving basiliximab induction therapy followed by steroid maintenance or withdrawal at 2 days post-transplant [99]. Maintenance therapy for all patients consisted of a calcineurin inhibitor and MMF or sirolimus. At 3 years, the incidence of biopsy-proven acute rejection, patients and graft survival, chronic allograft nephropathy, or graft function was not significantly different. Moreover, the steroid withdrawal group benefited from a lower rate of new-onset diabetes after transplantation.

Successful avoidance of steroids is contingent upon the use of calcineurin inhibitors. In 2006 Gelens and colleagues performed a single-center, randomized, trial of three parallel groups, which were: tacrolimus and sirolimus (group one), tacrolimus and MMF (group two), and sirolimus and MMF with daclizumab induction [100]. During an interim analysis when 50% of the patients were included, group one had a significantly increased rejection free survival (82%) compared to group three (34%, P=0.03) and between groups one and two (tacrolimus-based, 76%) and group three (34%, P=0.04). The study was halted prematurely. Despite the current armamentarium of antibody-depleting medications, steroid withdrawal seems feasible only with a calcineurin inhibitor-based regimen.

4.3. Induction therapy and steroid withdrawal

The possible minimization of maintenance immunosuppression has been studied using basiliximab and rATG without compromising allograft outcomes. In the Astellas Steroid Withdrawal Study, patients assigned to the steroid-withdrawal arm and treated with rATG experienced a lower cumulative incidence of biopsy-proven acute rejection at 5 years compared to patients treated with basiliximab [101]. Selection bias; however, may have marred this study, given that the investigators selected which antibody induction agent was used. Our transplant center's experience utilizing induction therapy to enable steroid withdrawal has been very successful in a diverse population, using rATG in the majority of patients [102] and basiliximab in well-matched living donor recipients [61]. In a study by Cantarovich et al., patients administered rATG and steroid-maintenance immunosuppression had significantly lower acute rejection rates compared to patients on a steroid-free immunosuppression regimen, although the incidence of malignancy, *de novo* diabetes, and hyperlipidemia were higher in steroid-maintenance group [103]. Patient survival, graft survival, and infection rates were not significantly different between the two groups at 1 year.

Alemetuzumab and steroid-free regimens have been compared to both basiliximab and rATG. In the study by Hanaway et al., acute rejection rates were relatively low in low-risk patients receiving alemtuzumab compared to basiliximab, although the reduced immunologic risk profile of alemtuzumab was not evident in high risk patients treated with rATG [54]. The overall rate of adverse events with alemtuzumab was similar to that of basiliximab or rATG over the 3 year study period (53% versus 50%, respectively; p=0.46). Moreover, the rate of cardiovascular events of all alemtuzumab treated patients compared to basiliximab or rATG was also similar (7% versus 10%, respectively; p=0.26), although the similarity was less evident in the high-risk immunologic group treated with rATG compared to alemtuzumab (12% versus 3%, respectively; p=0.06). Cai et al. analyzed the United Network for Organ Sharing registry and found that recipients of alemtuzumab in conjunction with steroid-maintenance therapy had the lowest risk of graft failure, while patients administered an interleukin-2 receptor antagonist on a steroid-free immunosuppression regimen had the highest risk of graft failure [104]. In a single-center, open-label randomized trial of 200 kidney transplant recipients, low dose dual induction therapy of rATG and daclizumab was compared to lose dose dual therapy of rATG and alemtuzumab in patients maintained on steroid-free maintenance immunosuppression [105]. Patient and graft survival rates as well as acute rejection and infectious complication rates were not significantly different. In addition, no patient developed post-transplant lymphoproliferative disorder.

5. New and experimental agents

5.1. Siplizumab (MEDI-507)

Originally described as BTI-322, siplizumab is a monoclonal humanized antibody to CD2. It is an IgG1k molecule derived from rat [106]. CD2, or lymphocyte function-associated antigen-2 (LFA-2) is an important T cell adhesion molecule that binds to CD58, or LFA-3. This is a transmembrane signal transduction molecule that facilitates T cell receptor binding. Early studies examined the use of siplizumab as an induction agent and treatment modality for acute rejection in solid organ transplantation as well as graft-versus-host disease [106, 107]. The first human study of siplizumab demonstrated the safety and feasibility in kidney transplantation, as compared to placebo; however, current endeavors are focused on investigating its use in nonmyeloablative conditioning regimens to achieve mixed chimerism [106, 108, 109]. In addition, it is being investigated for the treatment of plaque psoriasis [110].

5.2. Alefacept

Alefacept is a dimeric fusion protein (Fig.7) constituted from LFA-3 and the human Fc portion of IgG1. Studies have demonstrated inhibition of T cell proliferation and depletion of effector memory T cells [111, 112]. Currently, alefacept is approved to treat plaque psoriasis. Preclinical studies in nonhuman primates have demonstrated a survival benefit of alefacept, when used in conjunction with costimulatory blockade, but not alone; however in human trials have never shown a benefit [113].

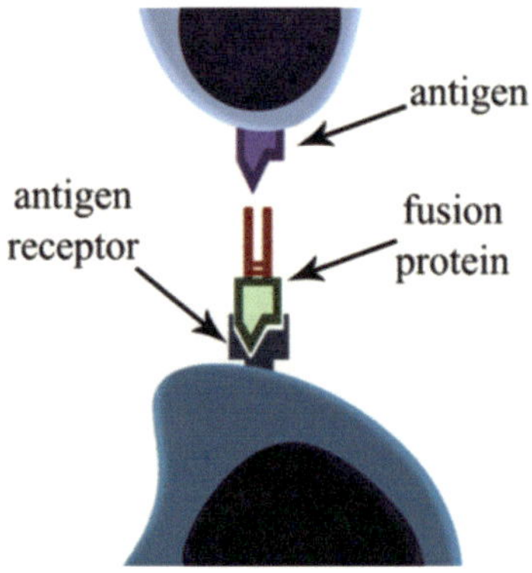

Figure 7. Mimicry. In this figure, the antibody is fused with a protein structural similar to the intended antigen, which can serve as activating or inhibitory.

5.3. Costimulatory blockade

5.3.1. Abatacept

Abatacept is a recombinant cytotoxic T-lymphocyte antigen 4 (CTLA4) fused with the Fc portion of IgG1 [114, 115]. Animal models demonstrated its ability to delay or even prevent the onset of allograft rejection, which is comparable to basiliximab and some polyclonal antibody therapies [114-116]. It has been approved for treatment of rheumatoid arthritis [117, 118]. Further investigations of this medication are not currently under development.

5.3.2. Belatacept

Belatacept is the improved version of abatacept, providing selective blockade of T cell activation as a fusion protein. Two amino acids have been changed to improve dissociation rates when binding to CD80 and CD86 [119, 120]. In the phase II trial comparing belatacept to cyclosporine, acute rejection rates were similar, while allograft function was significantly improved in patients receiving belatacept [119]. In the phase III trial of kidney transplantation, patients receiving belatacept experienced improved allograft function at 12 months; however, acute rejection rates and severity of acute rejection episodes were significantly higher in the belatacept arm of the study. Additionally, the incidence of PTLD was greater in patients receiving belatacept [120]. An additional study investigating the efficacy of belatacept in kidney transplantation of extended criteria donors demonstrated similar results, with a predilection towards central nervous system (CNS) forms of PTLD [121]. The novelty of costimulation blockade is the ability to avoid calcineurin inhibitors, especially in allografts at increased risk of delayed graft function. Belatacept has recently been approved for the prophylaxis of organ rejection in adult patients receiving a kidney transplant, in combination with basiliximab induction, mycophenolate mofetil, and corticosteroids [122]. Current recommendations include using it only in patients who are EBV seropositive; however, patients should be monitored for an increased risk of infectious complications and Progressive Multifocal Leukoencephalopathy.

5.4. Eculizumab

Recently, a new medication called eculizumab has emerged as a humanized monoclonal antibody to complement component 5 (C5) to mediate complement-mediated injury [123]. Blocking complement activation, especially the last step of the complement cascade, has important implications in kidney transplantation. However, the role of eculizumab appears to be more applicable to cases of clear complement-mediated destruction, such as antibody-mediated rejection and desensitization protocols [124]. Furthermore, the logistics of administration may further hinder its' use as a maintenance immunosuppression agent, as it must be administered biweekly or weekly intravenously at least for the first 1-2 months upon initiation of therapy. Currently, it is only approved for the treatment of patients with paroxysmal nocturnal hemoglobinuria [123].

Author details

Cheguevara Afaneh. Meredith J. Aull and Sandip Kapur
Department of Surgery, Division of Transplant Surgery, New York-Presbyterian Hospital- Weill Cornell Medical College, New York, NY, USA

Acknowledgement

The authors gratefully acknowledge the expert assistance of Ms. Johanna Martin in creating all figures depicted in this chapter.

6. References

[1] Cosimi, A.B. The clinical value of antilymphocyte antibodies. *Transplant Proc*, Vol.13, No.1, (March 1981), pp. 462-8.
[2] Henricsson, A.; Husberg, B., & Bergentz, S.E. The mechanism behind the effect of ALG on platelets in vivo. *Clin Exp Immunol*, Vol.29, No.3, (September 1977), pp. 515-22.
[3] Rosenberg, J.C.; Lekas, N.; Lysz, K., et al. (1975). Effect of antithymocyte globulin and other immune reactants on human platelets. *Surgery*, Vol.77, No.4, (April 1975), pp. 520-9.

[4] Niblack, G.; Johnson, K.; Williams, T., et al. Antibody formation following administration of antilymphocyte serum. *Transplant Proc*, Vol.19, No.1, (February 1987), pp. 1896-7.

[5] Prin Mathieu, C.; Renoult, E.; Kennel De March, A., et al. Serum anti-rabiit and anti-horse IgG, IgA, and IgM in kidney transplant recipients. *Nephrol Dial Transplant*, Vol.12, No.10, (October 1997), pp. 2133-9.

[6] Tatum, A.H.; Bollinger, R.R., & Sanfilippo, F. Rapid serological diagnosis of serum sickness from antilymphocyte globulin therapy using enzyme immunoassay. *Transplantation*, Vol.38, No.6, (December 1984), pp. 582-6.

[7] Kohler, G. & Milstein, C. Continuous cultures of fused cells secreting antibody of predefined specificity. *Nature*, Vol.256, No.5517, (August 1975), pp. 495-7.

[8] Cosimi, A.B.; Burton, R.C.; Colvin, R.B., et al.. Treatment of acute renal allograft rejection with OKT3 monoclonal antibody. *Transplantation*, Vol.32, No.6, (December 1981), pp. 535-9.

[9] Ortho Multicenter Transplant Study Group. A randomized clinical trial of OKT3 monoclonal antibody for acute rejection of cadaveric renal transplants. *N Engl J Med*, Vol. 313, No.6, (August 1985), pp. 337-42.

[10] Ponticelli, C.; Rivolta, E.; Tarantino, A., et al. Treatment of severe rejection of kidney transplant with OKT3.PAN. *Transplant Proc*, Vol.1, No.1, (February 1987), pp. 1908-9.

[11] Jaffers, G.J.; Fuller, T.C.; Cosimi, A.B., et al. Monoclonal antibody therapy: anti-idiotype and non-anti-idiotype antibodies to OKT3 arising despite intense immunosuppression. *Transplantation*, Vol.41, No.5, (May 1986), pp. 572-8.

[12] Vincenti, F.; Lantz, M.; Birnbaum, J., et al. A phase I trial of humanized anti-interleukin 2 receptor antibody in renal transplantation. *Transplantation*, Vol.63, No.1, (January 1997), pp. 33-8.

[13] Boulianne, G.L.; Hozumi, N.; Shulman, M.J., et al. Production of functional chimaeric mouse/human antibody. *Nature*, Vol.312, No.5995, (December 1984), pp. 643-6.

[14] Jones, P.T.; Dear, P.H.; Foote, et al. Replacing the complementarity-determining regions in human antibody with those from a mouse. *Nature*, Vol.321, No.6069, (May 1986), pp. 522-5.

[15] Morrison, S.L.; Johnson, M.J.; Herzenberg, L.A., et al. Chimeric human antibody molecules: mouse antigen-binding domains with human constant region domains. *Proc Natl Acad Sci U S A*, Vol.81, No.21, (November 1984), pp. 6851-5.

[16] Capra, J.D., & Edmundson, A.B. The antibody combining site. *Sci Am*, Vol.236, No.1, (January 1977), pp. 50-9.

[17] Tite, J.P.; Sloan, A.; Janeway, C.J. The role of L3T4 in T cell activation: L3T4 may be both an Ia-binding protein and a receptor that transduces a negative signal. *J Mol Cell Immunol*, Vol.2, No.4, (1986), pp. 179-90.

[18] Wong, J.T.; Eylath, A.A.; Ghobrial, I., et al. The mechanism of anti-CD3 monoclonal antibodies: mediation of cytolysis by inter-T cell bridging. *Transplantation*, Vol.50, No.4, (October 1990), pp. 683-9.

[19] Kerr, P.G. & Atkins, R.C. The effects of OKT3 therapy on infiltrating lymphocytes in rejecting renal allografts. *Transplantation*, Vol.48, No.1, (July 1989), pp. 33-6.

[20] Ferrant, J.L.; Benjamin, C.D.; Cutler, A.H., et al. The contribution of the Fc effector mechanisms in the efficacy of anti-CD154 immunotherapy depends on the nature of the immune challenge. *Int Immunol*, Vol.16, No.11, (Novemeber 2004), pp. 1583-94.
[21] Pearl, J.P.; Parris, J.; Hale, D.A., et al. Immunocompetent T-cells with a memory-like phenotype are the dominant cell type following antibody-mediated T-cell depletion. *Am J Transplant*, Vol.5, No.3, (March 2005), pp. 465-74.
[22] Szczech, L.A.; Berlin, J.A.; Aradhye, S., et al. Effect of anti-lymphocyte induction therapy on renal allograft survival: a meta-analysis. *J Am Soc Nephrol*, Vol.8, No.11, (November 1997), pp. 1771-7.
[23] Humar, A.; Ramcharan, T.; Denny, R., et al. Are wound complications after a kidney transplant more common with modern immunosuppression? *Transplantation*, Vol.72, No.12, (December 2001), pp. 1920-3.
[24] Singh, A.; Stablein, D., & Tejani, A. Risk factors for vascular thrombosis in pediatric renal transplantation: a special report of the North American Pediatric Renal Transplant Cooperative Study. *Transplantation*, Vol.63, No.9, (May 1997), pp. 1263-7.
[25] Bustami, R.T.; Ojo, A.O.; Wolfe, R.A., et al. Immunosuppression and the risk of post-transplant malignancy among cadaveric first kidney transplant recipients. *Am J Transplant*, Vol.4, No.1, (January 2004), pp. 87-93.
[26] Jamil, B.; Nicholls, K.; Becker, G.J., et al. Impact of acute rejection therapy on infections and malignancies in renal transplant recipients. *Transplantation*, Vol.68, No.10, (November 1999), pp. 1597-603.
[27] Meier-Kriesche, H.U.; Li, S.; Gruessner, R.W., et al. Immunosuppression: evolution in practice and trends, 1994-2004. *Am J Transplant*, Vol.6, No.5, (2006), pp. 1111-31.
[28] Hardinger, K.L. Rabbit antithymocyte globulin induction therapy in adult renal transplantation. *Pharmacotherpay*, Vol.26, No.12, (December 2006), pp. 1771-83.
[29] Bonnefoy-Berard, N.; Vincent, C., & Revillard, J. Antibodies against the functional leukocyte surface molecules in polyclonal antilymphocyte and antithymocyte globulins. *Transplantation*, Vol.51, No.3, (March 1991), pp. 669-73.
[30] Bourdage ,J.S. & Hamlin, D.M. Comparative polyclonal antithymocyte globulin and antilymphocyte/antilymphoblast globulin anti-CD antigen analysis by flow cytometry. *Transplantation*, Vol.59, No.8. (April 1995), pp. 1194-200.
[31] Bunn, D.; Lea, C.K.; Bevan, D.J., et al. The pharmacokinetics of anti-thymocyte globulin (ATG) following intravenous infusion in man. *Clin Nephrol*, Vol.45, No.1, (January 1996), pp. 29-32.
[32] Guttmann, R.D.; Caudrelier, P.; Alberici, G., et al. Pharmacokinetics, foreign protein immune response, cytokine release, and lymphocyte subsets in patients receiving thymoglobuline and immunosuppression. *Transplant Proc*, Vol.29, No.7A, pp. 24S–6.
[33] Brennan, D.C.; Flavin, K.; Lowell, J.A., et al. A randomized,double-blinded comparison of thymoglobulin versus Atgam for induction immunosuppressive therapy in adult renal transplant recipients. *Transplantation*, Vol.67, No.7, (April 1999), pp. 1011-8.
[34] Hardinger, K.L.; Schnitzler, M.A.; Miller, B., et al. Five–year follow up of thymoglobulin versus ATGAM induction in adult renal transplantation. *Transplantation* 2004; 78: 136.

[35] IMTIX–SangStat. Thymoglobuline (rabbit antithymocyte globulin) prescribing information. Lyon, France; 2003.

[36] Merion, R.; White, D.J.; Thiru, S., et al. Cyclosporine: five years experience in cadaveric renal transplantation. *N Engl J Med*, Vol.310, No.3, (January 1984), pp. 148-54.

[37] Shoskes, D.A. & Halloran, P.F. Delayed graft function in renal transplantation: etiology, management and long-term significance. *J Urol*, Vol.155, No.6, (June 1996), pp. 1831-40.

[38] Beiras-Fernandez, A.; Chappell, D.; Hammer, C., et al. Influence of polyclonal anti-thymocyte globulins upon ischemia reperfusion injury in a non-human primate model. *Transpl Immunol*, Vol.15, No.4, (April 2006), pp. 273-9.

[39] Cecka, J.M.; Gjertson, D., & Terasaki, P. Do prophylactic antilymphocyte globulins (ALG and OKT3) improve renal transplant in recipient and donor high-risk groups? *Transplant Proc*, Vol.25, No.1, (February 1993), pp. 548-9.

[40] Shield, C.F.; Edwards, E.B.; Davies, D.B., et al. Antilymphocyte induction therapy in cadaver renal transplantation. *Transplantation*, Vol.63, No.9, (May 1997), pp. 1257-63.

[41] Schaffer, D.; Langone, A.; Nylander, W.A., et al. A pilot protocol of a calcineurin-inhibitor free regimen of kidney transplant recipients of marginal donor kidneys or with delayed graft function. *Clin Transplant*, Vol.17, No.9, (2003), pp. 31-4.

[42] Debets, J.M.H.; Leunissen, K.M.L.; van Hooff, H.J., et al. Evidene of involvement of tumor necrosis factor in adverse reactions during treatment of kidney allograft rejection with antithymocyte globulin. *Transplantation*, Vol.47, No.3, (March 1989), pp. 487-92.

[43] Buchler, M.; Hurault de Ligny, B.; Madec, C., et al. Induction therapy by anti-thymocyte globulin (rabbit) in renal transplantation: a 1-yr follow-up of safety and efficacy. *Clin Transplant*, Vol.17, No.6, (December 2003), pp. 539-45.

[44] Mourad, G.; Garrigue, V.; Squifflet, J.P., et al. Induction versus noninduction in renal transplant recipients with tacrolimus-based immunosuppression. *Transplantation*, Vol.72, No.6, (September 2001), pp. 1050-5.

[45] Abott, K.C.; Hypolite, I.O.; Viola, R., et al. Hospitalizations for cytomegalovirus disease after renal transplantation in the United States. *Ann Epidemiol*, Vol.12, No.6, (August 2002), pp. 402-409.

[46] Gourishankar, S.; McDermid, J.C.; Jhangri, G.S., et al. Herpes zoster infection following solid organ transplantation: incidence, risk factors and outomes in the current immunosuppressive era. *Am J Transplant*, Vol.4, No.1, (January 2004), pp. 108-15.

[47] Hale, G.; Waldmann, H.; Friend, P., et al. Pilot study of CAMPATH-1, a rat monoclonal antibody that fixes human complement, as an immunosuppressant in organ transplantation. *Transplantation*, Vol.42, No.3, (September 1986), pp. 308-11.

[48] Hale, G. The CD52 antigen and development of the CAMPATH antibodies. *Cytotherapy*, Vol.3, No.3, (2001), pp. 137-43.

[49] Kirk, A.D.; Hale, D.A.; Mannon, R.B., et al. Results from a human renal allograft tolerance trial evaluating the humanized CD52-specific monoclonal antibody alemtuzumab (CAMPATH-1H). *Transplantation*, Vol.76, No.1, (July 2003), pp. 120-9.

[50] Gabardi, S.; Martin, S.T.; Roberts, K.L., et al. Induction immunosuppressive therapies in renal transplantation. *Am J Health Syst Pharm*, Vol.68, No.3, (February 2011), pp. 211-8.

[51] Clatworthy, M.R.; Friend, P.J.; Calne, R.Y., et al. Alemtuzumab (CAMPATH-1H) for the treatment of acute rejection in kidney transplant recipients: long-term follow-up. *Transplantation,* Vol.87, No.7, (April 2009), pp. 1092-5.
[52] Csapo, Z.; Benavides-Viveros, C.; Podder, H., et al. Campath-1H as rescue therapy for the treatment of acute rejection in kidney transplant patients. *Transplant Proc,* Vol.37, No.5, (June 2005), pp. 2032-6.
[53] Jirasiritham, S.; Khunprakant, R.; Techawathanawanna, N., et al. Treatment of simultaneous acute antibody-mediated rejection and acute cellular rejection with alemtuzumab in kidney transplantation: a case report. *Transplant Proc,* Vol.42, No.3, (April 2010), pp. 987-9.
[54] Hanaway, M.J.; Woodle, E.S.; Mulgaonkar, S., et al. Alemtuzumab induction in renal transplantation. *N Engl J Med,* Vol. 364, No.20, (May 2011), pp. 1909-19.
[55] Coles, A.J.; Wing, M.; Smith, S., et al. Pulsed monoclonal antibody treatment and autoimmune thyroid disease in multiple sclerosis. *Lancet,* Vol.354, No.9191, (Novemeber 1999), pp. 1691-5.
[56] Kirk, A.D.; Hale, D.A.; Swanson, S.J., et al. Autoimmune thyroid disease after renal transplantation using depletional induction with alemtuzumab. *Am J Transplant,* Vol.6, No.5, (May 2006), pp. 1084-5.
[57] Kahan, B.D.; Rajagopalan, P.R. & Hall, M. Reduction of the occurrence of acute cellular rejection among renal allograft recipients treated with basiliximab, a chimeric anti-interleukin-2-receptor monoclonal antibody. *Transplantation,* Vol.67, No.2, pp. 276-84.
[58] Nashan, B.; Moore, R.; Amlot, P., et al. Randomized trial of basiliximab versus placebo for control of acute cellular rejection in renal allograft recipients. CHIB201 International Study Group. *Lancet,* Vol.350, No.9086, (October 1997), pp. 1193-8.
[59] Lebranchu, Y.; Bridoux, F.; Buchler, M., et al. Immunoprophylaxis with basiliximab compared with antithymocyte globulin in renal transplant patients receiving MMF-containing triple therapy. *Am J Transplant,* Vol.2, No.1, pp. 48-56.
[60] Mourad, G.; Rostaing, L.; Legendre, C., et al. Sequential protocols using basiliximab versus antithymocyte globulins in renal-transplant patients receiving mycophenolate mofetil and steroids. *Transplantation,* Vol.78, No.4, (August 2004), pp. 584-90.
[61] Afaneh, C.; Halpern, J.; Cheng, E., et al. Steroid avoidance in two-haplotype-matched living donor renal transplants with basiliximab induction therapy. *Transplant Proc,* Vol.42, No.10, (December 2010), pp. 4526-9.
[62] Parrott, N.R.; Hammad, A.Q.; Watson, C.J., et al. Multicenter, randomized study of the effectiveness of basiliximab in avoiding addition of steroids to cyclosporine a monotherapy in renal transplant recipients. *Transplantation,* Vol.79, No.3, (February 2005), pp. 344-8.
[63] Vincenti, F.; Ramos, E.; Brattstrom, C., et al. Multicenter trial exploring calcineurin inhibitors avoidance in renal transplantation. *Transplantation,* Vol.71, No.9, (May 2011), pp. 1282-7.
[64] Cherikh, W.S.; Kauffman, H.M.; McBride, M.A., et al. Association of the type of induction immunosuppression with posttransplant lymphoproliferative disorder, graft

survival, and patient survival after primary kidney transplantation. *Transplantation*, Vol.76, No.9, (Novemeber 2003), pp. 1289-93.

[65] Kirkman, R.L.; Shapiro, M.E.; Carpenter, C.B., et al. A randomized prospective trial of anti-Tac monoclonal antibody in human renal transplantation. *Transplantation*, Vol.51, No.1, (January 1991), pp. 107-13.

[66] Hershberger, R.E.; Starling, R.C.; Eisen, H.J., et al. Daclizumab to prevent rejection after cardiac transplantation. *N Engl J Med*, Vol.352, No.26, (June 2005), pp. 2705-13.

[67] Nashan, B.; Light, S.; Hardie, I.R., et al. Reduction of acute renal allograft rejection by daclizumab. *Transplantation*, Vol.67, No.1, (January 1999), pp. 110-5.

[68] Deans, J.P.; Li, H.; Polyak, M.J., et al. CD20-mediated apoptosis: signaling through lipid rafts. Immunology, Vol.107, No.2, (October 2002), pp. 176-82.

[69] Grillo-Lopez, A.J.; White, C.A.; Varns, C., et al. Overview of the clinical development of rituximab: first monoclonal antibody approved for the treatment of lymphoma. Semin Oncol, Vol.26, No.5, (October 1999), pp. 66-73.

[70] Tyden, G.; Genberg, H.; Tollemar, J., et al. A randomized, double-blind, placebo controlled, study of single-dose rituximab as induction in renal transplantation. Transplantation, Vol.87, No.9, (May 2009), pp. 1325-9.

[71] Fuchinoue, S.; Ishii, Y.; Sawada, T., et al. The 5-year outcome of ABO-incompatible kidney transplantation with rituximab induction. Transplantation, Vol.91, No.18, (April 2011), pp. 853-7.

[72] Sonnenday, C.J.; Warren, D.S.; Cooper, M., et al. (2004). Plasmapheresis, CMV, hyperimmune globulin, and anti-CD20 allow ABO-incompatible renal transplantation without splenectomy. Am J Transplant, Vol.4, No.8, (August 2004), pp. 1315-22.

[73] Becker, Y.T.; Samaniego-Picota, M., & Sollinger, H.W. The emerging role of rituximab in organ transplantation. *Transpl Int*, Vol.19, No.8, (August 2006), pp. 621-8.

[74] Fehr, T.; Rüsi, B.; Fischer, A., et al. Rituximab and intravenous immunoglobulin treatment of chronic antibody-mediated kidney allograft rejection. Transplantation, Vol.87, No.12, (June 2009), pp. 1837-4.

[75] Svoboda, J.; Kotloff, R., & Tsai, D.E. Management of patients with post-transplant lymphoproliferative disorder: the role of rituximab. Transpl Int, Vol.19, No.4, (April 2006), pp. 259-69.

[76] Grim, S.A.; Pham, T.; Thielke, J., et al. Infectious complications associated with the use of rituximab for ABO-incompatible and positive cross-match renal transplant recipients. Clin Transplant, Vol.21, No.5, (September 2007), pp. 628-32.

[77] Kamar, N.; Milioto, O.; Puissant-Lubrano, B., et al. Incidence and predictive factors for infectious disease after rituximab therapy in kidney-transplant patients. Am J Transplant, Vol.10, No.1, (July 2009), pp. 89-98.

[78] Nishida, H.; Ishida, H.; Tanaka, T., et al. Cytomegalovirus infection following renal transplantation in patients administered low-dose rituximab induction therapy, Transpl Int, Vol.22, No.10, (July 2009), pp. 961-9.

[79] Bonvini, P.; Zorzi, E.; Basso, G., et al. Bortezomib-mediated 26S proteasome inhibition causes cell-cycle arrest and induces apoptosis in CD-30+ anaplastic large cell lymphoma. *Leukemia*, Vol.21, No.4 (April 2007), pp. 838–42.

[80] Perry, D.K.; Burns, J.M.; Pollinger, H.S., et al. Proteasome inhibition causes apoptosis of normal human plasma cells preventing alloantibody production. Am J Transplant, Vol.9, No.1, (January 2009), pp. 201-9.
[81] San Miguel, J.F.; Schlag, R.; Khuageva, N.K., et al. Bortezomib plus melphalan and prednisone for initial treatment of multiple myeloma. N Engl J Med, Vol.359, No.9, (August 2008), pp. 906-17.
[82] Trivedi, H.L.; Terasaki, P.I.; Feroz, A., et al. Abrogation of anti-HLA antibodies via proteasome inhibition. Transplantation, Vol.87, No.10, (May 2009), pp.1555-61.
[83] Jordan, S.C.; Toyoda, M.; Kahwaji, J., et al. Clinical Aspects of Intravenous Immunoglobulin Use in Solid Organ Transplant Recipients. Am J Transplant, Vol.11, No.2, (January 2011), pp. 196-202.
[84] Jordan, S.C.; Toyoda, M., & Vo, A.A. Intravenous immunoglobulin a natural regulator of immunity and inflammation. Transplantation, Vol.88, No.1, (July 2009), pp. 1-6.
[85] Kazatchkine, M.D. & Kaveri, S.V. Immunomodulation of autoimmune and inflammatory disease with intravenous immune globulin. N Engl J Med, Vol.345, No.10, (September 2001), pp. 747-55.
[86] Casadei, D.H.; del C Rial, M.; Opelz, G., et al. A randomized and prospective study comparing treatment with high-dose intravenous immunoglobulin with monoclonal antibodies for rescue of kidney grafts with steroid-resistant rejection. Transplantation, Vol.71, No.1, (January 2001), pp. 53-8.
[87] Lefaucheur, C.; Nochy, D.; Andrade, J., et al. Comparison of combination plasmapheresis/IVIG/Anti-CD20 versus high dose IVIG in the treatment of antibody-mediated rejection. Am J Transplant, Vol.9, No.5, (May 2009), pp. 1099-107.
[88] Shehata, N.; Palda, V.; Meyer, R., et al. The use of immunoglobulin therapy for patients undergoing solid organ transplantation: an evidence -based practice guideline. Transf Med Rev, Vol.24, No.1, (January 2010), pp. S7-27.
[89] Pisani, B.A.; Mullen, G.M.; Malinowska, K., et al. Plasma- pheresis with intravenous immunoglobulin G is effective in patients with elevated panel reactive antibody prior to cardiac transplantation. J Heart Lung Transplant, Vol.18, No.7, (July 1999), pp. 701-6.
[90] Kahwaji, J.; Barker, E.; Pepkowitz, S., et al. Acute hemolysis after high dose IVIG therapy in highly HLA sensitized patients. Clin J Am Soc Nephrol, Vol.4, No.12, (October 2009), pp. 1993-7.
[91] Knight, S.R. & Morris, P.J. Steroid avoidance or withdrawal after renal transplantation increases the risk of acute rejection but decreases cardiovascular risk: a meta analysis. *Transplantation*, Vol.89, No.1, (January 2010), pp. 785-94.
[92] Ojo, A.O.; Hanson, J.A.; Wolfe, R.A., et al. Long-term survival in renal transplant recipients with draft function. *Kidney Int*, Vol.57, No.1, (January 2000), pp.307-13.
[93] Griffin, P.J.; Da Costa, C.A.; Salaman, J.R. A controlled trial of steroids in cyclosporine-treated renal transplant recipients. *Transplantation*, Vol.43, No.4, (April 1987), pp. 505-8.
[94] Hricik, D.E.; Whalen, C.C.; Lautman, J., et al. Withdrawal of steroids after renal transplantation- clinical predictors of outcome. *Transplantation*, Vol.53, No.1, (January 1992), pp. 41-5.

[95] Hricik, D.E.; O'Toole, M.A.; Schulak, J.A., et al. Steroid-free immunosuppression in cyclosporine-treated renal transplant recipients: a meta-analysis. *J Am Soc Nephrol*, Vol.4, No., (1993), pp. 1300-5.

[96] Shapiro, R.; Jordan, M.L.; Scantlebury, V.P., et al. Outcome after steroid withdrawal in renal transplant patients receiving tacrolimus-based immunosuppression. Transplant Proc, Vol.30, No.4, (June 1998), pp. 1375-7.

[97] Pascual, J.; Querada, C.; Zamora, J., et al. Steroid withdrawal in renal transplant patients on triple therapy with a calcineurin inhibitor and mycophenolate mofetil: a meta-analysis of randomized, controlled trials. *Transplantation*, Vol.78, No.10, (November 2004), pp. 1548-56.

[98] Vanrenterghem, Y.; van Hooff, J.P.; Squifflet, J.P., et al. Minimization of immunosuppressive therapy after renal transplantation: results of a randomized controlled trial. Am J Transplant, Vol.5, No.1, (January 2005), pp. 87-95.

[99] Kumar, M.S.; Heifets, M.; Moritz, M.J., et al. Safety and efficacy of steroid withdrawal two days after kidney transplantation: analysis of results at three years. *Transplantation*, Vol.81, No.6, (March 2006), pp.832-9.

[100] Gelens, M.A.; Christiaans, M.H.; van Heurn, E.L., et al. High rejection rate during calcineurin inhibitor-free and early steroid withdrawal immunosuppression in renal transplantation. *Transplantation*, Vol.82, No.9, (November 2006), pp. 1221-3.

[101] Woodle, E.S.; First, M.R.; Pirsch, J., et al. A prospective, randomized, double-blind placebo-controlled multicenter trial comparing early (7 day) corticosteroid cessation versus long-term, low-dose corticosteroid therapy. *Ann Surg*, Vol.248, No.4, (October 2008), pp. 564-77.

[102] Aull, M.J.; Dadhania, D.; Afaneh, C., et al. Early corticosteroid withdrawal in high risk recipients of renal allografts: a single center report of ethnically diverse recipients and recipients of marginal deceased donor kidneys. *Transplantation*, 2012 Sep 20. DOI: 10.1097/TP.0b013e318265c461 [Epub ahead of print]

[103] Cantarovich, D.; Rostaing, L.; Kamar, N., et al. Corticosteroid avoidance in adult kidney transplant recipients under rabbit anti-T-lymphocyte globulin, mycophenolate mofetil and delayed cyclosporine microemulsion introduction. *Transpl Int*, Vol.23, No.3, (March 2010), pp. 313-24.

[104] Cai, J., & Terasaki, P.I. Induction immunosuppression improves long-term graft and patient outcome in organ transplantation: an analysis of united network for organ sharing registry data. *Transplantation*, Vol.90, No.12, (December 2010), pp. 1511-5.

[105] Ciancio, G.; Gaynor, J.J.; Sageshima, J., et al. Randomized trial of dual antibody induction therapy with steroid avoidance in renal transplantation. *Transplantation*, Vol.92, No.12, (December 2011), pp. 1348-57.

[106] Pruett, T.L.; McGory, R.W.; Wright, F.H., et al. Safety profile, pharmacokinetics, and pharmacodynamics of siplizumab, a humanized anti-CD2 monoclonal antibody, in renal allograft recipients. *Transplant Proc*, Vol.41, No.9, (November 2009), pp. 3655-61.

[107] Squifflet, J.P.; Besse, T.; Malaise, J., et al. BTI-322 for induction therapy after renal transplantation: a randomized study. *Transplant Proc*, Vol.29, No.1-2, (February 1997), pp. 317-9.

[108] Kawai, T.; Cosimi, A.B.; Spitzer, T.R., et al. HLA-mismatched renal transplantation without maintenance immunosuppression. *N Engl J Med*, Vol.358, No..4, (January 2008), pp. 353-61.

[109] Spitzer, T.R.; McAfee, S.L.; Dey, B.R., et al. Nonmyeloablative haploidentical stem-cell transplantation using anti-CD2 monoclonal antibody (MEDI-507)-based conditioning for refractory hematologic malignancies. *Transplantation*, Vol.75, No.10, (May 2003), pp. 1748-51.

[110] Langley, R.G.; Papp, K.; Bissonnette, R., et al. Safety profile of intravenous and subcutaneous siplizumab, an anti-CD2 monoclonal antibody, for the treatment of plaque psoriasis: results of two randomized, double-blind, placebo-controlled studies. Int J Dermatol, Vol.49, No.7, (July 2010), pp. 818-28.

[111] Ellis, C.N.; Krueger, G.G. & Alefacept Clinical Study Group. Treatment of chronic plaque psoriasis by selective targeting of memory effector T lymphocytes. N Engl J Med, *Vol.*345, No.4, (July 2001), pp. 248-55.

[112] Gordon, K.B.; Vaishnaw, A.K.; O'Gorman, J., et al. Treatment of psoriasis with alefacept: correlation of clinical improvement with reductions of memory T-cell counts. *Arch Dermatol*, Vol.139, No.12, (December 2003), pp. 1563-70.

[113] Weaver, T.A.; Charafeddine, A.H.; Agarwal, A., et al. Alefacept promotes co-stimulation blockade based allograft survival in nonhuman primates. *Nat Med*, Vol.15, No.7, (July 2009), pp. 746-9.

[114] Lenschow, D.J.; Zeng, Y.; Thistlethwaite, J.R., et al. Long-term survival of xenogeneic pancreatic islet grafts induced with CTLA4Ig. *Science*, Vol.257, No.5071, (August 1992), pp. 789-92.

[115] Turka, L.A.; Linsley, P.S.; Lin, H., et al. T-cell activation by the CD28 ligand B7 is required for cardiac allograft rejection in vivo. *Proc Natl Acad Sci U S A*, Vol.89, No.22, (November 1992), pp. 11102-5.

[116] Kirk, A.D.; Harlan, D.M.; Armstrong, N.N., et al. CTLA4-Ig and anti-CD40 ligand prevent renal allograft rejection in primates. *Proc Natl Acad Sci U S A*, Vol.94, No.16, (August 1997), pp. 8789-94.

[117] Genovese, M.C.; Becker, J.C.; Schiff, M., et al. Abatacept for rheumatoid arthritis refractory to tumor necrosis alpha inhibition. *N Engl J Med*, Vol.353, No.11, pp. 1114-23.

[118] Nogid, A. & Pham, D.Q. Role of abatacept in the management of rheumatoid arthritis.*Clin Ther*, Vol.28, No.11, (November 2006), pp. 1764-78.

[119] Vincenti, F.; Larsen, C.; Durrbach, A., et al. Costimulation blockade with belatacept in renal transplantation. N Engl J Med, Vol.353, No.8, (August 2005), pp. 770-81.

[120] Vincenti, F.; Charpentier, B.; Vanrenterghem, Y., et al. A phase III study of belatacept-based immunosuppression regimens versus cyclosporine in renal transplant recipients (BENEFIT study). *Am J Transplant*, Vol.10, No.3, (March 2010), pp. 535-46.

[121] Durrbach, A.; Pestana, J.M.; Pearson, T., et al. A phase III study of belatacept versus cyclosporine in kidney transplants from extended criteria donors (BENEFIT-EXT study). *Am J Transplant*, Vol.10, No.3, (March 2010), pp. 547-57.

[122] Bristol-Myers Squibb Company. Nulojix® (belatacept) prescribing information. Princeton, New Jersey, USA; (2011).

[123] Fehr, T. & Gaspert, A. Antibody-mediated kidney allograft rejection: therapeutic options and their experimental rationale. *Transpl Int*, Vol.25, No.6, (June 2012), pp. 623-32.
[124] Larrea, C.F.; Cofan, F.; Oppenheimer, F., et al. Efficacy of eculizumab in the treatment of recurrent atypical hemolytic-uremic syndrome after renal transplantation. Transplantation, Vol.89, No.7, (April 2010), pp. 903-4.

Chapter 8

Complications of Kidney Transplantation: Effects of Over-Immunosuppression

Meredith J. Aull, Cheguevara Afaneh and Sandip Kapur

Additional information is available at the end of the chapter

http://dx.doi.org/10.5772/53672

1. Introduction

Kidney transplantation is a relatively young field within medicine which continues to experience rapid advances in several areas. The number of immunosuppressive medications available to prevent and treat immunologic rejection of the transplanted organ has increased significantly since the late 1990's, however, there continues to be a great need for developing novel, less toxic medications. The fine balance between over- and under-immunosuppression is difficult to achieve in many transplant recipients, particularly as candidacy for kidney transplantation has expanded to include the elderly, patients with HIV and/or Hepatitis C infection, and sensitized transplant candidates. The relationship between infection and rejection remains closely intertwined, and can be a vicious cycle, with reduction of immunosuppression to manage infection potentially triggering rejection, and increased immunosuppression in the setting of rejection potentially leading to infectious complications. This chapter will focus on post-transplant complications resulting from over-immunosuppression, specifically infection and malignancy.

2. Infection

The occurrence of infection after transplantation is a significant determinant of transplant outcome [1]. The incidence of infections after solid-organ transplantation is dependent on several factors, including the degree of immunosuppression, the type of organ transplanted, technical or surgical complications, need for additional antirejection therapy, environmental exposures, and the time frame after transplantation. A comprehensive list of factors contributing the 'net state of immune deficiency' can be found in reference [2]. Most recent United States data shows that infectious complications cause 20.9% of kidney transplant recipient death with a functioning allograft [3]. Infection also accounts for a significant proportion of death-censored graft loss, accounting for 7.7% of graft losses in the U.S.

between 1990 and 2006 [4]. Using the leading cause of allograft loss, chronic rejection as a reference, risk factors for infection-related graft loss included prior acute rejection and utilization of any induction therapy. Older transplant recipients (> 65 years at transplant) had a higher risk of infection related graft loss (14.1%). In this series, the infections leading to graft loss were caused by infections associated with urological complications and polyomavirus associated nephropathy [4]. Other infections that directly contribute to death-censored graft loss include pyelonephritis and acute kidney injury in the setting of sepsis/critical illness.

The occurrence of infection after transplantation usually falls within 3 general time frames: the first month, the second through the sixth month, and more than 6 months after transplantation [2, 5, 6]. Infections that occur during the first month after transplantation are generally the same nosocomial infections seen in non-immunosuppressed patients after surgery. These infections include bacterial and candidal urinary tract infection (UTI), wound/surgical site infections, catheter-related infections, and pneumonia.

The period from the second to sixth month after transplantation is the time during which opportunistic infections "classically" associated with transplantation occur [1] , although the patterns have changed thanks to the availability of antimicrobial prophylaxis against some infections [2]. The most common infections during this period include cytomegalovirus (CMV), *Pneumocystis (carinii) jiroveci, Aspergillus* species, *Nocardia* species, *Toxoplasmosis, Listeria monocytogenes,* and fungal infections. In addition, reactivation of immunomodulating viruses will begin to manifest a clinically significant effect. These viruses include Epstein Barr virus (EBV), CMV, hepatitis B virus (HBV), hepatitis C virus (HCV), human herpesvirus type 6 (HHV-6), and human immunodeficiency virus (HIV) [1, 6]. Multi-drug resistant (MDR) bacteria such as *Klebsiella, Pseudomonas, Acinetobacter, Staphylococcus,* and *Enterococcus* can also be problematic during this period [5, 7-9].

More than 6 months after transplantation, most transplant recipients (80%) are doing well [6], and can be classified into one of three risk groups [5]:

1. Patients who have done well and immunosuppression is being tapered
2. Patients who have required increased immunosuppression exposure due to rejection
3. Patients at risk for late progressive viral reactivation (polyomavirus, CMV, HBV, HCV, HPV)

The most common infections seen during this period mimic those seen in the general community [6]. Such infections include influenza virus, UTIs, and pneumococcal pneumonia. Although opportunistic infections are rarely observed during this time period, reactivation of varicella zoster virus (VZV) or CMV can occur. In addition, transplant recipients who have had multiple rejection episodes requiring additional antirejection may be predisposed to opportunistic infections more commonly seen 2 to 6 months after transplantation. It is recommended that patients being treated for acute rejection be placed back on opportunistic infection prophylaxis [10]. Transplant recipients experiencing chronic infection due to HBV, HCV, CMV, EBV, or HIV, resulting in a greater degree of morbidity, are subsequently at an increased risk for other infections [1, 6]. In patients who undergo repeat transplantation, the typical timetable of infections may be altered. Infections characteristic of 1 of the 3 conventional time periods may occur simultaneously and with an increased severity [11]. In addition, modern immunosuppressive agents, as well as availability of prophylaxis against some infections has led to an altered timeline for many patients.

Although not addressed in this chapter due to space constraints, transplant centers should be aware of the newer emerging infectious diseases that may affect transplant recipients [12]. This is also a great concern due to increasing rates of transplant tourism, where patients travel to foreign countries to receive a transplant and may be exposed to infectious complications not typically seen in their home country, where they will receive their follow-up care. In addition, transplant recipients travelling for leisure should consult with a travel medicine specialist when possible [13].

2.1. Bacterial infection

Some of the most prevalent microbial pathogens observed after organ transplantation are bacteria. The specific bacterial infections that occur after transplantation can be divided into 4 categories [14]:

- Infections due to surgical or technical complications,
- Infections related to prolonged hospitalization (nosocomial infections),
- Infections associated with the degree of immunosuppression (opportunistic infections), and
- Infections occurring months after transplantation when the transplant recipient resumes normal activity (community-acquired infections).

Although transplant recipients are susceptible to common bacterial pathogens observed in normal hosts, the immunosuppressed state of the recipient after transplantation predisposes the patient to bacterial pathogens not commonly observed in the normal host. These opportunist pathogens include *Legionella* species, *Nocardia* species, *Rhodococcus* species, *L monocytogenes*, and *Mycobacteria* species. Following transplantation, disruption of anatomic barriers is commonly associated with bacterial infections. For instance, the upper airway is normally colonized with bacteria, and the lower respiratory tract is normally sterile. Endotracheal intubation creates a conduit between the upper and lower respiratory tract, introducing bacteria to the lower respiratory tract and resulting in disease of the bronchial tubes or lung parenchyma. Indwelling urinary and vascular catheters may become colonized with nosocomial bacteria or cutaneous flora and introduce these pathogens into the urinary tract, transplant kidney, or bloodstream.

2.1.1. Urinary tract infection

The most common infections occurring after kidney transplantation are UTIs, which may include asymptmatic bacteriuria, cystitis, and/or pyelonephritis. The reported incidence of

UTI in kidney recipients is 7.3% to to 90% [15-18] with the variation likely due to differences in definitions of infection and prophylactic strategies. Predisposing factors include renal insufficiency, ischemic changes of the graft, decreased urine flow through the urinary epithelium, prolonged urinary catheterization, ureteral stenting, post-transplant diarrhea, and underlying medical conditions such as diabetes mellitus, female gender, urinary tract abnormalities, bladder dysfunction, and bladder outlet obstruction [17-20]. In pediatric kidney transplant recipients, age less than 5 at the time of transplant and lower urinary tract abnormalities may be risk factors for post-transplant UTI [21]. Studies analyzing whether the utilization of double-J ureteral stents during a kidney transplant procedure increases the risk of post-transplant UTI have produced conflicting results [22-24]. It has been suggested that a shorter duration (3 weeks versus 6 weeks) of ureteral stent placement may reduce the incidence of UTI [24].

The most common pathogens implicated in UTIs include *E. coli*, *Staphylococci*, *Enterococci*, *Enterobacter* and *Pseudomonas aeruginosa* [20, 25]. Despite routine treatment of asymptomatic bacteriuria, patients still develop symptomatic cystitis and pyelonephritis, and recurrent asymptomatic bacteriuria has been shown to be an independent risk factor for transplant pyelonephritis [16]. Recurrent UTI can also contribute to inflammation and fibrosis of the allograft [16, 26]. Bloodstream infections, the majority (75%) of which were due to a urinary source (*E. Coli* in 50% of infections) have also been shown to lead to allograft failure (either directly or by causing death) and all-cause mortality [27]. It is recommended that all UTI's in kidney transplant recipients be considered complicated, and thus short-term treatment regimens are not recommended [20].

2.1.2. Clostridium difficile associated diarrhea and colitis

Clostridium difficile associated diarrhea (CDAD) and *C. difficile* colitis are an increasingly important cause of morbidity and mortality after solid organ transplantation, with reported incidence of 0.5% to 16.0% of kidney transplant recipients [28-30]. CDAD tends to occur early in the post-transplant period, although later cases related to exposure to antibiotics or increased immunosuppression due to allograft rejection also occur. Transplant recipients are also at higher risk for fulminant *C. difficile* colitis as compared to the general population. CDAD is often difficult to eradicate completely, leading to recurrent infection, due to the fact that it is a spore forming bacterium.

Risk factors for CDAD include older age, antimicrobial exposure, and rabbit anti-thymocyte globulin induction therapy [30, 31]. For patients developing fulminiant CDAD, risk factors identified include peak leukocyte count of 25,000/mm^3 or greater and evidence of pancolitis on CT scan. For those developing fulminant CDAD, colectomy has been associated with improved patient and graft survival when compared to patients managed with medical therapy alone [30]. Medications that suppress gastric acid production, commonly used in transplant recipients, may also increase risk of CDAD [31].

The most commonly utilized diagnostic test for CDAD is *C. difficile* toxin detection in the stool via ELISA [31]. Antimicrobial management of CDAD includes oral metronidazole (first line for mild to moderate CDAD) or oral vancomycin (for severe CDAD), with intravenous (IV) metronidazole added in severe cases [31]. It is important to note that IV vancomycin does not penetrate the intestinal lumen, and is therefore ineffective for managment of CDAD. The removal or reduction in other antibiotics is an important adjunctive step. Surgery is often necessary in fulminant cases, in order to avoid colonic rupture. Other adjunctive therapies sometimes employed but with less supporting data include vancomycin enema, *Lactobacillus* probiotic supplementation, and intravenous immune globulin (IVIG) [5, 31]. An algorithm for management of patients with *C. difficile* infection can be found in reference [31].

2.1.3. *Tuberculosis*

Worldwide, the estimated incidence of tuberculosis (TB) (*Mycobacterium tuberculosis*) in kidney transplant recipients is 20 to 70 times that of the general population [32]. Treatment of active TB infection in transplant recipients is complicated due to drug interactions, antimicrobial resistance, and toxicity of the antimicrobials used for treatment of TB. Extrapulmonary involvement, atypical presentation, and limitations of the tuberculin skin test make diagnsois difficult. Although newer methods are available, which measure release of interferon γ (such as Quantiferon Gold), more data is needed regarding utilization of these assays in kidney transplant candidates and recipients [33].

Identification of high risk patients (those living in endemic areas or those with prior infection or exposure) is essential in order to administer prophylaxis with isoniazid (INH). A meta analysis of INH prophylaxis in kidney transplant recipients found that the relative risk of TB infection was significantly reduced, while risk of toxicity (hepatitis) did not differ between patients that did or did not receive prophylaxis [33]. Current European [34] and U.S. [35] guidelines recommend 9 months of INH prophylaxis for those with latent TB infection, however, the optimal timing of prophylaxis is unclear, particularly for patients awaiting a deceased donor transplant. When treating transplant recipients with active tuberculosis, close monitoring of calcineurin inhibitor levels with concomitant dose increase is needed due to presence of rifampin or related drugs in the anti-tuberculosis regimen [35].

2.1.4. *Prophylaxis of bacterial infection*

Trimethoprim/sulfamethoxazole (TMP/SMX), traditionally used for prophylaxis against *Pneumocystis jiroveci* pneumonia, has proven efficacy in reducing the incidence of UTIs, as well as bacteremias after transplantation [36, 37], although resisitance to common urinary tract pathogens is increasingly common in more recent years [16, 38]. TMP/SMX is also effective in preventing infections by *L monocytogenes*, *Nocardia* species, and *Toxoplasmosis gondii*, leading to recommendations for its use in all patients without contraindication to its use [2]. Therapy should continue for at least 6 months after transplantation, although the duration varies from center to center. In sulfa-allergic patients, alternatives to TMP/SMX include atovaquone, pentamidine, and dapsone. For patients not on TMP/SMX, ciprofloxacin (x 3 to 6 months) has been recommeded as UTI prophylaxis [20].

To prevent surgical wound and abdominal infections, the local perioperative antibacterial prophylaxis should be administered. The prophylactic antibiotic of choice should be determined by the resident flora of the transplanted, the prevalent bacterial flora identified in wound infections and the institutional antibiotic susceptibility pattern [39]. In kidney transplant recipients, the target pathogens include uropathogens and staphylococci; hence either a first-generation cephalosporin or ampicillin/sulbactam is an appropriate prophylactic agent. More recently, it has been suggested that due to the low incidence of surgical site infection observed in the absence of peri-operative antimicrobial prophylaxis, prophylaxis should only be used in higher risk patients (> 65 years of age and/or obese (defined as body mass index > 35)) in order to reduce resistance, adverse events, and cost [40]. Obesity, an established risk factor for wound complications, is often targeted prior to transplant. Interestingly, significant pre-transplant weight loss has also been identified as a risk factor for wound complications, attributed to body contour changes resulting in an unfavorable abdominal panniculus [41].

2.1.5. *Treatment of bacterial infection*

The antibiotic of choice for the treatment of infection after renal transplantation is largely dependent on the susceptibility of the bacteria identified in the urine, blood, or wound culture, and is very important due to increasing bacterial resisitance to commonly used antimicrobials. Fluoroquinolones, cephalosporins, or penicillins are commonly used to treat UTIs. For infections due to coagulase-negative staphylococci or ampicillin-resistant enterococci, vancomycin is utilized. Critically ill patients require intial broad spectrum antimicrobials, which should then be narrowed as culture results become available. Nephrotoxic agents (such as aminoglycosides) should be avoided whenever possible, relying on effective non-nephrotoxic alternatives instead.

Treatment duration depends on the origin and severity of infection. Wound infections and most UTIs require treatment for 5 to 7days, whereas pyelonephritis usually requires 2 weeks of therapy or longer. Imaging to rule out obstruction or anatomic abnormalities should be considered in cases of recurrent UTIs. In addition, wound infections may require debridement with an adjunctive antibiotic regimen. Patients with neutropenic fever may receive granulocyte colony stimulating growth factors, which have been shown not to increase the risk of acute rejection [5]. Depending on the severity of the infection, reduction in immunosuppression, with close monitoring of graft function, may also play an important role in clearing the infection.

2.2. Fungal infection

Invasive fungal infections are a significant infectious complication among solid-organ transplant recipients and remain a major cause of morbidity and mortality. Among all solid-organ transplant recipients, kidney transplantation is currently associated with the lowest rate of fungal infections, with a one-year cumulative incidence of 1.3% [46]. *Candida, Aspergillus,* and *Cryptococcus* are the most common fungal pathogens in solid-organ transplantation [42]. The Transplant-Associated Infection Surveillance Network (TRANSNET) reports that leading invasive fungal infections are candidiasis (49%), Cryptococcus (15%), Aspergillosis (14%), and endemic mycoses (10%) [43]. In this report, Pneumocystis represented only 1% of invasive fungal infections, likely demonstrating the effectiveness of prophylactic strategies.

Pneumocystis jiroveci pneumonia (PJP) usually occurs within the first 6 months after transplantation without prophylaxis. Risk factors for PJP include prior CMV infection, underlying pulmonary disease, allograft dysfunction, net state of immunosuppression, allograft rejection, and prolonged neutropenia [44, 45]. Recently, a nosocomial cluster of PJP was reported, spread via exposure in clinic waiting areas [44]. Universal prophylaxis against PJP is recommended for 6 to 12 months after transplant [45].

The most common pathogen is the *Candida* species, mostly *Candida albicans* or less commonly, *Candida glabrata, C. tropicalis, or C. parapsilosis* [43, 46]. Identifying the species of *Candida* is important for choosing appropriate antifungal agents, and *C. glabrata* should be tested for antifungal susceptibility, especially in areas with known resistance or if the infection is not responding to the initial therapy [43]. The majority of these infections occur within the first 2 months after transplantation, and occur as candidemia, UTI, or peritonitis [43]. Asymptomatic candiduria is generally not treated unless the patient is neutropenic or will be undergoing a urologic procedure, while symptomatic candiduria is usually treated [43, 47]. Imaging of the transplant kidney to rule out abscess in the collecting system or presence of fungus ball(s) is also recommended [43, 47]. Fluconazole is the only azole to concentrate in the urine, and so has an important role in the treatment of *Candida* UTI's.

Infections due to endemic fungi typically occur in the mid to late posttransplantation period, although some do occur within 2 months of transplant. Endemic fungal infections are associated with pathogens like *Histoplasma capsulatum, Blastomyces dermatitidis,* and *Coccidioides immitis*. For detailed review of the various types of fungal infections in solid organ transplantation, the reader is referred to references [42, 45, 46, 48-51]. Although rare, donor-derived fungal infections are important to consider; recent guidelines outline occurrence and management of such infections [48].

2.2.1. Prevention and treatment of fungal infections

Systemic prophylaxis of fungal infection is generally not required for kidney transplant recipients. Prevention of oral candidiasis is achieved through use of topical nystatin or clotrimazole. Multiple options are available for the treatment of invasive fungal infections in solid-organ transplantation, including amphotericin B (liposomal formulations preferred due to less nephrotoxicity), azole antifungals (fluconazole, itraconazole, voriconazole, posiconazole) and echinocandins (caspofunginm micafungin, anidulafungin). The optimal regimen should be based on antifungal susceptibility testing. Detailed review of these agents is beyond the scope of this chapter, however, a brief discussion of drug-drug interactions between antifungal agents and immunosuppressants is warranted, as well as mention of toxicities of concern in kidney transplant recipients (see Section 2.5).

2.3. Viral infection

Many factors affect the development of viral infection after solid-organ transplantation. These factors include recipient and donor serostatus, recipient comorbidities (eg, diabetes mellitus), immunosuppression regimen, organ(s) transplanted, ischemia-reperfusion injury to graft, and community-acquired infection. Viral infection can be particularly devastating to transplant recipients because of the immunosuppressive properties of the viral pathogens themselves, which may increase the patients' susceptibility to other opportunistic infection (particularly fungal infection), or posttransplant lymphoproliferative disease (PTLD).

2.3.1. Cytomegalovirus

Cytomegalovirus (CMV), a herpesvirus, is the most important viral infection in solid-organ transplantation because of its broad effects on immunocompromised patients [6]. Active infection produces not only signs and symptoms associated with the viral syndrome itself, but also has other widespread effects associated with cytokine-mediated inflammatory response and generation of cross-reactive T cells [52]. These effects may lead to allograft injury and/or acute rejection, systemic immunosuppression from the virus, and EBV-associated PTLD [6]. Risk factors for CMV infection/disease include CMV donor-positive/recipient-negative (D+/R-) serostatus pairs, recent treatment for acute rejection, recent completion of prophylactic antiviral therapy, and rabbit anti-thymocyte globulin induction therapy [53, 54]. In CMV D+/R- pairs, there may be an association between the use of CMV prophylaxis and improved graft survival and lower acute rejection rates [55].

Clinical Manifestations

Differentiation between CMV infection and CMV disease is important when assessing a patient for CMV. A patient with CMV infection has active viral replication in the blood or other body fluids, but does not necessarily experience systemic signs and symptoms such as malaise, fever, and pancytopenia. Patients with CMV disease, however, most commonly have a viral syndrome with fever or have invasive infection that has affected an organ system, such as colitis, hepatitis, or pneumonitis [56].

Diagnosis and Monitoring

CMV serology of the donor and recipient are useful for estimating the recipient's risk of CMV developing after transplantation, but is not useful for diagnosing CMV infection/disease because seroconversion often does not occur until after symptoms are resolved [10, 53, 57]. Rather, methods that quantify the extent of the CMV infection are necessary to make the diagnosis. Two common methods include CMV antigenemia (stain circulating neutrophils for CMV antigen) and CMV DNA polymerase chain reaction (PCR) (quantitative viral load) [58]. A major limitation of antigenemia is the need for sufficient quantities of neutrophils to perform the test, which is often not possible because of the neutropenia caused by the CMV virus itself. Therefore, the CMV viral load is a key diagnostic tool; trends in viral loads are more valuable than individual levels [57]. Viral load assays vary between laboratories, however, and assay standardization is needed. Another limitation includes the fact that peripheral viral load may be undetectable in patients with invasive CMV disease, particularly when the gastrointestinal tract and lungs are sites of infection. In these cases, biopsy of the infected tissue and/or bronchial alveolar lavage is often necessary to confirm diagnosis [57].

Prevention

Several strategies have been used to prevent and treat CMV. Some centers routinely provide antiviral prophylaxis (called universal prophylaxis) to patients at risk for CMV (particularly D+/R- pairs), whereas others employ preemptive strategies, in which patients are routinely monitored and receive prophylaxis only if laboratory markers become positive. Each method has benefits and drawbacks. Benefits of universal prophylaxis include preventing both CMV and other herpes viruses and lack of need for intensive monitoring. Drawbacks include the risk of developing ganciclovir-resistant CMV (although a small risk), adverse effects of the medications, the fact that late CMV disease may occur despite early prophylaxis (delayed onset), and the fact that the disease may have atypical features.

For preemptive strategies, benefits include decreasing the use of antivirals and their associated adverse effects and costs. However, the logistically demanding monitoring schedule, requirement for strict compliance to the costly surveillance methods, potential to develop CMV disease before detection, and development of drug resistance are disadvantages of preemptive strategies [57]. CMV-related morbidity is also a significant risk when adherence to monitoring guidelines is poor [59]. Drug resistance can occur if ganciclovir is used in a patient with active viral replication, owing to its poor oral bioavailability. A recent prospective randomized trial of pre-emptive therapy versus valganciclovir prophylaxis in CMV serostatus positive kidney transplant recipients found that both CMV infection and CMV disease were significantly higher in the pre-emptive group, in particular for D+/R+ patients [60]. The general consensus is that the highest risk patients (D+/R-) should receive universal prophylaxis [10, 61].

With the introduction of valganciclovir, a prodrug of ganciclovir with superior oral bioavailability, interest has focused on use of this agent to prevent and treat CMV infection and disease. For outpatients, valganciclovir 900 mg per day or ganciclovir 1000 mg three times per day are commonly used to prevent CMV [10]. Pharmacokinetic studies show that oral valganciclovir administration at 450 mg (given once daily) gives exposure that is equivalent to the standard oral regimen of ganciclovir (1 g administered 3 times a day) [62]. The manufacturer-recommended dose of valganciclovir for CMV prophylaxis is 900 mg/day, and this dose appears to be equivalent in efficacy to oral ganciclovir, with an increased incidence of neutropenia compared with ganciclovir [56]. In several studies, researchers have retrospectively evaluated the efficacy of low-dose valganciclovir (450 mg daily) as prophylaxis for CMV in kidney transplant recipients [63]. An analysis comparing 3 months of standard ganciclovir versus low dose valganciclovir in the prophylaxis of CMV in 129 kidney or pancreas transplant recipients revealed a 14% incidence of CMV disease at 1 year after transplantation (10% noninvasive and 4% invasive) [63]. The incidence was similar between patients receiving ganciclovir and valganciclovir, and risk factors for development of CMV disease included CMV D+/R- serostatus and use of thymoglobulin as part of immunosuppression regimen (incidence 25% in patients receiving thymoglobulin). The same investigators later reported outcomes in 37 kidney or pancreas recipients who received thymoglobulin induction and an extended course (6 months) of CMV prophylaxis with low-dose valganciclovir [64]. The incidence of CMV disease decreased in thymoglobulin-treated patients from 25% to 8% when prophylaxis was extended from 3 months to 6 months.

The duration of CMV prophylaxis also remains controversial; current recommendations suggest a minimum of 3 months of therapy [10]. Several studies have demonstrated a lower incidence of CMV disease after transplantation in patients receiving prophylaxis for 6 months, particularly in patients at highest risk for developing CMV [53, 64-67]. From a pharmacoeconomic perspective, prolonged (200 days vs. 100 days) valganciclovir prophylaxis for high-risk patients (D+/R-) has been shown to be cost-effective [68].

Treatment

Patients with CMV infection/disease should be treated with IV ganciclovir or oral valganciclovir; IV ganciclovir should be used in severe/life-threatening cases, and when gastrointestinal symptoms (such as diarrhea) may limit absorption of valganciclovir [10]. Ganciclovir (IV) is the gold standard for treatment due to the large body of experience with it and its lack of nephrotoxicity, which limits the use of other antiviral agents such as cidofovir and foscarnet. The treatment dose of 5 mg/kg IV every 12 hours must be adjusted for renal function; this adjustment should be done carefully, as subtherapeutic ganciclovir exposure in the setting of high CMV viral load may promote the development of resistance [57]. Because the bone marrow–suppressive effects of ganciclovir may further compound the neutropenia caused by the CMV virus itself, care should be exercised in adjusting the dose of ganciclovir to avoid these effects. Rather, use of white blood cell growth factors may be preferable in order to avoid the subtherapeutic ganciclovir exposure [57]. At a dose of 900 mg, valganciclovir provides exposure similar to that of 5 mg/kg body weight of IV ganciclovir, and can also be administered twice per day for treatment of active CMV infection [10, 62]. Thus, the cost of treating active CMV infection could be substantially lowered by its potential to treat with oral valganciclovir in the outpatient setting, for mild to moderate cases in patients not experiencing significant gastrointestinal symptoms (ie. diarrhea) [10]. Another key component of managing patients with CMV disease includes careful reduction in immunosuppression, taking into consideration patient and organ-specific factors. CMV immunoglobulin may also have an adjunctive role in treatment of severe CMV disease [10, 57].

Close monitoring of viral load is necessary to assess response to therapy; monitoring should begin 1 week after initiation of therapy and treatment should be continued until the viral load has been undetectable for 1 week [57]. The role of secondary prophylaxis after treatment is not clearly defined. When secondary prophylaxis is employed, viral load should be monitored for potential development of resistance and use of valganciclovir may be preferable owing to its superior bioavailability [57]. CMV disease recurs in approximately

15% to 35% of patients. Recurrence is due to incomplete suppression of CMV rather than the development of resistance. Patients at higher risk for recurrence include D+/R- pairs, multisystem CMV disease, those who receive treatment for acute rejection, patients with high viral loads at the time of initial diagnosis of the infection, and those who had a detectable viral load at the end of therapy for the initial infection [57].

Ganciclovir-resistant strains of CMV have developed in recent years, and are attributed to mutation of the UL97 +/- the UL54 gene(s), with the combined mutations leading to a high-level of ganciclovir resistance [10, 69]. Patients at highest risk for developing ganciclovir-resistant CMV include D+/R- pairs, as well as kidney-pancreas transplant recipients [57]. Utilization of pre-emptive strategies in D+/R- patients has been associated with development of GCV-resistance in more than 10% of patients [70]. Treatment of ganciclovir-resistant strains includes high-dose IV GCV, combination therapy with ganciclovir plus foscarnet, and CMV hyperimmunoglobulin [10, 57]. Increasing the ganciclovir dose (up to 10 mg/kg every 12 hours) with careful monitoring for toxic effects may also be useful in these patients [57]. An algorithm for management of ganciclovir resistance can be found in reference [10].

2.3.2. Varicella zoster virus

The adult seroprevalence rate for varicella zoster virus (VZV) in the United States is greater than 90%. Primary varicella infection is a risk for seronegative transplant recipients; adults are more likely to experience severe infection leading to complications such as hepatitis, pneumonitis, and encephalitis. In an analysis of herpes zoster (shingles) infection in the setting of modern immunosuppression, researchers evaluated 869 solid-organ transplants performed between 1994 and 1999, and the incidence of varicella zoster was 7.4% in kidney recipients. Herpes zoster infection occurred at a median of 9.0 months after transplantation and resulted in significant morbidity; 62.7% of cases were within 1 year of transplant. Independent risk factors for infection included induction therapy and antiviral therapy (other than >6 weeks of CMV prophylaxis with acyclovir or ganciclovir) [71].

Clinical Manifestations

Cutaneous scarring, defined as skin disfigurement (scarring or hypopigmentation), occurred in 18.7% of patients with herpes zoster, usually following a dermatomal pattern. Postherpetic neuralgia, defined as pain persisting more than 30 days after rash development, occurred in 42.7% of patients [71]. More serious manifestations of VZV infection may include pneumonitis, hepatitis, or encephalitis. This is especially true in primary infections, where morbidity and mortality may be high.

Diagnosis and Monitoring

Diagnosis of VZV infection typically involves clinical examination of skin lesions. Viral cultures, direct fluorescent antibody assays, or PCR testing may be used to confirm diagnosis when necessary [72].

Prevention

CMV prophylaxis with ganciclovir will most likely prevent VZV, although acyclovir is effective for those patients not receiving ganciclovir [72]. Patients who are VZV seronegative before transplantation should be vaccinated against varicella whenever possible, although pre-transplant administration of the herpes zoster vaccine, Zostavax is not recommended at this time due to a higher live-virus content [72]. The varicella vaccine should not be administered to patients receiving immunosuppressants, because the varicella vaccine is a live, attenuated vaccine that may cause infection in immunocompromised patients. After transplantation, seronegative patients exposed to VZV should receive postexposure prophylaxis, although this is not guaranteed to prevent infection. Postexposure prophylaxis consists of varicella zoster immunoglobulin if the patient arrives for treatment within 96 hours of initial exposure (preferred), or antiviral therapy if that 96-hour window has passed. However, the immunoglobulin preparation is no longer widely available to transplant centers, so IVIG may be utilized [72]. Although some centers have reported administration of the varicella vaccine after liver transplantation with minimal adverse effects [73], others have reported development of infection [74]. Therefore, this practice remains controversial and is not supported by existing guidelines [72].

Treatment

Patients with active, serious VZV infection should be treated with IV acyclovir, whereas less serious infections may be treated with oral acyclovir, valacyclovir, or famciclovir. In rare cases of acyclovir resistance, foscarnet may be used [72].

2.3.3. *Herpes simplex virus 1 and 2*

Adult seroprevalence rates for herpes simplex virus 1 and 2 in the U.S. are 62% and 22%, respectively. Most infections after transplantation are due to reactivation of latent virus.

Clinical Manifestations

Infection with herpes simplex virus generally is manifested by orolabial lesions or genital/perianal lesions, although more serious systemic infection can result in esophagitis, hepatitis, or pneumonitis.

Diagnosis and Monitoring

Diagnosis of infection with herpes simplex virus 1 or 2 typically involves clinical examination of skin lesions. Culture of scrapings/tissue from lesions may be necessary to confirm diagnosis in some cases, and PCR assays are increasingly being used [75].

Prevention and Treatment

CMV prophylaxis with ganciclovir will most likely prevent HSV; acyclovir is effective for those patients not receiving ganciclovir [59]. HSV infections are usually treated with oral acyclovir, valacyclovir, or famciclovir [75]. In more serious infections, IV acyclovir may be employed, although alternative therapy such as foscarnet may be required in cases of acyclovir resistance [75].

2.3.4. *Human herpesvirus 6, 7 and 8*

Human herpesvirus (HHV) 6 and 7 are viral pathogens that can cause significant morbidity and mortality in transplant recipients. Although HHV 6 infection has been most commonly reported among stem cell transplant recipients, cases have also been reported in solid-organ transplant recipients [76-78]. As with CMV, HHV 6 and 7 appear to have immunomodulatory effects and may predispose patients to secondary infection. Indeed, the mortality associated with HHV 6 appears to be related primarily to the development of secondary fungal infection [77, 78]. HHV 8 is also known as Kaposi sarcoma–associated herpesvirus because development of Kaposi sarcoma is driven by this virus. The seroprevalence of HHV 8 exhibits geographic variation; it is most common in the Mediterranean, Middle East, and some areas of Africa.

Clinical Manifestations

Transplant recipients with HHV 6 infection commonly have fever, bone marrow suppression, interstitial pneumonitis, and/or encephalitis. In addition, hepatitis and cutaneous rash have also been found in patients infected with HHV 6. Severe cases may progress to aplastic bone marrow and secondary infection with fungal and/or other viral pathogens. Symptoms associated with HHV 7 are not as well documented. Patients with HHV 8 may have cutaneous lesions, fever, and evidence of bone marrow suppression.

Diagnosis and Monitoring

Patients who are HHV 6–negative before transplantation appear to have a higher incidence of infection, although most cases are reactivations because more than 90% of patients are seropositive by adulthood. As with other viral illnesses, quantitative PCR is useful in diagnosis and in monitoring patients with this infection. HHV 8 serostatus of the donor and recipient may be assessed on the basis of geographic location. Patients who are seropositive before transplantation, who are at risk for primary infection, or who have Kaposi sarcoma can then be monitored after transplantation by means of HHV 8 viral loads [79].

Prevention and Treatment

Routine prophylaxis for HHV is not recommended [79]. Symptomatic patients may be treated with ganciclovir, foscarnet, or cidofovir, in combination with immunosuppression reduction [79]. For patients with Kaposi sarcoma, reduction and/or withdrawal of immunosuppression is first-line therapy, and conversion from calcineurin inhibitor therapy to sirolimus is also recommended due to regression of KS lesions after conversion [79]. Surgery, irradiation, and chemotherapy may be required in patients who do not respond to the reduction in immunosuppression.

2.3.5. *Epstein Barr virus*

EBV is a herpesvirus that infects most people at a young age and causes infectious mononucleosis. In immunocompromised patients, primary EBV infection or reactivation of latent infection can cause PTLD, a feared consequence of immunosuppressive therapy. Risk factors for the development of early PTLD include EBV seronegativity at the time of transplantation (leaving children at higher risk than adults), type of organ transplanted, type and degree of immunosuppression, CMV donor/recipient mismatch, CMV disease, and lymphocyte depleting antibody induction, while late PTLD may be related to duration of immunosuppression, type of organ transplanted, and older age of the recipient [80]. Kidney transplant recipients are considered low risk for development of PTLD (~1%). PTLD affects the transplant allograft in approximately 30% of cases. Lesions in the central nervous system are the most difficult to treat. In general, early occurrence of PTLD is polyclonal and easier to treat, whereas late PTLD is often monoclonal, and infected B cells may lose CD20 expression, making treatment difficult.

Clinical Manifestations

Signs and symptoms of PTLD may include those of a primary EBV infection/infectious mononucleosis, specifically fever, malaise, and swollen lymph nodes in the neck, tonsils, axilla, and/or groin. In addition, patients may have other nonspecific symptoms, depending on the type of organ transplanted.

Diagnosis and Monitoring

Diagnosis of PTLD is a combination of clinical assessment, blood tests, EBV-related blood tests, radiographic imaging, histology, and other adjunctive tests [80]. Pathological examination of tissue is the gold standard for the diagnosis of PTLD; excisional biopsies are preferred over needle biopsies. No specific staging system exists for PTLD; however, the current recommendation is to use the Ann Arbor staging classification system with Cotswold's modifications, which is used to stage non-Hodgkin lymphoma. Diagnosis is based on morphological classification, origin cell type, presence of EBV, and presence of CD20+ cells [80, 81].

Prevention

Because no definitive methods to prevent PTLD are known, diligent monitoring of high-risk patients is needed; this is done by performing serial EBV PCR. Risk is defined as high in D+/R- pairs, children, and patients receiving high dose and/or intensity immunosuppression [80, 81]. Utilization of ganciclovir/valganciclovir for CMV prophylaxis may give some protection, as ganciclovir has greater in vitro activity against EBV than acyclovir.

Treatment

Unfortunately, controlled trials in the treatment of PTLD are generally lacking. Key strategies for the management of patients with PTLD include reduction in immunosuppression, surgical resection, and local irradiation [80]. Secondary treatments may include antivirals, immunoglobulin, and monoclonal antibodies against B cells [80]. Anti-CD20 antibody (rituximab) is promising as first-line therapy after immunosuppression reduction because of its high specificity for B cells with a low adverse event profile. Cytotoxic chemotherapy (such as CHOP) is often used when first- and second-line therapies fail. Patients with CNS lesions may be treated with local radiotherapy, intrathecal anti-CD20 antibody, and/or interferon α [80]. EBV-specific cytotoxic T lymphocytes (CTL) may also have a role in the treatment of PTLD [82]. Patients may receive another transplant after successful treatment of PTLD; however, careful examination of patient-specific factors must occur.

2.3.6. Adenovirus

A concern mostly in children, adenovirus is a virus with many different serotypes that may cause diverse signs and symptoms during acute illness. Adenovirus is transmitted through respiratory secretions, fecal-oral route, and fomites; donor transmission has also been postulated in several reported cases. Adenovirus infection may occur in transplant recipients of any age; however, complications occur more commonly, and infections may be more severe in children [83].

Clinical Manifestations

Symptomatic disease can vary greatly, ranging from self-limiting febrile illness, to hemorrhagic cystitis or gastroenteritis, to severe infection with necrotizing hepatitis or pneumonia.

Diagnosis and Monitoring

The gold standard for diagnosis of adenovirus is by culture or antigen detection. In patients with invasive disease, tissue specimens can be examined for histology ("smudge cells" signaling cytopathic inclusions; the gold standard) or adenovirus PCR may be performed on the specimen [83].

Prevention and Treatment

No specific preventative measure is available, other than avoiding the spread of the virus via droplet and contact precautions for infected patients [83]. Supportive care, in conjunction with a decrease in immunosuppression is the standard of care for these patients. The use of antiviral agents such as ribavirin, ganciclovir, cidofovir, and respiratory syncytial virus immunoglobulin have been reported [83]. Cidofovir has the best data supporting its use, however its nephrotoxicity is an important concern in renal transplant recipients [83].

2.3.7. Human parvovirus B19

By adulthood, 30% to 60% of people are seropositive for parvovirus B19, an infection that usually is asymptomatic or manifests as a mild illness called erythema infectiosum in school-aged children and is commonly acquired through infected respiratory secretions. Parvovirus infects erythroid precursor cells, causing areticulocytic anemia in patients with severe infection.

Clinical Manifestations

Parvovirus infection develops in approximately 1% to 2% of transplant recipients, resulting in a pure red cell aplasia with a low or absent reticulocyte count. Other manifestations of the infection may include fever, arthralgia, rash, pancytopenia, and hepatitis.

Diagnosis and Monitoring

In transplant recipients, parvovirus B19 immunoglobulin M is a marker for ongoing infection, and parvovirus B19 DNA PCR may also be useful. Both have limitations, however, because transplant recipients may not be able to mount a response, making the serologic findings a less than ideal marker, whereas PCR may remain positive for up to 9 months after the initial infection. Therefore, the best diagnostic tool appears to be a positive PCR in a patient with pure red cell aplasia. Bone marrow biopsy may be considered for patients with signs and symptoms but negative serology and PCR [84].

Prevention and Treatment

No strategies are available to prevent parvovirus B19 infection in transplant recipients, although a vaccine is being developed [84]. The treatment of choice for parvovirus B19 infection is IVIG, although the optimal dosing regimen and duration of therapy are not clear. Current guidelines recommend 400 mg/kg/day for 5 days, possibly in conjunction with immunosuppression reduction [84].

2.3.8. Human papilloma virus

Patients with human papillomavirus (HPV) infection have an increased risk of cervical intraepithelial neoplasia (CIN) and cervical cancer, as well as risk for squamous cell cancers (SCC) of the anus, vulva, vagina, and penis [85]. The role of HPV in skin and oropharyngeal SCC is less clear [85]. The virus, in combination with exposure to ultraviolet radiation and the degree and length of immunosuppression are important factors in the development of cutaneous lesions. Viral warts may progress to these cancers in immunocompromised patients, with HPV DNA being found in 70% to 90% of cutaneous tissue in patients with SCC. Many strains of HPV exist, with HPV 5 and HPV 8 appearing to have a higher prevalence in transplant recipients with skin cancers.

Clinical Manifestations

Infected patients have cutaneous and anogenital warts (verruca vulgaris). Although less common, HPV may also be manifest as a respiratory tract infection.

Diagnosis and Monitoring

Diagnosis is made by examination of cutaneous warts during physical examination. Warts that look suspicious (eg, discolored) should be sampled by biopsy because of the known risk of malignant transformation of these lesions. In addition, suspicious anogenital warts should also be sampled, particularly as these lesions may be clinically indistinguishable from squamous epithelial lesions. Renal transplant candidates and recipients should have a pap smear yearly due to the increased risk of cervical cancer in this population [85]. HPV viral load by PCR is also utilized on clinical specimens.

Prevention

Patients with preexisting lesions should receive treatment before transplantation. An HPV vaccine has been developed, although its role prior to transplantation remains to be determined. Currently, it is recommended for use pre-transplant in the FDA-approved patient populations [85]. After transplantation, high-risk patients (those with a history of warts, keratoses, skin cancer, or long-term immunosuppression) should be followed up by a dermatologist every 3 to 6 months. Patients must be educated to avoid excessive sun exposure, to wear protective clothing when in the sun, and to use sunscreen to protect them. For those patients (or their partners) with anogenital lesions, sexual transmission should be avoided by abstinence or condoms (although condoms do not provide complete protection).

Treatment

It is recommended that warts causing physical and/or psychological signs or symptoms be treated with cytotoxic agents that destroy the infected epidermis, such as salicylic acid, lactic acid, or cryotherapy. In addition, surgical removal and physical ablation are often employed; a more rare treatment includes stimulation of the local immune response in the infected area [85].

2.3.9. Polyomavirus

Polyomavirus nephropathy (PVN) is a significant cause of morbidity and graft loss in renal transplant recipients, and is described in great detail in another chapter of this textbook.

2.3.10. Hepatitis B

Chronic hepatitis B virus (HBV) infection was traditionally considered a risk factor for poorer patient and graft survival after kidney transplantation [86]. In the more recent era, which is distinguished by the availability of oral anti-viral agents, analysis of OPTN/UNOS data has shown equivalent patient and graft survival in HBV(+) versus HBV(-) kidney transplant recipients [87]. The risk of liver failure does, however, continue to be increased in HBV(+) patients [87].

Diagnosis and Monitoring

HBV(+) patients on anti-viral therapy should be monitored every three months after transplantation, specifically for viral load (HBV DNA) and ALT, both to monitor efficacy as well as assess for development of resistance [88]. In addition, those with cirrhosis should be monitored yearly for development of hepatocellular carcinoma (HCC) via hepatic ultrasound and alpha fetoprotein [88].

Prevention and Treatment

All patients should be vaccinated against HBV, preferably before beginning dialysis due to poorer immune response to the vaccine in dialysis and transplant patients [89]. Re-vaccination should occur when hepatitis B surface antibody titers fall below 10 mIU/mL [88]. Utilization of nucleoside or nucleotide analogues to suppress HBV viral load in HBV-infected kidney transplant recipients has led to reduction in mortality, although development of hepatocellular carcinoma still exists and requires routine monitoring [90]. All HBV surface antigen positive transplant recipients should receive prophylaxis with tenofovir, entecavir, or lamivudine, although concerns over lamivudine resistance limit its use [88]. Use of interferon therapy after transplant is not recommended due to risk of precipitating rejection [88].

2.3.11. Hepatitis C

Hepatitis C is the leading indication for liver transplantation in the United States, and up to 38% of kidney transplant recipients worldwide have hepatitis C infection [91]. Hepatitis C infection is associated with poorer patient and graft survival after kidney transplantation as compared to Hepatitis C(-) patients, however, outcome after transplant is better than remaining on dialysis [92]. As with hepatitis B, it is important to clear the virus or decrease viral load before transplantation due to risk of rejection with post-transplant interferon.

Monitoring

After transplant, the ALT of HCV(+) patients should be monitored monthly for 6 months, and then every 3 to 6 months thereafter [88].

Treatment

Use of interferon therapy after kidney transplantation is not recommended due to risk of precipitating rejection, and should be used only when benefit clearly outweighs the risk of rejection [88]. This may include patients with fibrosing cholestatic hepatitis or life-threatening vasculitis. The use of newer oral agents for hepatitis C (including telaprevir and boceprevir) is contraindicated in transplant recipients due to lack of research studies [93]. Pharmacokinetic studies conducted in healthy volunteers have demonstrated significant drug interactions between telaprevir and cyclosporine or tacrolimus, which could lead to life-threatening toxicity [93, 94].

2.3.12. Less common but significant viral infections after transplantation

Novel Influenza A (H1N1) is a swine-origin influenza A virus that became a pandemic in 2009. In kidney transplant recipients, H1N1 caused significant morbidity and mortality [95-98], and mortality is higher in transplant recipients compared to the general population [97]. More severe cases develop pneumonia and may require ICU admission and ventilator support. Poorer outcomes are associated with delayed introduction of treatment; oseltamivir has been used to successfully treat transplant recipients with H1N1 [96-98].

West Nile Virus (WNV) is a single-stranded RNA virus of the Flaviviridae family that is transmitted to humans by mosquitoes. Since 1999, an increasing number of cases have occurred in North America. A limited number of severe cases have been reported in solid-organ transplant recipients, causing morbidity and mortality. Compared with the general population, where the infection rate for WNV was 5 per 100,000, the rate in transplant recipients was 200 per 100,000 ($P < .001$) [99]. A seroprevalence study found a 0.25% seroprevalence and a resultant 40% risk of meningoencephalitis in a transplant patient with community acquired WNV [100]. Similar studies of immunocompetent persons estimate the risk of meningoencephalitis to be less than 1%. Transmission through infected blood transfusion and/or transplanted organ is a risk [101]. Clinical signs and symptoms of infection in transplant recipients included fever, confusion, headache, weakness, encephalitis, and meningitis [99].

Based on the limited number of cases of WNV infection in transplant recipients, it appears that delayed seroconversion due to immunosuppression may occur, leading to delayed diagnosis. Other diagnostic methods such as PCR may be used, although that method is not useful in all patients [99]. Transplant recipients should be educated about the risks of WNV infection, particularly in endemic areas. Patients should be encouraged to use insect repellant and to avoid the outdoors during the periods of dawn and dusk, when mosquitoes are most active. Treatment of WMV in recipients of solid-organ transplants has generally been empiric and supportive. Both interferon and ribavirin have in vitro activity against WNV, but available data are not sufficient to associate use of these agents with clinical outcome. In addition, IVIG may be useful. Reduction or discontinuation of immunosuppression, based on the clinical situation, is most likely important adjunct treatment.

Lymphocytic choriomeningitis virus (LCMV) is a rodent-borne, Old World arenavirus. Four clusters of LCMV infection in solid-organ transplant recipients have been reported, with some cases specifically linked to donor transmission of the virus [102, 103]. Liver function and coagulation abnormalities, transplant organ dysfunction, fever, rash, diarrhea, hyponatremia, thrombocytopenia, hypoxia, and renal failure are manifestations of the infection that develop in transplant recipients of infected organs. The mortality rate is high. LCMV is very rare; no routine screening is performed on organ donors. LCMV antibodies, immunohistochemistry, PCR, and viral culture may be used for diagnosis in suspected cases [102]. Treatment with IV ribavirin, in combination with reduction in immunosuppression, may have been beneficial in the 1 surviving patient of the outbreak described in reference [102].

2.3.13. Vaccination in solid-organ transplant candidates and recipients

Because of the likelihood of poor response to vaccines after transplantation due to inability to mount an optimal effective response, it is very important to have all vaccinations up to date before transplantation, and to carefully consider timing of administration in the post-transplant period [104]. Influenza (inactivated) and pneumococcal vaccines should be given at their recommended schedules after transplantation, in order to confer as much protection to the patient as possible [105]. Household contacts of transplant patients should also receive the inactivated influenza vaccine on an annual basis. Live vaccines should be avoided in transplant recipients, however their household contacts may receive live vaccines if necessary, with the exception of smallpox and oral-poliovirus vaccines [105]. More details about vaccination can be found in other chapters within this book.

2.4. Parasitic infection

Reactivation of latent parasitic infection in previously infected patients or de novo infection by natural means or through the donated organs is of increasing concern in the transplant community. Multiple factors are contributing to increased incidence, including the presence of transplant centers in endemic areas, donor and/or recipient travel from endemic areas to Western countries for transplant, transplant tourism, immigrants with latent infection, leisure travel by recipients, and use of non-cyclosporine based immune regimens [106]. Parasitic diseases affecting transplant recipients are outlined in Table 1.

Classification	Parasitic Infection	Clinical Presentation in Transplant Recipients	Comments
Protozoa: Non-Intestinal	Toxoplasmosis (*Toxoplasma gondii*)	Brain abscess, chorioretinitis, pneumonitis, disseminated disease	PJP prophylaxis with TMP/SMX covers Toxoplasmosis
	Chagas Disease *Trypanosoma cruzi*	Panniculitis or other subcutaneous involvement; myocarditis and encephalitis less common	Donors from indiginous areas should be tested
	Leishmania (Old World and New World)	Visceral: fever, enlarged spleen, pancytopenia, malabsorption, interstitial pneumonitis	Mortality usually related to bacterial superinfection
	Malaria (*Plasmodium* species)	Fever, hemolysis, thrombocytopenia	Identification of species important for treatment due to resistance patterns
	Babesiosis (*Babesia* species)	Fever, malaise, hemolytic anemia, possible adult respiratory distress syndrome	May be difficult to distinguish babesiosis from malaria; morphology and DNA testing used to distinguish
	Acanthamoeba	Keratitis, granulomatous amoebic encephalitis, pulmonary lesions, cutaneous lesions, sinusitis, disseminated disease	Biopsy diagnosis of cutaneous lesions and cerebrospinal fluid examination essential for diagnosis
Protozoa: Intestinal	*Blastocystis hominis, Cryptosporidium, Cyclospora, Giardia, Isospora belli, Microsporidia*	Gastroenteritis, eosinophilia	Difficult to eradicate; reduction in immunosuppression may be important in clearing infection. Reduce risk by drinking only municipal or bottled water
	Entamoeba histolytica	Amebic colitis, liver abscess; less commonly pulmonary, cardiac, brain involvement	Reduce risk by drinking only municipal or bottled water
Intestinal Nematode	*Strongyloides stercoralis*	Pulmonary involvement, bacterial sepsis/meningitis (Gram negative GI organisms), acute, severe abdominal disease, eosinophilia	Difficult to eradicate; high mortality with disseminated infection

Classification	Parasitic Infection	Clinical Presentation in Transplant Recipients	Comments
Trematodes	Schistosomiasis (*Schistosoma* species)	Abdominal pain, anorexia, diarrhea; hematuria, dysuria, urinary frequency; fibrosis of liver or bladder and ureters	Reduce risk by avoiding fresh water in endemic regions
Cestodes	Echinococcosis (*Echinococcus*)	Liver failure; possible extrahepatic involvement in lungs, brain	May be difficult to distinguish from hepatic malignancy

Table 1. Parasitic diseases affecting transplant recipients

2.5. Drug-drug interactions and toxicities of anti-infective agents

There are a number of clinically significant drug interactions and toxicities that must be considered when treating infection in the transplant population (see Table 2). Drug levels of several of the primary immunosuppressants must therefore be monitored frequently and dose adjustment is needed to achieve the desired level of the immunosuppressant [107]. This is important to remember both when initiating and discontinuing therapy.

Anti-Infective Agent/Class	Drug Interactions or Important Toxicities in the Transplant Population	Additional Information
Azole Antifungals (systemic)	Increase levels of cyclosporine, tacrolimus, sirolimus and everolimus via Cytochrome P450 3A4 inhibition	Empiric dose adjustment of immunosuppressant is recommended when initiating azole therapy
Clotrimazole (topical) [108, 109]	Increase levels of tacrolimus (and possibly others) via Cytochrome P450 3A4 inhibition in the gut	Dose adjustment often necessary
Amphotericin B	Enhanced nephrotoxicity	When therapy needed for invasive fungal infection, liposomal formulations preferred to reduce risk of nephrotoxicity
Aminoglycosides	Enhanced nephrotoxicity	Avoid when possible
Macrolide antibiotics	Increase levels of cyclosporine, tacrolimus, sirolimus and everolimus via Cytochrome P450 3A4 inhibition Effect most pronounced with erythromycin and clarithromycin; more rare with azithromycin	Empiric dose adjustment of immunosuppressant is recommended when initiating macrolide therapy, particularly erythromycin or clarithromycin

Anti-Infective Agent/Class	Drug Interactions or Important Toxicities in the Transplant Population	Additional Information
Rifamycins	Decrease levels of cyclosporine, tacrolimus, sirolimus and everolimus via Cytochrome P450 3A4 induction	Empiric dose adjustment of immunosuppressant is recommended when initiating rifamycin therapy
Ganciclovir, Valganciclovir	Enhanced bone marrow suppression	Monitor WBC and platelet counts
Foscarnet, Cidofovir	Enhanced nephrotoxicity	Avoid when possible

Table 2. Important Drug Interactions and Toxicities with Anti-Infective Agents and Immunosuppressants

3. Malignancy

The net state of immunosuppression also affects the development of post-transplant malignancy. This includes not only *de novo* malignancy, but also recurrence of pre-transplant lesions. As seen in Table 3, a significant number of cancers are related to oncogenic viral infections. The Transplant Cancer Match Study assessed cancer risk in more than 175,000 solid organ transplant recipients, as compared to the general population [97]. It is important to note that this analysis includes only patients transplanted in the U.S., and the importance of biliary tract and bladder cancers due to parasitic infection outside of the U.S. are not represented in the analysis. In addition, non-melanoma skin cancers are not included in the analysis. Overall, transplant recipients had a cancer risk twice that of the general population. For kidney transplant recipients, the standardized incidence ratio for the most common malignancies seen across all transplant recipients regardless of organ was highest for kidney cancer (6.66), non-Hodgkin lymphoma (6.05) and lung cancer (1.46).

Non-melanoma skin cancers are the most common malignancy seen in the organ transplant population, and the incidence of these cancers is 3 to 5 times that of the general population. Although both basal (BCC) and squamous cell carcinoma (SCC) occur, SCC tends to occur more frequently in transplant recipients, as compared to a predominance of BCC in the general population. Both SCC and BCC occur at a younger age when compared to the general population. In addition, SCC tends to be more aggressive in transplant recipients as compared to the course in the general population [110]. This includes an increased number of primary tumors, deep tissue spread, perineural and lymphatic invasion, recurrence, and need for radiation or chemotherapy [110]. Guidelines for the management of transplant patients with SCC were published in 2004 [111]. Recurrent, de novo and donor-transmitted melanoma are also a concern in transplant recipients [112]. Guidelines for proposed reduction in immunosuppression for transplant patients with skin cancers are available [113].

Renal cell carcinoma (RCC) of the native kidney(s) is diagnosed in 0.3% to 4.8% of kidney transplant recipients [114, 115], and in the transplant kidney in approximately 0.2% [116].

Patients with pre-transplant cystic lesions are more likely to develop RCC by three years after transplant compared to those without (2.3% vs. 0.7%, respectively) [115]. Risk factors for developing RCC after transplant have included pre-transplant cystic disease/lesions, male gender, African-American race, older recipients (> 65 years at transplant), longer time on dialysis prior to transplant, older donor age (> 55 years), and treatment of acute rejection within 1 year of transplant [114, 115]. Most cases of RCC have papillary or clear cell histology, and RCC in one kidney is associated with RCC in the contralateral native kidney. Most cases are diagnosed incidentally, are low-grade, and are managed by native nephrectomy. More aggressive tumors may require chemotherapy, minimization or change in immunosuppression, and/or radiation. Interestingly, the mTOR inhibitor everolimus is FDA-approved as second line therapy for advanced RCC, and thus may be a preferred immunosuppressant in this setting.

Historically, post-transplant lymphoproliferative disorder (PTLD) has been a major concern for solid organ transplant recipients. A recent analysis of Scientific Registry of Transplant Recipients (SRTR) data for 156,740 kidney transplant recipients found an incidence of 0.7% at 5 years and 1.4% at 10 years [117]. This analysis, similar to prior reports, showed a clear distinction between early (less than 2 years after transplant) and late-onset (more than 2 years) PTLD. Risk factors for early PTLD on multivariate analysis include age 19 or younger at transplant, non-Hispanic white ethnicity, EBV negative serostatus at transplant, and CMV negative serostatus at transplant, while risk factors for late PTLD include age 19 or younger or 50 years or older at transplant and non-Hispanic white ethnicity. The use of induction therapy, including when the analysis was limited to T cell depleting agents, did not increase the risk of PTLD. In addition to PTLD, elderly transplant recipients are at increased risk for various hematologic malignancies [118]. Treatment of PTLD may include reduction in immunosuppression, surgery, anti-viral therapy, chemotherapy (including immunochemotherapy (rituximab)), and/or radiation.

Infectious Agent	Associated Sites/Types of Cancer
Epstein Barr Virus (EBV)	Non-Hodgkin Lymphoma, Hodgkin Lymphoma, PTLD, Nasopharyngeal
Human Papillomavirus	Cervix, Vulva, Vagina, Penis, Anus, Oropharynx
Hepatitis B and Hepatitis C	Liver
Human Herpesvirus 8 (HHV8)	Kaposi sarcoma
Helicobacter pylori	Stomach

Table 3. Oncogenic Infectious Agents

4. Conclusion

In summary, complications of over-immunosuppression after solid-organ transplantation can lead to significant morbidity and mortality if not promptly diagnosed and treated. However, the growing armamentarium of knowledge, diagnostic tools and therapeutic agents available for the prevention and treatment of these infections and malignancies will continue to improve the quality of care for these patients.

Author details

Meredith J. Aull, Cheguevara Afaneh and Sandip Kapur
Department of Surgery, Division of Transplant Surgery,
NewYork-Presbyterian Hospital/Weill Cornell Medical College, New York, NY, USA

5. References

[1] Snydman, D.R., *Infection in solid organ transplantation.* Transpl Infect Dis, 1999. 1(1): p. 21-8.

[2] Fishman, J.A. and A.S.T.I.D.C.o. Practice, *Introduction: infection in solid organ transplant recipients.* Am J Transplant, 2009. 9 Suppl 4: p. S3-6.

[3] *U S Renal Data System, USRDS 2011 Annual Data Report: Atlas of Chronic Kidney Disease and End-Stage Renal Disease in the United States, National Institutes of Health, National Institute of Diabetes and Digestive and Kidney Diseases, Bethesda, MD, 2011.*

[4] Parasuraman, R., et al., *Increasing trend in infection-related death-censored graft failure in renal transplantation.* Transplantation, 2011. 91(1): p. 94-9.

[5] Avery, R.K., *Infectious disease following kidney transplant: core curriculum 2010.* Am J Kidney Dis, 2010. 55(4): p. 755-71.

[6] Fishman, J.A. and R.H. Rubin, *Infection in organ-transplant recipients.* N Engl J Med, 1998. 338(24): p. 1741-51.

[7] van Delden, C., E.A. Blumberg, and A.S.T.I.D.C.o. Practice, *Multidrug resistant gram-negative bacteria in solid organ transplant recipients.* Am J Transplant, 2009. 9 Suppl 4: p. S27-34.

[8] Garzoni, C. and A.S.T.I.D.C.o. Practice, *Multiply resistant gram-positive bacteria methicillin-resistant, vancomycin-intermediate and vancomycin-resistant Staphylococcus aureus (MRSA, VISA, VRSA) in solid organ transplant recipients.* Am J Transplant, 2009. 9 Suppl 4: p. S41-9.

[9] Munoz, P. and A.S.T.I.D.C.o. Practice, *Multiply resistant gram-positive bacteria: vancomycin-resistant enterococcus in solid organ transplant recipients.* Am J Transplant, 2009. 9 Suppl 4: p. S50-6.

[10] Humar, A., D. Snydman, and A.S.T.I.D.C.o. Practice, *Cytomegalovirus in solid organ transplant recipients.* Am J Transplant, 2009. 9 Suppl 4: p. S78-86.

[11] Patel, R. and C.V. Paya, *Infections in solid-organ transplant recipients.* Clin Microbiol Rev, 1997. 10(1): p. 86-124.

[12] Nishi, S.P., V.G. Valentine, and S. Duncan, *Emerging bacterial, fungal, and viral respiratory infections in transplantation.* Infect Dis Clin North Am, 2010. 24(3): p. 541-55.

[13] Kotton, C.N., P.L. Hibberd, and A.S.T.I.D.C.o. Practice, *Travel medicine and the solid organ transplant recipient.* Am J Transplant, 2009. 9 Suppl 4: p. S273-81.

[14] Paya, C.V. and P.E. Hermans, *Bacterial infections after liver transplantation.* Eur J Clin Microbiol Infect Dis, 1989. 8(6): p. 499-504.

[15] Vidal, E., et al., *Bacterial urinary tract infection after solid organ transplantation in the RESITRA cohort.* Transpl Infect Dis, 2012 doi: 10.1111/j.1399-3062.2012.00744.x. [Epub ahead of print].

[16] Fiorante, S., et al., *Systematic screening and treatment of asymptomatic bacteriuria in renal transplant recipients.* Kidney Int, 2010. 78(8): p. 774-81.

[17] Peterson, P.K., et al., *Fever in renal transplant recipients: causes, prognostic significance and changing patterns at the University of Minnesota Hospital.* Am J Med, 1981. 71(3): p. 345-51.

[18] Wyner, L.M., *The evaluation and management of urinary tract infections in recipients of solid-organ transplants.* Semin Urol, 1994. 12(2): p. 134-9.

[19] Lorenz, E.C. and F.G. Cosio, *The impact of urinary tract infections in renal transplant recipients.* Kidney Int, 2010. 78(8): p. 719-21.

[20] Rice, J.C., N. Safdar, and A.S.T.I.D.C.o. Practice, *Urinary tract infections in solid organ transplant recipients.* Am J Transplant, 2009. 9 Suppl 4: p. S267-72.

[21] Esezobor, C.I., P. Nourse, and P. Gajjar, *Urinary tract infection following kidney transplantation: frequency, risk factors and graft function.* Pediatr Nephrol, 2012. 27(4): p. 651-7.

[22] Mathe, Z., et al., *Stented Ureterovesical Anastomosis in Renal Transplantation: Does it Influence the Rate of Urinary Tract Infections?* Eur J Med Res, 2010. 15(7): p. 297-302.

[23] Fayek, S.A., et al., *Ureteral stents are associated with reduced risk of ureteral complications after kidney transplantation: a large single center experience.* Transplantation, 2012. 93(3): p. 304-8.

[24] Huang, L., et al., *A comparative study of 3-week and 6-week duration of double-j stent placement in renal transplant recipients.* Urol Int, 2012. 89(1): p. 89-92.

[25] Villacian, J.S. and C.V. Paya, *Prevention of infections in solid organ transplant recipients.* Transpl Infect Dis, 1999. 1(1): p. 50-64.

[26] Ciszek, M., et al., *Urine cytokines profile in renal transplant patients with asymptomatic bacteriuria.* Transplantation, 2006. 81(12): p. 1653-7.

[27] Al-Hasan, M.N., et al., *Impact of Gram-negative bloodstream infection on long-term allograft survival after kidney transplantation.* Transplantation, 2011. 91(11): p. 1206-10.

[28] Stelzmueller, I., et al., *Clostridium difficile colitis in solid organ transplantation--a single-center experience.* Dig Dis Sci, 2007. 52(11): p. 3231-6.

[29] Apaydin, S., et al., *Prevalence of clostridium difficile toxin in kidney transplant recipients.* Scand J Infect Dis, 1998. 30(5): p. 542.

[30] Boutros, M., et al., *Clostridium difficile colitis: increasing incidence, risk factors, and outcomes in solid organ transplant recipients.* Transplantation, 2012. 93(10): p. 1051-7.

[31] Dubberke, E.R., D.J. Riddle, and A.S.T.I.D.C.o. Practice, *Clostridium difficile in solid organ transplant recipients.* Am J Transplant, 2009. 9 Suppl 4: p. S35-40.

[32] Munoz, P., C. Rodriguez, and E. Bouza, *Mycobacterium tuberculosis infection in recipients of solid organ transplants.* Clin Infect Dis, 2005. 40(4): p. 581-7.

[33] Currie, A.C., S.R. Knight, and P.J. Morris, *Tuberculosis in renal transplant recipients: the evidence for prophylaxis.* Transplantation, 2010. 90(7): p. 695-704.

[34] Transplantation, E.E.G.o.R., *European best practice guidelines for renal transplantation. Section IV: Long-term management of the transplant recipient.* Nephrol Dial Transplant, 2002. 17 Suppl 4: p. 1-67.

[35] Subramanian, A., S. Dorman, and A.S.T.I.D.C.o. Practice, *Mycobacterium tuberculosis in solid organ transplant recipients.* Am J Transplant, 2009. 9 Suppl 4: p. S57-62.

[36] Foxman, B., *Recurring urinary tract infection: incidence and risk factors.* Am J Public Health, 1990. 80(3): p. 331-3.

[37] Tolkoff-Rubin, N.E., et al., *A controlled study of trimethoprim-sulfamethoxazole prophylaxis of urinary tract infection in renal transplant recipients.* Rev Infect Dis, 1982. 4(2): p. 614-8.

[38] Giullian, J.A., K. Cavanaugh, and H. Schaefer, *Lower risk of urinary tract infection with low-dose trimethoprim/sulfamethoxazole compared to dapsone prophylaxis in older renal transplant patients on a rapid steroid-withdrawal immunosuppression regimen.* Clin Transplant, 2010. 24(5): p. 636-42.

[39] Soave, R., *Prophylaxis strategies for solid-organ transplantation.* Clin Infect Dis, 2001. 33 Suppl 1: p. S26-31.

[40] Laftavi, M.R., et al., *Universal perioperative antimicrobial prophylaxis is not necessary in kidney transplantation.* Clin Transplant, 2012. 26(3): p. 437-42.

[41] Kuo, J.H., et al., *Renal transplant wound complications in the modern era of obesity.* J Surg Res, 2012. 173(2): p. 216-23.

[42] Singh, N., G. Forrest, and A.S.T.I.D.C.o. Practice, *Cryptococcosis in solid organ transplant recipients.* Am J Transplant, 2009. 9 Suppl 4: p. S192-8.

[43] Pappas, P.G., et al., *Invasive fungal infections among organ transplant recipients: results of the Transplant-Associated Infection Surveillance Network (TRANSNET).* Clin Infect Dis, 2010. 50(8): p. 1101-11.

[44] Phipps, L.M., et al., *Nosocomial Pneumocystis jirovecii pneumonia: lessons from a cluster in kidney transplant recipients.* Transplantation, 2011. 92(12): p. 1327-34.

[45] Martin, S.I., J.A. Fishman, and A.S.T.I.D.C.o. Practice, *Pneumocystis pneumonia in solid organ transplant recipients.* Am J Transplant, 2009. 9 Suppl 4: p. S227-33.

[46] Pappas, P.G., F.P. Silveira, and A.S.T.I.D.C.o. Practice, *Candida in solid organ transplant recipients.* Am J Transplant, 2009. 9 Suppl 4: p. S173-9.

[47] Pappas, P.G., et al., *Clinical practice guidelines for the management of candidiasis: 2009 update by the Infectious Diseases Society of America.* Clin Infect Dis, 2009. 48(5): p. 503-35.

[48] Singh, N., et al., Donor-Derived Fungal Infections in Organ Transplant Recipients: Guidelines of the American Society of Transplantation, Infectious Diseases Community of Practice(dagger). Am J Transplant, 2012 doi: 10.1111/j.1600-6143.2012.04100.x. Epub 2012 Jun 13.

[49] Singh, N., S. Husain, and A.S.T.I.D.C.o. Practice, *Invasive aspergillosis in solid organ transplant recipients.* Am J Transplant, 2009. 9 Suppl 4: p. S180-91.

[50] Proia, L., R. Miller, and A.S.T.I.D.C.o. Practice, *Endemic fungal infections in solid organ transplant recipients.* Am J Transplant, 2009. 9 Suppl 4: p. S199-207.

[51] Kubak, B.M., S.S. Huprikar, and A.S.T.I.D.C.o. Practice, *Emerging & rare fungal infections in solid organ transplant recipients.* Am J Transplant, 2009. 9 Suppl 4: p. S208-26.

[52] Kotton, C.N. and J.A. Fishman, *Viral infection in the renal transplant recipient.* J Am Soc Nephrol, 2005. 16(6): p. 1758-74.
[53] Luan, F.L., et al., *Choice of induction regimens on the risk of cytomegalovirus infection in donor-positive and recipient-negative kidney transplant recipients.* Transpl Infect Dis, 2010. 12(6): p. 473-9.
[54] Razonable, R.R., et al., *Allograft rejection predicts the occurrence of late-onset cytomegalovirus (CMV) disease among CMV-mismatched solid organ transplant patients receiving prophylaxis with oral ganciclovir.* J Infect Dis, 2001. 184(11): p. 1461-4.
[55] Opelz, G., B. Dohler, and A. Ruhenstroth, *Cytomegalovirus prophylaxis and graft outcome in solid organ transplantation: a collaborative transplant study report.* Am J Transplant, 2004. 4(6): p. 928-36.
[56] Paya, C., et al., *Efficacy and safety of valganciclovir vs. oral ganciclovir for prevention of cytomegalovirus disease in solid organ transplant recipients.* Am J Transplant, 2004. 4(4): p. 611-20.
[57] Preiksaitis, J.K., et al., *Canadian society of transplantation consensus workshop on cytomegalovirus management in solid organ transplantation final report.* Am J Transplant, 2005. 5(2): p. 218-27.
[58] Snydman, D.R., *Posttransplant microbiological surveillance.* Clin Infect Dis, 2001. 33 Suppl 1: p. S22-5.
[59] Kunzle, N., et al., *Preemptive treatment approach to cytomegalovirus (CMV) infection in solid organ transplant patients: relationship between compliance with the guidelines and prevention of CMV morbidity.* Transpl Infect Dis, 2000. 2(3): p. 118-26.
[60] Witzke, O., et al., *Valganciclovir prophylaxis versus preemptive therapy in cytomegalovirus-positive renal allograft recipients: 1-year results of a randomized clinical trial.* Transplantation, 2012. 93(1): p. 61-8.
[61] Fishman, J.A., *Prophylaxis, preemption and drug resistance in CMV infection: too little, too much or just right?* Am J Transplant, 2012. 12(1): p. 13-4.
[62] Pescovitz, M.D., et al., *Valganciclovir results in improved oral absorption of ganciclovir in liver transplant recipients.* Antimicrob Agents Chemother, 2000. 44(10): p. 2811-5.
[63] Akalin, E., et al., *Cytomegalovirus disease in high-risk transplant recipients despite ganciclovir or valganciclovir prophylaxis.* Am J Transplant, 2003. 3(6): p. 731-5.
[64] Akalin, E., et al., *Decreased incidence of cytomegalovirus infection in thymoglobulin-treated transplant patients with 6 months of valganciclovir prophylaxis.* Am J Transplant, 2004. 4(1): p. 148-9.
[65] Gabardi, S., et al., *Efficacy and safety of low-dose valganciclovir for prevention of cytomegalovirus disease in renal transplant recipients: a single-center, retrospective analysis.* Pharmacotherapy, 2004. 24(10): p. 1323-30.
[66] Taber, D.J., et al., *Valganciclovir prophylaxis in patients at high risk for the development of cytomegalovirus disease.* Transpl Infect Dis, 2004. 6(3): p. 101-9.
[67] Doyle, A.M., et al., *24-week oral ganciclovir prophylaxis in kidney recipients is associated with reduced symptomatic cytomegalovirus disease compared to a 12-week course.* Transplantation, 2006. 81(8): p. 1106-11.

[68] Blumberg, E.A., et al., *Prolonged prophylaxis with valganciclovir is cost effective in reducing posttransplant cytomegalovirus disease within the United States.* Transplantation, 2010. 90(12): p. 1420-6.

[69] Hantz, S., et al., *Drug-resistant cytomegalovirus in transplant recipients: a French cohort study.* J Antimicrob Chemother, 2010. 65(12): p. 2628-40.

[70] Couzi, L., et al., *High incidence of anticytomegalovirus drug resistance among D+R- kidney transplant recipients receiving preemptive therapy.* Am J Transplant, 2012. 12(1): p. 202-9.

[71] Gourishankar, S., et al., *Herpes zoster infection following solid organ transplantation: incidence, risk factors and outcomes in the current immunosuppressive era.* Am J Transplant, 2004. 4(1): p. 108-15.

[72] Pergam, S.A., A.P. Limaye, and A.S.T.I.D.C.o. Practice, *Varicella zoster virus (VZV) in solid organ transplant recipients.* Am J Transplant, 2009. 9 Suppl 4: p. S108-15.

[73] Khan, S., J. Erlichman, and E.B. Rand, *Live virus immunization after orthotopic liver transplantation.* Pediatr Transplant, 2006. 10(1): p. 78-82.

[74] Levitsky, J., et al., *Varicella infection following varicella vaccination in a liver transplant recipient.* Am J Transplant, 2002. 2(9): p. 880-2.

[75] Zuckerman, R., A. Wald, and A.S.T.I.D.C.o. Practice, *Herpes simplex virus infections in solid organ transplant recipients.* Am J Transplant, 2009. 9 Suppl 4: p. S104-7.

[76] Singh, N. and D.L. Paterson, *Encephalitis caused by human herpesvirus-6 in transplant recipients: relevance of a novel neurotropic virus.* Transplantation, 2000. 69(12): p. 2474-9.

[77] Rossi, C., et al., *Fatal primary infection due to human herpesvirus 6 variant A in a renal transplant recipient.* Transplantation, 2001. 71(2): p. 288-92.

[78] Benito, N., et al., *Infection with human herpesvirus 6 after kidney-pancreas transplant.* Am J Transplant, 2004. 4(7): p. 1197-9.

[79] Razonable, R.R., D.M. Zerr, and A.S.T.I.D.C.o. Practice, *HHV-6, HHV-7 and HHV-8 in solid organ transplant recipients.* Am J Transplant, 2009. 9 Suppl 4: p. S100-3.

[80] Allen, U., J. Preiksaitis, and A.S.T.I.D.C.o. Practice, *Epstein-barr virus and posttransplant lymphoproliferative disorder in solid organ transplant recipients.* Am J Transplant, 2009. 9 Suppl 4: p. S87-96.

[81] Preiksaitis, J.K. and S. Keay, *Diagnosis and management of posttransplant lymphoproliferative disorder in solid-organ transplant recipients.* Clin Infect Dis, 2001. 33 Suppl 1: p. S38-46.

[82] Davis, J.E. and D.J. Moss, *Treatment options for post-transplant lymphoproliferative disorder and other Epstein-Barr virus-associated malignancies.* Tissue Antigens, 2004. 63(4): p. 285-92.

[83] Ison, M.G., M. Green, and A.S.T.I.D.C.o. Practice, *Adenovirus in solid organ transplant recipients.* Am J Transplant, 2009. 9 Suppl 4: p. S161-5.

[84] Eid, A.J., K.M. Posfay-Barbe, and A.S.T.I.D.C.o. Practice, *Parvovirus B19 in solid organ transplant recipients.* Am J Transplant, 2009. 9 Suppl 4: p. S147-50.

[85] Kwak, E.J., K. Julian, and A.S.T.I.D.C.o. Practice, *Human papillomavirus infection in solid organ transplant recipients.* Am J Transplant, 2009. 9 Suppl 4: p. S151-60.

[86] Fabrizi, F., et al., *HBsAg seropositive status and survival after renal transplantation: meta-analysis of observational studies.* Am J Transplant, 2005. 5(12): p. 2913-21.

[87] Reddy, P.N., et al., *Impact of pre-existing hepatitis B infection on the outcomes of kidney transplant recipients in the United States.* Clin J Am Soc Nephrol, 2011. 6(6): p. 1481-7.
[88] Kasiske, B.L., et al., *KDIGO clinical practice guideline for the care of kidney transplant recipients: a summary.* Kidney Int, 2010. 77(4): p. 299-311.
[89] Vallet-Pichard, A., et al., *Viral hepatitis in solid organ transplantation other than liver.* J Hepatol, 2011. 55(2): p. 474-82.
[90] Cosconea, S., et al., *Benefits associated with antiviral treatment in kidney allograft recipients with chronic hepatitis B virus infection.* J Hepatol, 2012. 57(1): p. 55-60.
[91] Fabrizi, F., P. Martin, and C. Ponticelli, *Hepatitis C virus infection and renal transplantation.* Am J Kidney Dis, 2001. 38(5): p. 919-34.
[92] Rostami, Z., et al., *The impact of Hepatitis C virus infection on kidney transplantation outcomes: A systematic review of 18 observational studies: The impact of HCV on renal transplantation.* Hepat Mon, 2011. 11(4): p. 247-54.
[93] Charlton, M., *Telaprevir, boceprevir, cytochrome P450 and immunosuppressive agents--a potentially lethal cocktail.* Hepatology, 2011. 54(1): p. 3-5.
[94] Garg, V., et al., *Effect of telaprevir on the pharmacokinetics of cyclosporine and tacrolimus.* Hepatology, 2011. 54(1): p. 20-7.
[95] Troppmann, C., et al., *Rapidly progressive lethal infection with novel influenza A (H1N1) 2009 virus in a kidney recipient: a cautionary tale.* Transplantation, 2010. 89(3): p. 369-70.
[96] Watcharananan, S.P., et al., *Influenza A/H1N1 2009 pneumonia in kidney transplant recipients: characteristics and outcomes following high-dose oseltamivir exposure.* Transpl Infect Dis, 2010. 12(2): p. 127-31.
[97] Smud, A., et al., *Pandemic influenza A/H1N1 virus infection in solid organ transplant recipients: a multicenter study.* Transplantation, 2010. 90(12): p. 1458-62.
[98] Kumar, D., et al., *Outcomes from pandemic influenza A H1N1 infection in recipients of solid-organ transplants: a multicentre cohort study.* Lancet Infect Dis, 2010. 10(8): p. 521-6.
[99] Kumar, D., et al., *Community-acquired West Nile virus infection in solid-organ transplant recipients.* Transplantation, 2004. 77(3): p. 399-402.
[100] Kumar, D., et al., *A seroprevalence study of west nile virus infection in solid organ transplant recipients.* Am J Transplant, 2004. 4(11): p. 1883-8.
[101] Centers for Disease, C. and Prevention, *West Nile virus transmission via organ transplantation and blood transfusion - Louisiana, 2008.* MMWR Morb Mortal Wkly Rep, 2009. 58(45): p. 1263-7.
[102] Centers for Disease, C. and Prevention, *Lymphocytic choriomeningitis virus infection in organ transplant recipients--Massachusetts, Rhode Island, 2005.* MMWR Morb Mortal Wkly Rep, 2005. 54(21): p. 537-9.
[103] Macneil, A., et al., *Solid Organ Transplant-associated Lymphocytic Choriomeningitis, United States, 2011.* Emerg Infect Dis, 2012. 18(8): p. 1256-1262.
[104] Kotton, C.N., *Vaccinations in kidney transplant patients: searching for optimal protection.* Clin J Am Soc Nephrol, 2011. 6(9): p. 2099-101.
[105] Danzinger-Isakov, L., D. Kumar, and A.S.T.I.D.C.o. Practice, *Guidelines for vaccination of solid organ transplant candidates and recipients.* Am J Transplant, 2009. 9 Suppl 4: p. S258-62.

[106] Kotton, C.N., R. Lattes, and A.S.T.I.D.C.o. Practice, *Parasitic infections in solid organ transplant recipients.* Am J Transplant, 2009. 9 Suppl 4: p. S234-51.
[107] Thomas, L.D., G.G. Miller, and A.S.T.I.D.C.o. Practice, *Interactions between antiinfective agents and immunosuppressants.* Am J Transplant, 2009. 9 Suppl 4: p. S263-6.
[108] Mieles, L., et al., *Interaction between FK506 and clotrimazole in a liver transplant recipient.* Transplantation, 1991. 52(6): p. 1086-7.
[109] Vasquez, E.M., et al., *Concomitant clotrimazole therapy more than doubles the relative oral bioavailability of tacrolimus.* Ther Drug Monit, 2005. 27(5): p. 587-91.
[110] Lott, D.G., et al., *Aggressive behavior of nonmelanotic skin cancers in solid organ transplant recipients.* Transplantation, 2010. 90(6): p. 683-7.
[111] Stasko, T., et al., *Guidelines for the management of squamous cell carcinoma in organ transplant recipients.* Dermatol Surg, 2004. 30(4 Pt 2): p. 642-50.
[112] Zwald, F.O., et al., *Melanoma in solid organ transplant recipients.* Am J Transplant, 2010. 10(5): p. 1297-304.
[113] Otley, C.C., et al., *Reduction of immunosuppression for transplant-associated skin cancer: expert consensus survey.* Br J Dermatol, 2006. 154(3): p. 395-400.
[114] Klatte, T. and M. Marberger, *Renal cell carcinoma of native kidneys in renal transplant patients.* Curr Opin Urol, 2011. 21(5): p. 376-9.
[115] Hurst, F.P., et al., *Incidence, predictors, costs, and outcome of renal cell carcinoma after kidney transplantation: USRDS experience.* Transplantation, 2010. 90(8): p. 898-904.
[116] Leveridge, M., et al., *Renal cell carcinoma in the native and allograft kidneys of renal transplant recipients.* J Urol, 2011. 186(1): p. 219-23.
[117] Quinlan, S.C., et al., *Risk factors for early-onset and late-onset post-transplant lymphoproliferative disorder in kidney recipients in the United States.* Am J Hematol, 2011. 86(2): p. 206-9.
[118] Quinlan, S.C., et al., *Increased risk for lymphoid and myeloid neoplasms in elderly solid-organ transplant recipients.* Cancer Epidemiol Biomarkers Prev, 2010. 19(5): p. 1229-37.

Chapter 9

BK Virus Infection in Renal Allograft Recipients

Darshana Dadhania

Additional information is available at the end of the chapter

http://dx.doi.org/10.5772/54615

1. Introduction

BK virus infection is a challenging complication in renal allograft recipients and has been associated with hematuria, ureteral stenosis, nephropathy and malignancy. BK virus infection occurs early during childhood and the virus lays dormant in uroepithelial cells. Reactivation of the virus in renal transplant recipients is particularly worrisome because of its propensity to cause local damage and incite an inflammatory response leading to acute kidney injury and possible graft loss. Recent, OPTN (Organ Procurement and Transplant Network) registry analysis suggests that the incidence of BK virus related complications are rising and between June 2004 and December 2008, 823 grafts were lost secondary to BK virus related complications [1]. This review will focus on BKV nephropathy (BKVN) in renal allograft recipients.

2. Early history of BKV replication

BK virus (BKV) is a non-enveloped DNA virus that is a member of the polyomavirus family. It shares >70% homology to the other polyomaviruses such as JC virus, a human pathogen, and simian virus 40, an unclear pathogen originally identified in monkeys [2]. BKV was first isolated by Gardner and his colleagues in 1971 from the ureter of a renal transplant recipient who presented with acute renal failure and ureteral stenosis [3]. It was not until 1995, that the second case was identified in the kidney biopsy of a renal allograft recipient at the University of Pittsburgh [4]. In both cases, the patients were treated for rejection prior to detection of the BK virus infection. The case from Pittsburgh illustrates the complexity of this problem. The biopsy of the patient demonstrated virus infection and acute rejection. Attempts at treatment of rejection with steroids only resulted in partial response. This was followed by IVIG therapy and a trial of reduction in immunosuppression. Eighteen weeks following the initial diagnosis, the patient lost his graft. The nephrectomy specimen showed "moderate acute rejection, chronic vascular rejection and scattered viral inclusions." BKV replication in immunosuppressed individuals has also been reported to cause native kidney pathology [5-7].

3. Natural history of BKV replication

By the age of 15, greater than 90% of individuals have evidence of past exposure to BKV as detected by BKV specific antibody response. The primary infection is associated with mild symptoms at best, mild upper respiratory infection or mild cystitis. The virus lies dormant in the uroepithelial cells in normal hosts where the intact immune system effectively prevents viral replication. When the host immune system is compromised, the virus, consisting of viral capsid proteins (VP1, VP2 & VP3) and circular double stranded DNA of approximately 5000 base pairs, begins its lytic life cycle [2, 8]. The virus capsid protein, VP1, attaches to the cell membrane via glycoproteins/gangliosides and is endocytosed via caveolae-mediated endocytosis. The virus is then transported to the nucleus where VP2&3 facilitate its entry and the virus utilizes host machinery to facilitate transcription of early and late genes. Early gene proteins, large T antigen, truncated T antigen and small t antigen, facilitate DNA replication and transcription of late genes, virus capsid protein. The virus capsid proteins are synthesized in the cytoplasm and transported back to the nucleus for final virus assembly containing the dsDNA virus copy. Intranuclear assembly of multiple virions causes cell rupture and release of virions into the extracellular space and possible entry into the circulation via peritubular capillaries.

In renal transplant recipients, BKV replication can be detected in the urine within weeks of transplantation. In our studies using BKV VP1 mRNA levels, we found the incidence of BKV replication to be 10% at 1 month, 20% at 3 months, 30% at 6 months which plateaued at 12 month post-transplantation. Similarly other studies identified viruria rates of 19% to 49% within the first year post-transplantation using DNA based assays [9, 10]. Hirsch and colleagues detected BKV replication using decoy cells in the urine in 30% of their study population [11]. Following the detection of viruria, some patients develop viremia. The incidence of BK viremia is less common, varying from 11% to 29% [12, 13]. Viremia is believed to result from a more extensive infection leading to severe tubular injury with rupture of tubular basement membranes and entry of the virus into the blood stream via peritubular capillaries. Ultimately, sustained viremia is associated with BKVN in 1% to 8% of individuals [14]. According to recent analysis of OPTN registry data, the cumulative incidence of BKVN increases from 2% at one year to 3.5% at two years to 6.6% at five years [1].

4. Risk factors for BKV replication and nephropathy

Risk factors for BKV replication and nephropathy include these that affect the recipient's immune response as well as other donor and recipient factors that have been linked through epidemiological studies. Modifiers of the immune response include immunosuppressive therapies, recipient humoral and cellular immunity as well as properties of the virus that may lead to increased virulence and immune evasion. Current data suggest that early recognition of BKV replication and modulation of immune therapy, allowing for effective recipient response against the virus, would reduce the risk of BKV nephropathy significantly [15]. [Table 1]

Modifiers of Effective Immune Response	Other Risk Factors
1. Therapy affecting immune response	1. Donor graft factors
Induction therapy (ATG)	Seropositive donor
Tacrolimus / MMF combination maintenance therapy	High donor BKV antibody titer
High dose tacrolimus therapy	Greater number of HLA mismatches
Treatment of rejection post-transplantation	Lack of HLA -C7 antigen
Steroid maintenance (triple drug therapy)	Ischemic injury / DGF
2. Recipient immune memory	Placement of ureteral stent
BKV specific humoral immunity / response	2. Recipient factors
BKV specific cellular immunity / response	Older age
3. Virus factors	Male gender
Virulence / Serotype(s)	History of Diabetes
Immune evasion	History of BKVN in previous graft

Table 1. Risk Factors for BKV Nephropathy (BKVN)
ATG, anti-thymocyte globulin; HLA, human leukocyte antigen; DGF, delayed graft function ; Adopted from Medeiros M, Dadhania D, and Velásquez-Jones L, "Nefropatía por virus BK" in Infecciones en el paciente receptor de trasplante renal (Alberú J, Morales JL; Publicaciones Permanyer; 2012) In press.

5. Immunosuppressive agents

The intensity of immunosuppression is the major risk factor for BKV replication and subsequent development of BKV nephropathy. Our center performed a prospective study to identify risk factors for BKV replication using BKV VP1 mRNA measurements in the urine and found that ATG induction (OR=5.8; P=0.008) and prednisone maintenance (OR=8.3; P=0.003) were independent risk factors for BKV replication in individuals maintained on tacrolimus and MMF [16]. In addition to potent induction therapies, treatment of acute rejection with steroids was also found to be an independent risk factor for BKV replication and nephropathy[11][17].

Type of maintenance immunosuppressive therapies may be an important risk factor for BKV nephropathy. As evidenced by low acute rejection rates, the combination of tacrolimus and mycophenolate mofetil is currently the most potent combination of maintenance immunosuppressive therapies [18-20]. Brennan and colleagues performed a prospective randomized controlled trial of 200 renal allograft recipients who received either tacrolimus or cyclosporine in combination with azathioprine (AZA) in the low risk group and MMF in the high risk group and found the incidence of BKV replication (viruria and viremia) to be highest in the tacrolimus /MMF combination (46% viruria and 13% viremia) [21].

The dose of maintenance immunosuppressive therapies may also be an important factor. In another retrospective review of 575 renal allograft recipients, Cosio and colleagues evaluated the impact of tacrolimus dose on the incidence of BKV nephropathy [22]. The historical cohort received higher tacrolimus doses (12-15ng/ml in first month, 10-12ng/ml month 1 to 4, 8-10ng/ml month 4 to 12 and then 6-8ng/ml) while the recent cohort received lower tacrolimus doses (10-12ng/ml in first month, 8-10ng/ml month 1-4 and 6-8ng/ml thereafter). The authors found a significantly lower incidence of BKV nephropathy with lower tacrolimus doses (3.6% in the low vs. 12.7% in the high tacrolimus group; $P<0.001$). In a recent case-controlled analysis of 99 renal allograft recipients (33 cases and 66 controls), the authors found higher tacrolimus levels and prednisone doses during the three months preceding the diagnosis of BKV nephropathy compared to the controls who had undergone a biopsy and did not have BKV nephropathy [23]. They performed random effects logistic modeling and found tacrolimus level (OR=1.3; P=0.03) and prednisone dose (OR=1.22; P=0.02) to be independently associated with BKVN diagnosis. MMF dose was not different between the two groups.

A recent study evaluated the treatment trends for BKV replication in a cohort of 48,292 solitary kidney transplant recipients transplanted from January 2003 to December 2006 [1]. In their analysis, the authors found a rising trend in treatment of BKV replication, corresponding to an increased use of ATG (anti-thymocyte13 globulin) induction therapy and tacrolimus based maintenance immunosuppression. Independent risk factors for BKV replication include ATG induction, tacrolimus, mycophenolate mofetil (MMF) and prednisone maintenance therapies and treatment of acute rejection within the first six months after transplant. In contrast, interleukin 2 receptor (IL-2R) antibody and alcmtuzumab induction were not associated with increased incidence of BKV associated treatment. mTOR inhibitor use was associated with a protective effect (HR=0.69; P=0.005) and may be associated with be associated with a decreased incidence of BKV nephropathy [1, 24]. In-vitro studies suggest that mTOR inhibitors may inhibit BKV replication via inhibition of large T antigen [25]. A large randomized controlled trial of everolimus with low dose cyclosporine versus MMF with standard cyclosporine dose suggested a lower incidence of BKV viruria and viremia in the everolimus treated group [26]. However, other studies have not demonstrated a protective effect and as a result larger prospective studies are needed to evaluate the role of mTOR inhibitors on BKV replication [18].

6. Recipient humoral and cellular immunity

BKV-specific antibody response may play an important role in the risk for developing BKV nephropathy. Epidemiological studies suggest greater than 90% of adults have been exposed to BK virus during the early years [27] and have measurable humoral immunity. It has also been noted that the antibody titers increase with the development of BKV viremia/nephropathy in the post-transplant period [28]. A study of 70 renal allograft recipients demonstrated that pre-transplant serum anti-BKV IgG titers were lower in patients who went on to develop BKV viremia compared to the 17 patients who never developed BKV viremia. In those that developed BKV infection, the magnitude of the rise in antibody titer post-transplant correlated with intensity of BKV infection [29]. The same authors demonstrated that the donor BKV seropositive status and the magnitude of the antibody titer was significantly associated with BKV replication in the recipient [30]. Together these data suggest that BKV-specific memory immune response is important for controlling BKV replication and preventing BKV nephropathy especially when the donor has had significant exposure to BKV as measured by BKV antibody titers.

Recent studies have focused on measuring cellular immune response to the BK virus. Similar to the antibody response, BKV specific INFγ secreting T cells increase with the development of BKV viremia. Detection of this cellular immune response early after development of BKV viremia is associated with self-limited BKV infection and the prevention of BKV nephropathy [31, 32]. In addition, tacrolimus therapy inhibits BKV specific T cell immune response and reduction of immunosuppressive therapies does lead to an increase in the BKV specific cellular immune response [33]. Recipients who are not able to increase BKV specific cellular immune response promptly with BKV replication may be at increased risk for nephropathy and kidney damage.

7. Other associated risk factors

Several studies have identified the HLA type of donor and recipient to be important risk factors for BKV nephropathy. Although not all of the studies have found a significant association between HLA mismatches and risk of BKV nephropathy, Awadalla and colleagues found 5-6 HLA mismatches as a significant independent risk factor for BKVN (OR=7.6; P=0.004) in a large study cohort (n=440) with 40 BKVN patients [34]. Although no association was found with HLA mismatches, Bohl and colleagues found an increased risk of BKVN if the donor lacked HLA-Cw7 allele (RR=3.6; P=0.008) [30]. In addition, they also found a significantly increased risk of BKVN with positive donor serostatus for BKV IgG (RR=3.1. P=0.007).

Additional recipient risk factors that have been identified are a history of diabetes, older age and male gender [1, 17, 35, 36]. Transplant surgery associated variables such as delayed graft function (DGF), ischemia, deceased donor grafts and use of ureteral stents have also been identified as risk factors for BKV viremia/nephropathy [1, 37, 38].

8. Diagnosis of BKV replication and BKVN

8.1. Noninvasive assays for diagnosis of BKV replication

There are several assays available for the diagnosis of BKV replication in renal allograft recipients. One of the earliest assays was the use of decoy cells in the urine. In this assay urine was examined under the microscope to look for virus infected cells that showed the typical ground glass appearance of the nucleus resulting from intranuclear viral inclusion bodies [39]. Evaluation of "negatively-stained" urine specimens using electron microscopy (EM) identified the typical icosahedral shaped virions [40]. In the current era, the most commonly used noninvasive assay for diagnosis of BKV replication is urine or plasma BKV DNA copy numbers using real-time quantitative PCR assays.

Our center has developed and validated a noninvasive assay for the diagnosis of BKV replication and BKV nephropathy using urinary cell mRNA assay. In a cohort of 89 patients, urinary cell mRNA levels of BKV VP1 copies above 6.5×10^5 (copies/ng total RNA) diagnosed BKVN with 100% sensitivity and 97% specificity with a positive predictive value of 86% for BKVN [41]. More recently, urinary Haufen was introduced as an accurate predictor of BKVN by a group from the University of North Carolina. Urinary Haufen are "cast-like polyomavirus aggregates" that are detected in the urine using EM [42]. In their investigation, the authors compared the diagnostic utility of current noninvasive tests in clinical practice to urinary Haufen and found that urinary Haufen was associated with the highest specificity and positive predictive value. Table 2 lists the results from this study as well as our center's study of urinary cell BKV VP1 assay to provide a comprehensive view of all the noninvasive diagnostic assays available for BKVN.

University of North Carolina – Singh et al. JASN 2009					
Test	N	Sensitivity	Specificity	PPV	NPV
Haufen	32	100%	99%	97%	100%
Decoy Cells	32	100%	36%	40%	100%
Urine BKV load – DNA >1,000 K	32	100%	47%	44%	100%
Plasma BKV load >10 K	32	72%	88%	74%	88%
Weill Cornell Medical Center – Dadhania et al. Transplantation 2010					
Test	N	Sensitivity	Specificity	PPV	NPV
Urinary cell BKV VP1 mRNA	88	100%	97%	86%	100%

Table 2. Non-Invasive Diagnosis of BKV Replication
PPV: Positive Predictive Value; NPV: Negative Predictive Value

8.2. Histological diagnosis of BKV nephropathy

Although noninvasive assays are commonly used as a screening tool to identify BKV replication early, the gold standard is still the renal allograft biopsy. The diagnosis of BKVN is made based on the presence of typical viral cytopathic changes in the renal tubular epithelial cells. The presence of BKV is confirmed using an immunohistochemical (IC) staining of the nucleus using an antibody against the large T antigen of SV40 virus which cross reacts with BK and JC viruses [43]. Recently a more sophisticated assay, fluorescence in situ hybridization (FISH) has been developed to identify BK virus within the kidney. In a recent study, a side by side comparison demonstrates no clear advantage of FISH over IC staining [44]. BKVN progresses from early lesions demonstrating normal renal parenchyma with scattered tubular epithelial cells with BK associated cytopathic changes, to significant tubular damage and an inflammatory response associated with tubulitis, to an advanced lesion where there is considerable tubular atrophy and interstitial fibrosis with chronic inflammation and only scattered cytopathic changes.

A large retrospective review of BKVN associated biopsies performed by the group at the University of Maryland has led the way in developing the diagnostic criteria for different patterns of BKVN [45]. They identified three patterns of histological injury: Pattern A with viral cytopathic changes and almost normal parenchyma, Pattern B with viral cytopathic changes and significant inflammation and tubulitis with varying degrees of interstitial fibrosis and tubular atrophy, and Pattern C with diffuse fibrosis and tubular atrophy associated with some inflammation and very little viral cytopathic changes. Pattern B was divided into B1, B2 & B3 based on the degree of interstitial fibrosis and tubular atrophy. In their evaluation, they noted that Pattern A was associated with 15% risk of graft loss, Pattern B was associated with 25-75% risk of graft loss and Pattern C was associated with >80% risk of graft loss. It is important to note that in their investigation, they also found a 37% discordance rate between two cores of renal allograft tissue obtained from the same biopsy procedure within the same patient, suggesting that the pathological changes can be patchy in nature and a renal allograft biopsy can miss the diagnosis of BKVN.

Recently, the Banff 2009 meeting group has collapsed these patterns into three simple stages – A (early), B (florid) and C (late sclerosing stage) and semiquantified the histological viral loads based on the cytopathic changes. At this time, there are no large studies correlating the use of this system with clinical outcomes [46]. However, a side by side comparison of this schema with an older schema demonstrated no clear advantage of the new staging system compared to the one developed by University of Maryland [47]. Overall, BKVN diagnosis associated with minimal inflammation and minimal scarring has the best prognosis and less than 15% risk of graft loss. The majority of patients with significant inflammation and/or scarring are at risk for persistent allograft dysfunction or progressive decline in renal function.

The presence of the BKV associated cytopathic changes with interstitial inflammation and tubulitis has been the topic of discussion for some time as tubulitis is a hallmark of acute rejection diagnosis. Some support the notion that it represents concurrent acute rejection process within the allograft. However, others feel that it is difficult to separate the anti-viral response from the anti-allograft response. Previous studies suggested that HLA-DR staining of renal allograft would distinguish BKVN with rejection from BKVN alone. However, these data have not been validated in subsequent studies and HLA-DR staining is not used routinely to identify concurrent acute rejection [48, 49]. In patients with BKVN, renal tubules with intense cytopathic changes demonstrated positive C4d staining of the tubular basement membrane but not in peritubular capillaries. In a study of 113 biopsies of renal allograft from recipients with BKV replication, PTC (peritubular capillary) C4d staining was found to be a valid marker for antibody mediated rejection [50]. In patients with BKVN, renal tubules with intense cytopathic changes demonstrated positive C4d staining of the tubular basement membrane but not in peritubular capillaries.

The makeup of cellular infiltration in a renal allograft with BKVN is very similar to those with acute rejection [51]. Our group feels it is difficult to distinguish the anti-viral cellular response from the anti-allograft cellular response. Using the urinary cell mRNA profiles, we found that the granzyme B mRNA levels of BKVN patients were heterogeneous [41]. Those with poor graft function following BKVN had levels that were similar to those with acute rejection while those with stable function had granzyme B mRNA levels that were similar to stable patients with normal protocol biopsies. Furthermore, we found a positive relationship between elevated granzyme B levels and the risk for decline in graft function and a trend towards increased graft loss in individuals with the highest levels of urinary cell granzyme B mRNA.[Figure1]

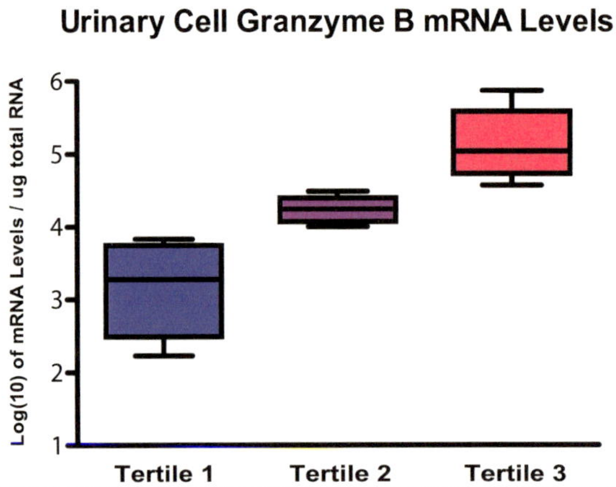

	(n=6)	(n=6)	(n=6)	P value
Declining Function	0%	50%	83%	0.014
Graft Loss	0%	33%	67%	0.20

Figure 1. Baseline Urinary Cell Granzyme B mRNA Levels Predict Graft Function in BKVN
Data derived from original study published by Dadhania et al. in *Transplantation* 2010;90(2):189-97

9. Management of BKV replication and BKVN

Routine monitoring of BKV replication is essential for the prevention of BKVN and improving renal allograft outcomes in individuals with BKVN. BKV infection progresses in stages, from viruria to viruria+viremia to viruria+viremia+nephropathy to graft loss. To prevent progression to nephropathy, intervention should begin at the stage of significant viruria and/or viremia. Intervention in this early stage prior to development of BKVN has been termed "preemptive" strategy and generally involves stepwise reduction in immunosuppressive therapies [15].

9.1. Preemptive reduction in immunosuppressive therapies

In the current era, noninvasive monitoring for BKV replication has become a routine practice. Most centers have developed thresholds for initiating preemptive reduction in immunosuppressive therapies in the hopes of preventing BKVN. In a prospective study of 62 renal allograft recipients, Ginevri and colleagues found the incidence of viruria to be 64% and viremia 22%. Of the the 13 individuals with viremia (2,460 to 170,000 copies/ml), 100% had clearance of viremia by median of 2 months follow up [52]. In another study of 123 patients, 13 developed viremia in which 2 had evidence of BKVN and the remaining 11 did not. With reduction in immunosuppression, 10 of 11 patients without BKVN had clearance of viremia by median of 5 months follow up [10]. Schaub and colleagues evaluated the impact of a three step protocol for reduction in immunosuppression in patients with viremia, presumptive BKVN and biopsy confirmed BKVN. In their study, step 1 was reduction in tacrolimus to target trough of 6-8ng/ml, step 2 was further reduction in tacrolimus to 4-6ng/ml and step 3 was 50% reduction in MMF (mycophenolate mofetil). In their prospective study of 206 patients, they found step 1 cleared viremia in 100% of patients (n=8) with less than 10,000 copies/ml of BKV, 47% (8/17) of those with presumptive BKVN (>10,000 copies/ml of BKV) and 15% (2/13) of those with BKVN. Step 1 & 2 cleared BKV viremia in 88% (15/17) of those with presumptive BKVN and 61% (8/13) of those with BKVN. Finally, Step 1,2&3 cleared BKV viremia in 92% of individuals with biopsy proven BKVN. However, they found the incidence of acute rejection (subclinical + clinical) to be 24% in those with presumptive BKVN and 38% in those with biopsy proven BKVN [49]. These data suggest that even with systematic monitoring for BKV viremia, a small percentage of patients will present with biopsy confirmed BKVN and clearance of BKV viremia is achieved easily in those with low copies of BKV. In those with high copies of BKV or presumptive BKVN, clearance of BK viremia is possible with systematic reduction in immunosuppressive therapies but at the expense of subclinical or clinical acute rejection episodes. As a result, patients who develop BKV viremia should be monitored closely, not only during the viremic phase but also after clearance of viremia.

10. Management of biopsy confirmed BKVN

The cornerstone of managing patients with BKVN is reduction in immunosuppressive therapies. However this strategy is associated with increased risk of acute rejection episodes and shorter graft survival times. Vasudev and colleagues evaluated their experience with BKVN by dividing their cohort into those recipients who did not have screening for BKV replication (n=16) and those who were diagnosed with BK viremia and subsequently found to have BKVN on biopsy (n=25). Renal allograft recipients were managed with reduction in immunosuppressive therapies and they found a three year actuarial graft survival rate of 58%. In those who retained their grafts, the stabilization of renal function correlated with reduction in calcineurin inhibitors.

The optimal management for those individuals that have BKVN with tubulitis is unclear. University of Pittsburgh performed a retrospective evaluation of individuals with BKVN and tubulitis who received initial increase in immunosuppression (pulse steroids) followed by reduction in immunosuppression, reduction in immunosuppression only and no change in immunosuppression. In their study, reduction in immunosuppression compared to pulse steroids was associated with reduction in cytopathic changes (83% vs. 20%; P=0.004) [53]. Pulse steroids did result in greater improvement in tubulitis (55% vs. 26%) but this effect was not associated with improvement in renal function. Reduction in immunosuppression resulted in lower rates of graft loss in individuals with BKVN and clearance of viremia was associated with improved graft survival (46% vs. 25%) [47]. However, greater than 30-50% of individuals continue to have significant decrease in renal function [54].

IVIG has also been used to manage BKV replication because of its anti-inflammatory activity as well as the presence of humoral immunity to BKV [55, 56]. Studies indicate that treatment with IVIG in combination with reduction in immunosuppression is associated with clearance of viremia and histological clearance. Recently, a case report suggested that the use of IVIG was associated with increase in BKV copies [57]. Since IVIG has anti-inflammatory properties, it is possible that use of IVIG is actually associated with an increase in total immunosuppression and thus results in a rise in BKV. To evaluate the use of IVIG as an anti-inflammatory agent that does not result in an increase in BKV replication requires controlled prospective trials.

To date there are no antiviral drugs that have been proven to effectively inhibit BKV replication and associated graft damage. Various antivirals as well as anti-inflammatory agents have been used for management of BKVN in single center studies and have been reviewed by Rinaldo and Hirsch [58]. Cidofovir, a nucleoside analogue used for treatment of numerous viruses, has been used for management of BKV replication in HSCT (hematopoietic stem cell transplant) recipients as well in those with kidney transplants [59]. Treatment with cidofovir is limited by its potential for nephrotoxicity and currently, a newer agent that is a lipid conjugate of cidofovir, CXM001, is being studied for management of BKV associated hemorrhagic cystitis and BKVN [60]. Fluoroquinolones, anti-bacterial drug that inhibits DNA gyrase, have also been suggested to have activity against BK virus. Single center studies suggest that use of fluoroquinolones do result in decrease BKV replication [61]. However, its use in the management of BKVN has not been prospectively studied.

In addition to anti-viral/anti-bacterial agents, agents with immunosuppressive properties have also been used to inhibit BKV replication. Leflunomide, an anti-inflammatory agent used in rheumatoid arthritis, is another agent whose metabolite inhibits protein kinase activity and pyrimidine synthesis. This drug has been shown to reduce BKV replication in some studies and the efficacy is linked to achieving drug levels above 40ug/ml. However, there are no randomized controlled trials demonstrating its effectiveness and it has been associated with significant liver toxicity. FK778 is a drug that is closely related to the active metabolite of leflunomide. A phase 2 randomized controlled trial that compared MMF or FK778 based maintenance immunosuppression did not demonstrate a benefit in preventing BK viruria or viremia [62]. Epidemiological studies also suggest that rapamycin, a maintenance immunosuppressive agent, may be associated with lower incidence of BKV replication. Preliminary data suggests that initiation of rapamycin to manage BKV replication may be associated with faster clearance of BKV viremia [63]. Larger studies are necessary to clarify the role of rapamycin in the management of BKVN.

When the patient presents with BKVN, one is obligated to intervene to avoid progression to graft loss. At this time, the main strategy that is employed for BKVN is reduction in immunosuppression. Johnston and colleagues pooled all the existing data on three different strategies to manage BKVN - reduction in immunosuppressive therapies (IS) alone versus cidofovir plus reduction in IS versus leflunomide with reduction in IS [64]. They found that the graft failure rate was not significantly different between the three groups. They concluded that there is no convincing evidence that the use of adjuvant therapies provides additional benefit to reduction in IS alone for management of BKVN patients.

11. Re-transplantation in renal allograft recipients with BKVN

Most reports indicate that risk of graft loss and persistent graft dysfunction following BKVN diagnosis is high [47]. Having suffered a graft loss, many of these patients return to the wait list with higher PRA (panel reactive antibodies) and as a result wait longer for a kidney transplant [65]. However, graft loss due to BKVN is not a contraindication to re-transplantation. The most important factor in preventing BKVN in the subsequent graft is clearance of BKV viremia/viruria prior re-transplantation [66]. Furthermore, at this time there are no recommendations for avoiding any specific immunosuppressive therapy at the time of subsequent transplant. Most recipients with failed graft due to BKVN have been re-transplanted with the centers' standard immunosuppressive protocols. Of the 126 individuals who underwent re-transplantation following graft loss attributable to BKV, BKV replication occurred in 17% with only 1 graft loss attributable to BKVN [65].

12. Summary

BKV infection and development of BKVN in renal allograft recipients is a growing concern given the use of more potent immunosuppressive agents. The lack of effective anti-viral therapy for BKV results in a challenging management problem for transplant physicians. At this time, data suggest that prevention of BKVN through prospective monitoring and preemptive reduction in immunosuppression is a reasonable approach. Laskin and colleagues suggested that viruria measurement every 3 months followed by viremia measurement if viruria is detected is as cost-effective as viremia monitoring every 3 months. Patients with BKV replication or nephropathy should be monitored very closely (every two weeks) until viremia has cleared. Persistent viremia should lead to a kidney biopsy to assess the histological stage of BKV and to determine prognosis.

The risk of graft loss remains high in individuals with BKVN and concurrent inflammation. There is an urgent need for randomized controlled trials to evaluate novel therapies and their potential advantage over reduction in immunosuppressive therapies alone. In addition, development and validation of noninvasive biomarkers to monitor BKV replication and associated inflammatory response are necessary to enhance the management of allograft recipients with BKVN.

Author details

Darshana Dadhania

Department of Transplantation Medicine and Extracorporeal Therapy, Division of Nephrology and Hypertension, Department of Medicine

NewYork-Presbyterian Hospital- Weill Cornell Medical College, New York, NY, USA

Acknowledgement

The author would like to thank Sue Pino for her careful review of the manuscript.

13. References

[1] Dharnidharka VR, Cherikh WS, Abbott KC. An OPTN analysis of national registry data on treatment of BK virus allograft nephropathy in the United States. Transplantation 2009; 87 (7): 1019.

[2] van Aalderen MC, Heutinck KM, Huisman C, ten Berge IJ. BK virus infection in transplant recipients: clinical manifestations, treatment options and the immune response. Neth J Med; 70 (4): 172.

[3] Gardner SD, Field AM, Coleman DV, Hulme B. New human papovavirus (B.K.) isolated from urine after renal transplantation. Lancet 1971; 1 (7712): 1253.

[4] Purighalla R, Shapiro R, McCauley J, Randhawa P. BK virus infection in a kidney allograft diagnosed by needle biopsy. Am J Kidney Dis 1995; 26 (4): 671.

[5] Crum-Cianflone N, Quigley M, Utz G, Hale B. BK virus-associated renal failure among HIV patients. AIDS 2007; 21 (11): 1501.

[6] Egli A, Helmersen DS, Taub K, Hirsch HH, Johnson A. Renal failure five years after lung transplantation due to polyomavirus BK-associated nephropathy. Am J Transplant; 10 (10): 2324.

[7] O'Donnell PH, Swanson K, Josephson MA, et al. BK virus infection is associated with hematuria and renal impairment in recipients of allogeneic hematopoetic stem cell transplants. Biol Blood Marrow Transplant 2009; 15 (9): 1038.

[8] Randhawa P, Brennan DC. BK virus infection in transplant recipients: an overview and update. Am J Transplant 2006; 6 (9): 2000.

[9] Babel N, Fendt J, Karaivanov S, et al. Sustained BK viruria as an early marker for the development of BKV-associated nephropathy: analysis of 4128 urine and serum samples. Transplantation 2009; 88 (1): 89.

[10] Almeras C, Foulongne V, Garrigue V, et al. Does reduction in immunosuppression in viremic patients prevent BK virus nephropathy in de novo renal transplant recipients? A prospective study. Transplantation 2008; 85 (8): 1099.

[11] Hirsch HH, Knowles W, Dickenmann M, et al. Prospective study of polyomavirus type BK replication and nephropathy in renal-transplant recipients. N Engl J Med 2002; 347 (7): 488.
[12] Agha I, Brennan DC. BK virus and immunosuppressive agents. Adv Exp Med Biol 2006; 577: 174.
[13] Bressollette-Bodin C, Coste-Burel M, Hourmant M, Sebille V, Andre-Garnier E, Imbert-Marcille BM. A prospective longitudinal study of BK virus infection in 104 renal transplant recipients. Am J Transplant 2005; 5 (8): 1926.
[14] Hirsch HH, Brennan DC, Drachenberg CB, et al. Polyomavirus-associated nephropathy in renal transplantation: interdisciplinary analyses and recommendations. Transplantation 2005; 79 (10): 1277.
[15] Ramos E, Drachenberg CB, Wali R, Hirsch HH. The decade of polyomavirus BK-associated nephropathy: state of affairs. Transplantation 2009; 87 (5): 621.
[16] Dadhania D, Snopkowski C, Ding R, et al. Epidemiology of BK virus in renal allograft recipients: independent risk factors for BK virus replication. Transplantation 2008; 86 (4): 521.
[17] Prince O, Savic S, Dickenmann M, Steiger J, Bubendorf L, Mihatsch MJ. Risk factors for polyoma virus nephropathy. Nephrol Dial Transplant 2009; 24 (3): 1024.
[18] Gralla J, Wiseman AC. Tacrolimus/sirolimus versus tacrolimus/mycophenolate in kidney transplantation: improved 3-year graft and patient survival in recent era. Transplantation 2009; 87 (11): 1712.
[19] Johnson C, Ahsan N, Gonwa T, et al. Randomized trial of tacrolimus (Prograf) in combination with azathioprine or mycophenolate mofetil versus cyclosporine (Neoral) with mycophenolate mofetil after cadaveric kidney transplantation. Transplantation 2000; 69 (5): 834.
[20] Vacher-Coponat H, Moal V, Indreies M, et al. A randomized trial with steroids and antithymocyte globulins comparing cyclosporine/azathioprine versus tacrolimus/mycophenolate mofetil (CATM2) in renal transplantation. Transplantation; 93 (4): 437.
[21] Brennan DC, Agha I, Bohl DL, et al. Incidence of BK with tacrolimus versus cyclosporine and impact of preemptive immunosuppression reduction. Am J Transplant 2005; 5 (3): 582.
[22] Cosio FG, Amer H, Grande JP, Larson TS, Stegall MD, Griffin MD. Comparison of low versus high tacrolimus levels in kidney transplantation: assessment of efficacy by protocol biopsies. Transplantation 2007; 83 (4): 411.
[23] Manitpisitkul W, Drachenberg C, Ramos E, et al. Maintenance immunosuppressive agents as risk factors for BK virus nephropathy: a case-control study. Transplantation 2009; 88 (1): 83.
[24] Benavides CA, Pollard VB, Mauiyyedi S, Podder H, Knight R, Kahan BD. BK virus-associated nephropathy in sirolimus-treated renal transplant patients: incidence, course, and clinical outcomes. Transplantation 2007; 84 (1): 83.

[25] Liacini A, Seamone ME, Muruve DA, Tibbles LA. Anti-BK virus mechanisms of sirolimus and leflunomide alone and in combination: toward a new therapy for BK virus infection. Transplantation; 90 (12): 1450.

[26] Tedesco Silva H, Jr., Cibrik D, Johnston T, et al. Everolimus plus reduced-exposure CsA versus mycophenolic acid plus standard-exposure CsA in renal-transplant recipients. Am J Transplant; 10 (6): 1401.

[27] Stolt A, Sasnauskas K, Koskela P, Lehtinen M, Dillner J. Seroepidemiology of the human polyomaviruses. J Gen Virol 2003; 84 (Pt 6): 1499.

[28] Hariharan S, Cohen EP, Vasudev B, et al. BK virus-specific antibodies and BKV DNA in renal transplant recipients with BKV nephritis. Am J Transplant 2005; 5 (11): 2719.

[29] Bohl DL, Brennan DC, Ryschkewitsch C, Gaudreault-Keener M, Major EO, Storch GA. BK virus antibody titers and intensity of infections after renal transplantation. J Clin Virol 2008; 43 (2): 184.

[30] Bohl DL, Storch GA, Ryschkewitsch C, et al. Donor origin of BK virus in renal transplantation and role of HLA C7 in susceptibility to sustained BK viremia. Am J Transplant 2005; 5 (9): 2213.

[31] Comoli P, Hirsch HH, Ginevri F. Cellular immune responses to BK virus. Curr Opin Organ Transplant 2008; 13 (6): 569.

[32] Schachtner T, Muller K, Stein M, et al. BK virus-specific immunity kinetics: a predictor of recovery from polyomavirus BK-associated nephropathy. Am J Transplant; 11 (11): 2443.

[33] Egli A, Kohli S, Dickenmann M, Hirsch HH. Inhibition of polyomavirus BK-specific T-Cell responses by immunosuppressive drugs. Transplantation 2009; 88 (10): 1161.

[34] Awadalla Y, Randhawa P, Ruppert K, Zeevi A, Duquesnoy RJ. HLA mismatching increases the risk of BK virus nephropathy in renal transplant recipients. Am J Transplant 2004; 4 (10): 1691.

[35] Trofe J, Gaber LW, Stratta RJ, et al. Polyomavirus in kidney and kidney-pancreas transplant recipients. Transpl Infect Dis 2003; 5 (1): 21.

[36] Ramos E, Drachenberg CB, Papadimitriou JC, et al. Clinical course of polyoma virus nephropathy in 67 renal transplant patients. J Am Soc Nephrol 2002; 13 (8): 2145.

[37] Siparsky NF, Kushnir LF, Gallichio MH, Conti DJ. Ureteral stents: a risk factor for polyomavirus BK viremia in kidney transplant recipients undergoing protocol screening. Transplant Proc; 43 (7): 2641.

[38] Thomas A, Dropulic LK, Rahman MH, Geetha D. Ureteral stents: a novel risk factor for polyomavirus nephropathy. Transplantation 2007; 84 (3): 433.

[39] Nickeleit V, Klimkait T, Binet IF, et al. Testing for polyomavirus type BK DNA in plasma to identify renal-allograft recipients with viral nephropathy. N Engl J Med 2000; 342 (18): 1309.

[40] Howell DN, Smith SR, Butterly DW, et al. Diagnosis and management of BK polyomavirus interstitial nephritis in renal transplant recipients. Transplantation 1999; 68 (9): 1279.

[41] Dadhania D, Snopkowski C, Ding R, et al. Validation of noninvasive diagnosis of BK virus nephropathy and identification of prognostic biomarkers. Transplantation; 90 (2): 189.

[42] Singh HK, Andreoni KA, Madden V, et al. Presence of urinary Haufen accurately predicts polyomavirus nephropathy. J Am Soc Nephrol 2009; 20 (2): 416.

[43] Drachenberg CB, Hirsch HH, Ramos E, Papadimitriou JC. Polyomavirus disease in renal transplantation: review of pathological findings and diagnostic methods. Hum Pathol 2005; 36 (12): 1245.

[44] Wang Z, Portier BP, Hu B, et al. Diagnosis of BK viral nephropathy in the renal allograft biopsy: role of fluorescence in situ hybridization. J Mol Diagn; 14 (5): 494.

[45] Drachenberg CB, Papadimitriou JC, Hirsch HH, et al. Histological patterns of polyomavirus nephropathy: correlation with graft outcome and viral load. Am J Transplant 2004; 4 (12): 2082.

[46] Sar A, Worawichawong S, Benediktsson H, Zhang J, Yilmaz S, Trpkov K. Interobserver agreement for Polyomavirus nephropathy grading in renal allografts using the working proposal from the 10th Banff Conference on Allograft Pathology. Hum Pathol; 42 (12): 2018.

[47] Masutani K, Shapiro R, Basu A, Tan H, Wijkstrom M, Randhawa P. The Banff 2009 Working Proposal for polyomavirus nephropathy: a critical evaluation of its utility as a determinant of clinical outcome. Am J Transplant; 12 (4): 907.

[48] Nickeleit V, Hirsch HH, Zeiler M, et al. BK-virus nephropathy in renal transplants-tubular necrosis, MHC-class II expression and rejection in a puzzling game. Nephrol Dial Transplant 2000; 15 (3): 324.

[49] Schaub S, Hirsch HH, Dickenmann M, et al. Reducing immunosuppression preserves allograft function in presumptive and definitive polyomavirus-associated nephropathy. Am J Transplant; 10 (12): 2615.

[50] Batal I, Zainah H, Stockhausen S, et al. The significance of renal C4d staining in patients with BK viruria, viremia, and nephropathy. Mod Pathol 2009; 22 (11): 1468.

[51] Rogers NM, Russ GR, Cooper J, Coates PT. Immunophenotyping of interstitial infiltrate does not distinguish between BK virus nephropathy and acute cellular rejection. Nephrology (Carlton) 2009; 14 (1): 118.

[52] Ginevri F, Azzi A, Hirsch HH, et al. Prospective monitoring of polyomavirus BK replication and impact of pre-emptive intervention in pediatric kidney recipients. Am J Transplant 2007; 7 (12): 2727.

[53] Celik B, Shapiro R, Vats A, Randhawa PS. Polyomavirus allograft nephropathy: sequential assessment of histologic viral load, tubulitis, and graft function following changes in immunosuppression. Am J Transplant 2003; 3 (11): 1378.

[54] Wadei HM, Rule AD, Lewin M, et al. Kidney transplant function and histological clearance of virus following diagnosis of polyomavirus-associated nephropathy (PVAN). Am J Transplant 2006; 6 (5 Pt 1): 1025.

[55] Sbrana S, Ruocco L, Vanacore R, Azzara A, Ambrogi F. In vitro effects of an immunoglobulin preparation for intravenous use (IVIG) on T-cells activation. Allerg Immunol (Paris) 1993; 25 (1): 35.

[56] Sener A, House AA, Jevnikar AM, et al. Intravenous immunoglobulin as a treatment for BK virus associated nephropathy: one-year follow-up of renal allograft recipients. Transplantation 2006; 81 (1): 117.
[57] Maggiore U, Medici MC, Vaglio A, Buzio C. Increased viral load after intravenous immunoglobulin therapy for BK virus-associated nephropathy. Transpl Infect Dis; 12 (5): 470.
[58] Rinaldo CH, Hirsch HH. Antivirals for the treatment of polyomavirus BK replication. Expert Rev Anti Infect Ther 2007; 5 (1): 105.
[59] Araya CE, Lew JF, Fennell RS, Neiberger RE, Dharnidharka VR. Intermediate dose cidofovir does not cause additive nephrotoxicity in BK virus allograft nephropathy. Pediatr Transplant 2008; 12 (7): 790.
[60] Gosert R, Rinaldo CH, Wernli M, Major EO, Hirsch HH. CMX001 (1-O-hexadecyloxypropyl-cidofovir) inhibits polyomavirus JC replication in human brain progenitor-derived astrocytes. Antimicrob Agents Chemother; 55 (5): 2129.
[61] Chandraker A, Ali S, Drachenberg CB, et al. Use of fluoroquinolones to treat BK infection in renal transplant recipients. American Journal of Transplantation 2004; 4: 587.
[62] Guasch A, Roy-Chaudhury P, Woodle ES, Fitzsimmons W, Holman J, First MR. Assessment of efficacy and safety of FK778 in comparison with standard care in renal transplant recipients with untreated BK nephropathy. Transplantation; 90 (8): 891.
[63] Sanchez Fructuoso AI, Calvo N, Perez-Flores I, et al. Mammalian target of rapamycin signal inhibitors could play a role in the treatment of BK polyomavirus nephritis in renal allograft recipients. Transpl Infect Dis; 13 (6): 584.
[64] Johnston O, Jaswal D, Gill JS, Doucette S, Fergusson DA, Knoll GA. Treatment of polyomavirus infection in kidney transplant recipients: a systematic review. Transplantation; 89 (9): 1057.
[65] Dharnidharka VR, Cherikh WS, Neff R, Cheng Y, Abbott KC. Retransplantation after BK virus nephropathy in prior kidney transplant: an OPTN database analysis. Am J Transplant; 10 (5): 1312.
[66] Geetha D, Sozio SM, Ghanta M, et al. Results of repeat renal transplantation after graft loss from BK virus nephropathy. Transplantation; 92 (7): 781.

Section 3

Selected Topics in Kidney Transplantation

Chapter 10

Cold Ischaemic Injury in Kidney Transplantation

Sarah A. Hosgood, James P. Hunter and Michael L. Nicholson

Additional information is available at the end of the chapter

http://dx.doi.org/10.5772/50666

1. Introduction

Kidney transplantation is considered the best treatment for end stage renal failure (ESRF) with longer life expectancy and superior quality of life compared to dialysis therapy [1-3]. However, a major constraint to transplantation is the lack of suitable organ donors. To increase the number of available organs there has been an incentive to use 'marginal' donors such as donation after cardiac death (DCD) and expanded criteria donors (ECD), in addition to kidneys from the traditional living and deceased donors [4,5]. Although an important source of organs for transplantation, once transplanted a significant proportion of these kidneys have early graft dysfunction.

There are many attributing factors that influence the outcome of the transplanted graft. Donor and recipient age, creatinine clearance, history of hypertension, poor human leukocyte antigen (HLA) matching, cause of death, ethnicity, the cold ischaemic (CI) time and in the case of DCD donors the warm ischaemic insult have all been described as major determinants of graft function and graft survival [6]. The CI time is perhaps the only modifiable factor that significantly affects graft outcome.

Since the 1970s organ preservation has relied on hypothermic conditions to allow an organ to be preserved outside the body from the time of retrieval until transplantation. This allows the organ to be allocated nationally, to the most suitable and immunologically matched recipient. Nonetheless, hypothermic preservation has its limitations and viability cannot be sustained for an indefinite period of time. Hypothermic preservation has been described as 'a compromise between the benefits and detriments of cooling' [7].

2. Standard criteria donor (SCD)

Deceased organ donors fall into three categories. A standard criteria donor is a deceased donor who is declared brain dead after a stroke or other brain injury. Brain death means that there is the irreversible loss of function of the brain.

3. Donation after cardiac death (DCD) donor

Donation after cardiac death donors (DCD) are donors from which the organs are retrieved after the cessation of circulation due to a cardiac arrest. These organs are regarded as marginal organs due to the warm ischaemic (WI) insult that they receive before the onset of preservation. This WI interval causes a degree of injury that can lead to irreversible damage, resulting in an unfavourable outcome after transplantation. Four classifications of DCD donors have been categorised depending on the circumstances of death and when the organs are retrieved [8,9] (Table 1).

Category	Definition	Type
1	Dead on arrival	Uncontrolled
2	Unsuccessful resuscitation	Uncontrolled
3	Awaiting cardiac arrest	Controlled
4	Cardiac arrest while brain death	Controlled/uncontrolled

Table 1. Maastricht categories of donation after cardiac death donors.

Maastricht type 1 and 2 donors are patients who have died suddenly from a cardiac event or trauma and therefore are usually based in the Accident & Emergency department. After a failed resuscitation, the patient is pronounced dead and a 5 minute 'hands off' period allowed to lapse. The organs are perfused *in-situ* through aortic cannulas inserted through the femoral artery [10].

Maastricht type 3 and 4 are patients who are based on an intensive care unit after a severe brain injury. The patient does not meet the criteria for brain stem death and will maintain spontaneous ventilation. Under controlled conditions with no possibility of recovery withdrawal of treatment is planned. After the cessation of the heartbeat the patient is transferred to the operating theatre and the kidneys retrieved after *in-situ* cooling. In the uncontrolled situation an unexpected cardiac arrest follows brain stem death. The WI time is usually within the region of 15 minutes for controlled donors but can be considerably longer in the uncontrolled situation.

4. Expanded criteria donors (ECD)

Expanded criteria donors (ECD) are defined as any brain dead donor aged ≥ 60 years or over 50 years with ≥ 2 of the following conditions; Hypertension, terminal serum creatinine equal or greater than 132μmol/L or death resulting from an intracranial haemorrhage.

5. Cold ischaemic injury

Hypothermic preservation is based on the principle that cooling an organ inhibits the enzymatic processes. There is a 2-3 fold decrease in metabolism for every 10°C reduction in temperature [11,12]. This slows the depletion of adenosine triphosphate (ATP) and also inhibits the degrading processes (phospholipid hydrolysis). Nonetheless, under hypothermic conditions the metabolic rate remains at about 10% and therefore over time, the hypoxic conditions cause substantial injury [12] this is termed CI injury.

The depletion of ATP due to the inhibition of oxidative metabolism increases levels of adenosine, inosine and hypoxanthine within the cell leading to the formation of lactic acid [13]. This lowers the intracellular pH causing lysosomal instability and the activation of lytic enzymes [14,15]. The depletion of ATP also reduces a large number of cellular processes. Inactivation of the Na+/K+ ATPase pump allows the accumulation of calcium, sodium and water within the cell causing cellular swelling [15]. The binding of transition metals such as iron to their carrier proteins (transferrin, ferritin) is also inhibited which increases the intracellular concentration of free iron [16,17]. This is a strong catalyst for the generation of oxygen free radicals which promotes the production of other free radicals [14]. The impact of CI injury is evident immediately after transplantation when oxygenated blood is re-introduced into the kidney. The downstream effects of ischaemia reperfusion (I/R) injury results in tubular and vascular damage with the impairment of blood flow to the kidney and reduced urine output after transplantation. The kidney can withstand CI times up to 48 hours. Nonetheless, attempts have been made to reduce CI injury and on average the CI time now falls below 24 hours in most transplant centres.

6. Impact

6.1. Delayed graft function

Renal graft function after transplantation is typically measured as incidence of delayed graft function (DGF). There are several definitions of DGF however the majority of centres define DGF as the requirement for dialysis within the first week after transplantation. The diagnosis is based on low urine output, slow decline in serum creatinine levels and increased metabolic instability. Acute tubular injury, otherwise termed acute tubular necrosis (ATN) caused by ischaemic injury is the main cause of DGF after transplantation [18]. DGF is associated with complications such as acute rejection, increased fibrosis and the risk of poorer long term graft survival. It also has a significant economic cost, can complicate patient treatment and prolong hospital stay [19]. Rates of DGF typically range from 5 to 40% in deceased donor kidney transplants [20]. Rates of DGF in live donor transplantation are significantly less (2-5%) due to the short CI time and healthy younger donors [21].

Many experimental studies have shown that the duration of CI directly influences graft function. Several studies suggest that even after 6 hours of CI, significant injury occurs [22,23]. Clinically, the CI time has been clearly shown as an independent risk factor for DGF and reducing the CI time can reduce the incidence of DGF. In an analysis of a series of DBD transplants the risk of DGF was found to increase by 23% for every 6 hours of CI [24] and Locke *et al* found that limiting the CI time to less than 12 hours reduced the risk of DGF by 15% [25]. Other studies have shown that the risk of DGF is increased by 3.3 and 4.4 fold by increasing the CI time by 5 and 10 hours [26].

6.2. Graft survival

The CI time is regarded as an independent risk factor for DGF and DGF is associated with reduced graft survival [27,28]. However, recent evidence suggests that the association of CI time and DGF may have less of an impact on graft survival than previously thought. A multicentre analysis of kidney preservation found that only when the preservation period exceeded 18 hours was the CI time associated with reduced graft survival [29]. A large analysis of registry data of paired deceased donor kidneys found that DGF induced by CI injury had a limited impact on the long term outcome. Nonetheless, in other studies the CI time has been found to independently influence graft survival even in live donor transplantation and in young deceased donors [30,31].

The disparity between DGF and survival is perhaps due to the lack of sensitivity of DGF in determining the severity of kidney injury. DGF is a simple and standard method of reporting early graft dysfunction. However, dialysis within the first week after transplantation can be used to correct metabolic instability without the presence of significant kidney injury. As such, it is difficult to determine the impact of DGF. DGF due to CI can be reversible and therefore have no effect on long term outcome [32]. However, in severe cases, DGF can lead to incomplete recovery and reduced graft survival due to the loss of nephron mass [33]. Giral-Classe *et al* reported that rather than the incidence of DGF, the duration of DGF was the important factor with DGF over six days associated with reduced long term graft survival [34]. More recently, urinary biomarkers have been used to determine the severity of acute kidney injury with cystatin C, neutrophil gelatinase-associated lipocalin (NGAL), interleukin-18 (IL-18] and kidney injury molecule-1 (KIM-1) emerging as the most reliable and sensitive markers of injury [35-37]. Although, not readily used as a diagnostic tool in clinical practice, they may be applied more frequently in the future.

7. Acute rejection

Acute rejection (AR) following renal transplantation can be split into two categories, cell mediated rejection and antibody mediated rejection (also termed vascular rejection). Acute cellular rejection is the more common of the two types and with the introduction of modern immunosuppressive agents rates have dropped from 50% a decade ago to 15-20% today. The typical stimulus for cellular rejection is the presence of so-called 'passenger leucocytes' which are immune cells carried within the blood vessels and tissues of the donor organ. Following transplantation they are exposed to the recipient immune system which recognises them as foreign and results in activation of host lymphocytes which attack the donor kidney. Antibody mediated rejection is less common and usually more severe and if left untreated can rapidly destroy the graft.

Acute rejection is an important factor in early outcomes of transplantation and is closely associated with delayed graft function (DGF) [38-41]. The precise link between DGF, acute rejection and CI time is difficult to fully elucidate. Prolonged CI has been shown to be one of the main risk factors for DGF and DGF is an independent risk factor for AR [42]. However, DGF is a result of a number of factors and it is over simplistic to ascribe acute rejection to just one of those factors. Nonetheless there is evidence that the CI time, alongside other factors, including duration of dialysis, number of HLA mismatches, panel reactive antibodies more than 5% are independent predictors of AR. A large retrospective analysis of 611 transplants demonstrated that CI time was the strongest predictor of DGF [42]. The risk of DGF increased from 9.6% with 12 hours CI time to 21.5% with 24 hours CI time. In the same analysis the risk of AR was increased by 4% for each additional hour of CI time and the risk of rejection in patients receiving kidneys with less than 24 hours CI time was 14.1% compared to 29.3% in kidneys with greater than 24 hours CI time. Furthermore, death-censored graft survival is significantly reduced in patients in whom AR complicates DGF. In addition CI duration of greater than 24 hours has a significantly reduced death-censored graft survival in comparison with durations of less than 24 hours [42].

8. Donor specific effects

Kidneys from DCD and ECD donors commonly present with high rates of DGF compared to SCD and live donors. [43]. DGF typically ranges from 22% to 84% in DCD kidneys compared to 14% to 40% in DBD donors [25, 44-47]. Evidence suggests that the outcome of kidneys from uncontrolled DCDs is poorer when compared to the controlled DCDs with significantly higher rates of DGF, as a response to the longer duration of warm ischaemic (WI) injury under the uncontrolled situation [48].

Kidneys from ECD have a 70% increased risk of graft loss and higher rates of DGF [25,49,50]. The prognosis is even poorer in DCD kidneys from older donors (over 50 years) with the risk of graft failure rising to 80% [25].

In addition to DGF, a small but significant proportion of kidneys from DCD donors also have primary non function (PNF) with rates reported to range from 4 to 19% amongst transplant centres over the last 30 years [51,52]. PNF is particularly detrimental as the patient is exposed to surgery and immunosuppressive therapies without benefit. Furthermore, they may become sensitized to donor antigens, reducing the opportunity for future transplants.

The WI insult in DCD kidneys and the reduced capacity of kidneys from ECDs to recover and regenerate are certainly major contributing factors for early graft dysfunction. Experimental evidence suggests that the combined effect of WI and CI injury exacerbates the injury during reperfusion and the duration of CI has been found to have a strong influence on graft outcome [53]. However, the impact of CI in clinical transplantation is again varied. It appears that as in SCDs, long term graft survival is not necessarily affected by DGF and CI not necessarily an independent predictor of graft survival. Recent evidence from clinical DCD and DBD programmes have reported similar rates of graft survival after 5 and 10 years [45,54-57]. In a series of 112 uncontrolled DCD kidneys, DGF rates were 84% compared to 22% in DBD donors [54]. Nevertheless, the graft survival rates were similar in both groups of patients, 69.3% versus 75.5% at 5 years and 50.3% versus 57.9% at 10 years, respectively. The link between WI, CI and graft survival is not well documented. However, it appears that prolonged CI after a period WI may not be as detrimental to graft survival as previously thought and that kidneys can recover from ischaemic injury with no long term effects [58].

9. Preservation techniques

Organ preservation was first introduced into clinical transplantation in the 1960s. Until this time without proper preservation conditions, kidneys were transplanted as soon as possible after retrieval to minimize the injury. It was then recognized that in order to improve the outcome of transplantation, better methods of preservation were required. Experimental studies in the 1950s by Lapchinsky [59] in the Soviet Union and the early work by Carrel and Lindbergh, showed that ischaemic injury could be minimized by reducing the temperature [60]. In 1963, Calne *et al* used the concept of hypothermic temperatures to extend the preservation time and successfully transplant canine kidneys after 12 hours of storage [61]. This led to the application and development of preservation techniques and solutions that are used today.

10. Static cold storage

Static cold storage (CS) is undoubtedly the simplest and most widely utilised method of hypothermic preservation. The kidney is flushed with cold preservation solution to remove the blood and cool the organ. The kidney is then stored in solution surrounded by crushed ice. Preservation solutions have been designed to counteract the detrimental effects of CI injury. There are a number of commercially available preservation solution, which all contain the same basic formula. This includes an impermeant to minimise swelling and provide stability to the ultra-structure of the cell. A buffer and a balanced electrolyte composition with either a high or low Na+ / K+ ratio to prevent the build up of intracellular acidosis and further minimize cellular swelling (Table 2). Solutions with a high potassium concentration are classified as intracellular and those with a high sodium concentration extracellular solutions.

Components	
Impermeants	glucose, lactobionate, mannitol, raffinose, sucrose
Colloid	hydroxyethyl starch (HES), polyethylene glycol (PEG)
Buffers	citrate, histidine, phosphate
Electrolytes	calcium, chloride, magnesium, magnesium sulphate, potassium, sodium
Anti-oxidants	allopurinol, glutathione, mannitol, trytophan
Additives	adenosine, glutamic acid, ketoglutarate

Table 2. Components commonly used in preservation solutions

11. Static cold storage solutions

11.1. Euro Collins

In 1969 Geoffrey Collins developed the first acellular preservation solution (Collins solution) containing a high concentration of potassium and glucose [62]. Collins solution was later modified omitting some of the ingredients such as magnesium, heparin, procain and replacing glucose with mannitol to provide better osmotic properties and lower the viscosity [63-65]. It was renamed Euro Collins solution and was widely used amongst the transplant community.

11.2. Hyperosmolar citrate

Hyperosmolar citrate (HOC) or more commonly known as Soltran or Marshall's solution was first developed in the 1970s as an alternative to Collins solution [66,67]. It is has a high potassium content and contains basic ingredients using citrate as a buffer. Its hypertonicity is designed to prevent fluid entry into cells. It is a relatively inexpensive, non-viscose solution that is still commonly used throughout the UK in kidney transplantation. It is not recommended for DCD or marginal kidneys despite the fact that there is little evidence to support this view.

12. University of Wisconsin solution

University of Wisconsin (UW) solution has a high potassium concentration to maintain the intracellular ionic balance. It is a more complex preservation solution compared to Euro Collin and HOC, containing trisaccharide raffinose and the anion lactobionate as osmotic impermeants, a phosphate buffer, anti-oxidants (glutathione) to scavenge oxygen free radicals, allopurinol to block the activity of xanthine oxidase and adenosine, an ATP precursor. It also contains the colloid hydroxyethyl starch (HES), to prevent cellular swelling [68]. However, it is debatable whether this is it necessary in a static storage solution and there is some evidence showing that HES can increase tubular damage and cause red blood cell aggregation. Another potential disadvantage of UW solution is the high concentrations of potassium. Although thought important in the prevention of the build up of intracellular calcium, potassium can induce cellular depolarization, reduce cellular 5'-triphosphate content and activate voltage-dependent channels, such as calcium channels [69]. Nonetheless, due to its composition UW solution had, and still has, a significant advantage over other preservation solutions enabling kidneys to be stored for longer periods with better function and less histological injury after transplantation. It is still considered the 'gold standard' preservation solution today.

13. Histidine-Tryptophan-Ketoglutarate (HTK)

HTK was originally developed as a cardioplegic solution but because of its low viscosity was quickly adopted for clinical preservation of the kidney, pancreas and liver [70-72]. It is an extracellular solution and uses the impermeant mannitol and histidine as a buffer. It also contains 2 amino acids, tryptophan, to stabilize cellular membranes and prevent oxidant damage and ketoglutararate, a substrate to support anaerobic metabolism. Recent concerns have been raised regarding its use for ECD and DCD kidneys or for kidneys with prolonged storage times [73]. Some clinical studies have associated its use with the increased risk of PNF and early graft loss [74]. Nonetheless, it is a popular preservation solution widely used throughout Europe and the UK.

14. Celsior solution

Celsior is an extracellular solution and was initially designed for heart transplantation. It contains a high sodium concentration with histidine as a buffer, lactobionate and mannitol to prevent oedema and glutathione as an antioxidant. The solution has proved beneficial in heart, liver, pancreas and in kidney transplantation [75-78].

15. Outcome

An abundance of experimental studies have investigated the efficacy of one solution over another with the majority of studies labelling UW solution as the most superior. However, clinically the evidence is sparse. UW, HTK and Celsior appear to be the better preservation solutions with little difference in rates of DGF between the solutions its usage. Euro Collin solution is not widely used and is regarded as inferior with the suggestion of increasing the risk of DGF [79]. The outcome of individual preservation solutions is more apparent when the CI time is extended beyond 24 hours with UW fairing significantly better than other solutions.

16. Hypothermic machine perfusion

Since the introduction of CS techniques in the 1970s there has been much debate about whether CS or hypothermic machine perfusion (HMP) is the best method of kidney preservation. Undoubtedly, the simplicity of CS has a significant advantage over HMP. However, HMP is it thought to be a better method of preservation in that it allows a continual flush of the microcirculation, prevents the accumulation of waste products, sustains a higher metabolic rate, protects against depolarization of the endothelial cell membrane and reduces free radical formation [80].

Folkert O Belzer was the first to develop a portable HMP system [81,82] in the 1960s. However, with the introduction and success of CS in the 1970s there was little development of this technique in subsequent decades. Nonetheless, with the increasing use of DCD and ECD kidneys over the last decade, there has been renewed interest into the use of HMP. New simpler and portable systems have been developed such as the Lifeport Kidney Transporter (Organ Recovery System, US) which has encouraged the use of this technology. Many experimental studies have found HMP to improve preservation [7,12] and the quality of the kidney. The largest multicentre clinical trial conducted in Europe comparing CS and HMP in deceased donors found that HMP reduced the risk of DGF compared to CS (adjusted odds ratio, 0.57; P=0.01] and improved 1 and 3 year graft survival [83,84]. Although the overall rate of DGF was only reduced by 6%.

The evidence suggests that HMP may be more beneficial in reducing DGF rates in marginal kidneys. In a sub-analysis of 82 pairs of DCD kidneys from the European trial, the DGF rate in the HMP group was 53.7% compared to 69.5% in kidneys that were statically stored [85]. However, there was no significant difference in graft survival at 1 or 3 years. In a further sub-analysis of ECD donors in this trial, HMP reduced rates of DGF from 29.7% to 22% and also improved 1 and 3 year graft survival in ECD kidneys [84,86]. In contrast to this support for HMP, a multicentre UK trial found no beneficial effects of HMP. 45 pairs of controlled DCD kidneys were randomized to HMP or CS [87]. The DGF rates were 58% vs 56% in the HMP and CS groups respectively. However, this trial has been criticised for the sequential design and the small number of patients [88].

HMP techniques are still open to criticism with the suggestion of increased endothelial injury, as found in a recent study of porcine livers [89], risk of trauma to the vessels and the question of cost effectiveness compared to static storage techniques [90]. Nonetheless, it appears that HMP may hold a significant advantage in reducing CI injury compared to CS techniques. The experimental evidence is strong and there is a growing abundance of evidence from clinical studies to suggest an advantage. However, the evidence is not conclusive and there is a need for more clinical trials to determine the superior method of preservation.

17. Normothermic machine perfusion

Maintaining an organ under normothermic conditions is an alternative technique of preservation. Continuous perfusion of the kidney at warmer temperatures with the delivery of nutrients and oxygen has the advantage of avoiding hypothermic injury and hypoxia. In addition, it also may aid recovery and prevent further injury.

Early attempts at normothermic preservation were generally unsuccessful due to the inability to maintain cellular integrity and support renal metabolism. However, advances have been made over the last few decades with the use of technology borrowed from cardiac surgery. The development of less traumatic perfusion pumps and the recognition of the necessity for the delivery of nutrients and oxygen to achieve successful perfusion has made normothermic preservation a realistic contender in clinical transplantation.

Normothermic perfusion can be applied in various ways. The concept of extracorporeal membrane oxygenation (ECMO) to maintain extracorporeal circulation at normal room or body temperature with hyperoxygenated blood can be used to maintain tissue perfusion after the heart has stopped. Normothermic recirculation has proved beneficial in the retrieval of hearts, lungs and abdominal organs. Valero *et al* assessed the effects of implementing this technique in clinical practice in small group of DCD donors [91]. Circulation was maintained for 60 minutes before total body cooling. The incidence of DGF and PNF was reduced after normothermic recirculation compared to standard *in situ* or total body cooling. Gravel *et al* described a DGF rate of 11% in controlled DCD donors [92] and Lee *et al* found similar 5 year graft survival rates to DBD and living donors [93]. Maintaining circulation before retrieval is thought to condition the organs by up-regulating adenosine receptors which may protect against preservation injury [91]. Reznik *et al*, recently reported the application of extracorporeal normothermic recirculation in uncontrolled DCD donors using leukocyte depleted blood [94,95]. Initial graft function was achieved in 6 out of the 16 patients. In the kidney, more evidence is needed to determine how normothermic recirculation before retrieval correlates with early and longer term graft function.

In consideration of the logistical problems of prolonged preservation a great deal of research has focused on using normothermic preservation in combination with hypothermic techniques. Experimentally, intermediate periods of normothermic preservation have been used to restored energy metabolism with replenishment of adenosine levels, effectively 'resuscitating' the organ and retaining viability compared to kidneys stored under hypothermic conditions [96,97].

Brasile *et al* found that a period of warm *ex-vivo* perfusion at the end of the preservation period could resuscitate the kidney after warm and cold ischaemic injury [98,99]. More prolonged normothermic preservation periods have also been more beneficial than hypothermic techniques [100,101]. The only report of a normothermic kidney perfusion technique in clinical practice is by Hosgood and Nicholson [102]. In this single case report of a short period of normothermic perfusion of a marginal kidney with an oxygenated packed red blood cell based solution, the recipient had immediate graft function compared to DGF in the recipient of the paired CS kidney. Further results of the ongoing series at Leicester are awaited. Nonetheless, despite the potential benefits, normothermic preservation is logistically difficult to carry out requiring technical support and expensive perfusion systems.

18. Biomarkers

Measuring the amount of ischaemic injury during preservation would be advantageous as the quality of the kidney could be assessed and a decision made upon its viability. This would be particularly beneficial for marginal kidneys to reduce the likelihood of PNF. Viability is normally assessed by numerous factors including donor history, duration of cardiac arrest, the quality of in-situ perfusion, CI interval and visual inspection of the kidney. Ultimately this relies on the judgement of an experienced surgeon. To avoid PNF, surgeons are typically cautious and therefore many kidneys are deemed unsuitable for transplantation and are discarded [57]. HMP has been used to assess viability. Two aspects can be measured; Firstly, the continuous recirculation of preservation solution through the kidney allows the perfusate flow to be measured and intra-renal resistance can be calculated. Secondly, the perfusate can be sampled to measure cellular injury.

Clinically, the perfusion flow index (PFI) has been used as a measure of flow and resistance [103,104]. This is based on a minimum flow being obtained for a given pressure. The Transplant Group at Newcastle, UK recommend that a PFI of greater than 0.6ml/min/mmHg/100 gram of kidney is needed for a kidney to be deemed suitable for transplantation [105]. However, the ability of these parameters to predict DGF or PNF in clinical practice is limited. Jochman *et al* recently reported that although renal resistance (RR) at the end of HMP was an independent risk factor for DGF and 1 year graft survival, it had a low predictive power and could not be relied on as a sole measure of viability [106]. This is in agreement with other small clinical studies by Sonnenday [107] and Guarrera [108] *et al* that showed that kidneys with poor perfusion parameters had a similar outcome to those with good parameters.

Viability can also be measured by sampling the perfusate for biomarkers of cellular injury. Markers such as redox free iron, glutathione S-transferase (GST), total glutathione S-transferase (tGST), lactate dehydrogenase (LDH), N-acetyl-β-D-glucosaminidase (NAG), heart-type fatty acid binding protein (H-FABP) and alanine aminopeptidase (Ala-AP) have all been used to determine injury [104-106,109]. There is little information on their predictive value. However, Jochman *et al* recently published the results from the European HMP trial in which perfusate samples were taken for the assessment of biomarkers at the end of HMP [106]. GST, NAG, and H-FABP were found to be independent predictors for DGF but not for graft survival in the first year after transplantation. LDH, ASAT, and Ala-AP were found to have no predictive potential for post transplant outcome. Furthermore, the biomarkers did not correlate with intra renal resistance. The evidence suggests that viability assessment during HMP cannot be used independently but may be used collectively with the kidney characteristics and donor demographics to determine the suitability of a kidney for transplantation.

Normothermic preservation techniques may hold more promise in the assessment of viability compared to HMP techniques. During normothermic perfusion renal function and metabolism are restored. In experimental models, low levels of blood flow, reduced renal function and low oxygen consumption have been associated with increased ischaemic injury. Furthermore, these functional measures could be combined with injury biomarkers to assess the quality of the kidney.

19. Experimental studies

19.1. Oxygenation

There is a growing body of evidence in support of recovering ischaemically damaged organs with oxygenated preservation techniques at low temperatures. Historically, oxygenation was considered an essential component of hypothermic kidney preservation in order to support mitochondrial resynthesis of ATP and to delay the injury process. However, with the introduction of the modern day preservation solutions, and the rapid adoption of simple CS techniques, oxygen was not thought to be a vital ingredient and as such is not commonly applied in the clinical setting. Various techniques have been used to apply oxygen under CS and HMP conditions.

Retrograde oxygen persufflation is a simple technique whereby filtered and humidified oxygen is bubbled directly through the renal vasculature during CS. The gas is then allowed to escape through small perforations in the surface of the organ. Reports of its application date back to the 1970s [110,111]. Experimentally, there has been renewed interest in this technique showing a beneficial effect on graft function when compared to CS and HMP techniques [112,113].

Hyperbaric oxygenation is the delivery of oxygen under increased atmospheric pressure. Hyperbaric oxygenation is normally used to treat decompression sickness, carbon monoxide poisoning, gas embolism, circulatory disorders and to promote wound healing [114-116]. However, it has been used in organ preservation. Under normal atmospheric pressure there is a limit to the amount of oxygen that can be carried in the blood. Increasing the atmospheric pressure at which it is delivered, increases the amount of dissolved oxygen in the plasma allowing deeper penetration into the tissue (Henry's Law). Therefore, tissues can be adequately oxygenated in the absence of a blood flow, a particular advantage in organ preservation [114,115]. Although an interesting concept and benefits have been demonstrated in liver and bowel transplantation, there has been little evidence of its use in kidney preservation in recent times.

Oxygen can also be added during HMP. At present, HMP is not supplemented with oxygen based on the presumption that air equilibration in perfusates sufficiently supports energy metabolism and that oxygen consumption at 4ºC is around 5% of that found at body temperature [117]. However, ATP can be restored in part, with the addition of oxygen and energy substrates during perfusion [118]. Short periods of oxygenated perfusion after CS have also been used to resuscitate and condition organs, correcting ATP loss, reducing levels of oxidative stress and improving organ viability [119]. The addition of free radial scavengers such as superoxide dismutase (SOD) to the preservation solution has been found to be beneficial [119,120] in preventing the generation of oxygen free radicals in this highly oxygenated environment.

20. Oxygenated solutions

Oxygen can also be effectively administered during preservation by the use of artificial oxygen carriers. Perfluorocarbons (PFC) are inert solutions that have a high capacity for dissolving oxygen. They release oxygen down a concentration gradient creating a highly oxygenated environment which is not affected by temperature [121,122]. They can be added simply during CS in a technique called the two layer method (TLM). The density of the PFC allows two layers to be formed, PFC on the bottom and the preservation solution on top. The organ is placed in the solution and remains between the two layers. Oxygen can be continuously added allowing adequate diffusion through the organ. TLM has been particularly beneficial for pancreas preservation, allowing a sufficient amount of ATP to be generated to improve organ viability [121,123]. The use of TLM has shown potential in other organs but has failed to gain much support as the ability of oxygen to penetrate deep into tissue in more densely capsulated organs has been questioned. In the kidney its beneficial effect was found in a rat model, however, when applied in a porcine model the results showed no advantage [121,124-126].

PFC can also be formulated as an emulsion for continuous perfusion and was applied during early attempts at machine perfusion [126-129]. However, the instability and adverse effects of the emulsions at that time prevented their continued application [121].

Other novel oxygen carriers have recently been applied experimentally in kidney preservation. Hemarina-M101 (M101] is a respiratory pigment derived from a marine invertebrate, *Arenicola marina* [130]. It has an extremely high affinity for oxygen and functions over a large range of temperatures (4-37ºC) releasing oxygen against a gradient. Using a porcine kidney model Thuiller *et al* recently showed in that adding M101 to UW or HTK solution during CS for 24 hours improved renal function and reduced fibrosis after transplantation. Micro-bubbles derived from Dodecafluoropentane (DDFPe) are also being investigated as oxygen replacement therapies and may in the future be applied during organ preservation [131,132].

In addition to hypothermic conditions, perfluorochemical and haemoglobin solutions can also be used to deliver oxygen at normothermic temperatures [133]. Brasile *et al* originally developed an acellular normothermic solution based on a modified cell culture medium and PFC emulsion (Perflubron) [134]. The perfusate was made up of a highly enriched tissue culture-like medium containing essential and non-essential amino acids, lipids, carbohydrates.

Historically, haemoglobin based solutions such as Stroma-free haemoglobin failed to demonstrate benefit experimentally because of toxic effects on the kidney. However, a newly developed solution, pyridoxalated haemoglobin-polyoxyethylene (PHP) has been deemed to be a more stable solution [133]. New more stable 2nd and 3rd generation PFCs are being developed and several are undergoing clinical trials to assess their safety. Humphreys *et al* recently used a commercially made PFC 'Oxygent' to provide oxygenation and reduced ischaemic injury to the kidney during a period of warm ischaemia by retrograde infusion through the urinary collecting system [135].

Other solutions such as Lifor, a new artificial preservation medium containing a non protein oxygen carrier that can be used at room temperature may also be used for preservation [136, 137]. These new solutions may hold more promise for future development of normothermic preservation perfusates. Nonetheless, the use of these normothermic perfusates in clinical practice is still awaited.

21. Experimental agents

I/R injury involves a cascade of events centralised by activated endothelial cells immediately after transplantation. One of the first inflammatory responses is the infiltration of neutrophils into the tissue. Cell adhesion molecules are recognised by leukocytes which interact with tissue cells to allow the movement of immune cells and mediators to the injury site [138,139]. This is mainly mediated through the up-regulation of endothelial adhesion molecules (ICAM-1, VCAM-1 and E-Selectin) [138]. The release of pro-inflammatory cytokines and chemokines, activation of the complement system and production of reactive oxygen species (ROS) [139] also cause significant cellular injury.

A vast number of therapies have been investigated to ameliorate the detrimental effects of I/R injury such as vasodilatory agents [140,141], antioxidants [142-144], anti-inflammatory agents [145,146] and growth factors [147] and in the experimental setting many of these have proved beneficial. Of particular interest are the therapies that collectively target several mechanisms of I/R injury, these include the endogenous gaseous molecules nitric oxide (NO) [148,149], carbon monoxide (CO) [150,151] and hydrogen sulphide (H_2S) [152,153]. Experimental models have shown their ability to reduce inflammation, oxidative damage, apoptosis and promote smooth muscle relaxation causing vasodilation to enhance renal blood flow. However, their application into clinical practice is awaited.

There is no single agent used as standard clinical practice to treat I/R injury and reduce DGF. Nonetheless, there are several agents of interest that have recently been examined in clinical trials. Recombinant human erythropoietin (EPO) is a treatment for anaemia in renal patients however it also has cytoprotective properties and has been shown to protect against kidney injury in experimental models [154, 155]. However, the results from two clinical trials contradict the majority of animal studies and showed no benefit of EPO in reducing rates of DGF [156,157]. Furthermore, in one trial concerns of the increase in the incidence of graft thrombosis where raised [157]. Other trials to assess the effects of EPO are ongoing and the results are pending. It has been suggested that EPO mediates protection through a tissue receptor that is distinct from the classical EPO-receptor that is known to mediate erythropoiesis [158]. A new compound has been formulated, pyroglutamate helix B surface peptide (pHBSP) that has the tissue-protective properties similar to those of EPO but without causing erythropoiesis [158]. Early experimental models suggest that this agent is beneficial in reducing kidney injury and may hold promise for future clinical trials.

Several volatile anaesthetic agents sevoflurane and desflurane are also being trialled in clinical transplantation to reduce kidney injury. These agents are thought to have a conditioning effect that up-regulates protective mechanisms to reduce the I/R injury response [159]. The conditioning effect can also be applied by short intervals of ischaemia either directly to the organ or remotely to a limb [160]. It can be applied to the donor or recipient and again experimental models have shown the benefits of conditioning techniques. They are particularly attractive for clinical transplantation in that no pharmacological intervention is required and therefore the technique is expected to have a high safety profile. The results of several clinical trials are eagerly awaited. Propofol is another anaesthetic agent that may reduce I/R injury [161,162]. Experimental models have highlighted the anti-oxidant and anti-apoptotic properties of the agent [161,162].

There has been a great deal of emphasis on stem cell therapy to reduce kidney injury. The ability of stem cells to differentiate into multiple lineages with the capacity to stimulate the regeneration of renal tissue is particularly attractive in kidney transplantation. Bone marrow derived mesenchymal stem cells have been used in the rat kidney to reduce inflammation and oxidative damage [163-165]. However, there has been no clinical application of this therapy in kidney transplantation.

Immunosuppressant therapies used on induction can be used to reduce I/R injury and DGF. They suppress leukocyte infiltration and reduce endothelial injury. Anti-CD25 [166] and antithymocyte globulin (ATG) [167] are amongst some of the agents being currently being studied to reduce the incidence of DGF.

22. Conclusion

CI injury is detrimental to early graft function and as such early graft dysfunction is associated with reduced graft survival and complications after transplantation. However, the direct impact of CI on long term graft survival is less clear. Clinical studies suggest that CI may not necessarily be an independent risk factor for reduced graft survival. Nonetheless, further evidence is needed to examine the relationship between CI injury and graft survival. Hypothermic preservation techniques are designed to counteract the detrimental effect of CI injury and hypothermic machine perfusion is emerging as a superior method of preservation compared with static cold storage. Other preservation techniques are being developed such as normothermic perfusion and the addition of oxygen and oxygen carriers during hypothermic preservation. These techniques may hold promise for the future to limit the damage caused by CI injury. Therapeutic agents administered to the recipient may also prove beneficial in reducing early graft dysfunction. Nonetheless, translation of these therapies from animal models to clinical practice remains difficult and the search for the optimal agent or therapy is ongoing.

Author details

Sarah A. Hosgood, James P. Hunter and Michael L. Nicholson
University of Leicester, Department of Infection,
Immunity and Inflammation, Transplant Group. Leicester General Hospital, UK

23. References

[1] Rao PS, Schaubel DE, Wei G, Fenton SS. Evaluating the survival benefit of kidney retransplantation. Transplantation 2006 Sep 15;82(5):669-674.

[2] Schnuelle P, Lorenz D, Trede M, Van Der Woude FJ. Impact of renal cadaveric transplantation on survival in end-stage renal failure: evidence for reduced mortality risk compared with hemodialysis during long-term follow-up. J Am Soc Nephrol 1998 Nov;9(11):2135-2141.

[3] Wolfe RA, Ashby VB, Milford EL, Ojo AO, Ettenger RE, Agodoa LY, et al. Comparison of mortality in all patients on dialysis, patients on dialysis awaiting transplantation, and recipients of a first cadaveric transplant. N Engl J Med 1999 Dec 2;341(23):1725-1730.

[4] Daemen JW, Oomen AP, Kelders WP, Kootstra G. The potential pool of non-heart-beating kidney donors. Clin Transplant 1997 Apr;11(2):149-154.

[5] Alvarez J, del Barrio R, Arias J, Ruiz F, Iglesias J, de Elias R, et al. Non-heart-beating donors from the streets: an increasing donor pool source. Transplantation 2000 Jul 27;70(2):314-317.

[6] Nyberg G, Nilsson B, Norden G, Karlberg I. Outcome of renal transplantation in patients over the age of 60: a case-control study. Nephrol Dial Transplant 1995;10(1):91-94.

[7] Taylor MJ, Baicu SC. Current state of hypothermic machine perfusion preservation of organs: The clinical perspective. Cryobiology 2010 Jul;60(3 Suppl):S20-35.

[8] Terasaki PI, Cho YW, Cecka JM. Strategy for eliminating the kidney shortage. Clin Transpl 1997:265-267.

[9] Kootstra G, Daemen JH, Oomen AP. Categories of non-heart-beating donors. Transplant Proc 1995 Oct;27(5):2893-2894.
[10] Snoeijs MG, Dekkers AJ, Buurman WA, van den Akker L, Welten RJ, Schurink GW, et al. In situ preservation of kidneys from donors after cardiac death: results and complications. Ann Surg 2007 Nov;246(5):844-852.
[11] Mitchell T, Saba H, Laakman J, Parajuli N, MacMillan-Crow LA. Role of mitochondrial-derived oxidants in renal tubular cell cold-storage injury. Free Radic Biol Med 2010 Nov 1;49(8):1273-1282.
[12] Fuller BJ, Lee CY. Hypothermic perfusion preservation: the future of organ preservation revisited? Cryobiology 2007 Apr;54(2):129-145.
[13] Kosieradzki M, Rowinski W. Ischemia/reperfusion injury in kidney transplantation: mechanisms and prevention. Transplant Proc 2008 Dec;40(10):3279-3288.
[14] Salahudeen AK. Cold ischemic injury of transplanted kidneys: new insights from experimental studies. Am J Physiol Renal Physiol 2004 Aug;287(2):F181-7.
[15] Weinberg JM. The cell biology of ischemic renal injury. Kidney Int 1991 Mar;39(3):476-500.
[16] Carden DL, Granger DN. Pathophysiology of ischaemia-reperfusion injury. J Pathol 2000 Feb;190(3):255-266.
[17] Pizanis N, Gillner S, Kamler M, de Groot H, Jakob H, Rauen U. Cold-induced injury to lung epithelial cells can be inhibited by iron chelators - implications for lung preservation. Eur J Cardiothorac Surg 2011 Oct;40(4):948-955.
[18] Kwiatkowski A, Wszola M, Perkowska-Ptasinska A, Ostrowski K, Domagala P, Fesolowicz S, et al. Influence of preservation method on histopathological lesions of kidney allografts. Ann Transplant 2009 Jan-Mar;14(1):10-13.
[19] Brook NR, Waller JR, Richardson AC, Andrew Bradley J, Andrews PA, Koffman G, et al. A report on the activity and clinical outcomes of renal non-heart beating donor transplantation in the United Kingdom. Clin Transplant 2004 Dec;18(6):627-633.
[20] Yarlagadda SG, Coca SG, Formica RN,Jr, Poggio ED, Parikh CR. Association between delayed graft function and allograft and patient survival: a systematic review and meta-analysis. Nephrol Dial Transplant 2009 Mar;24(3):1039-1047.
[21] Gok MA, Shenton BK, Pelsers M, Whitwood A, Mantle D, Cornell C, et al. Reperfusion injury in renal transplantation: comparison of LD, HBD and NHBD renal transplants. Ann Transplant 2004;9(2):33-34.
[22] Dragun D, Hoff U, Park JK, Qun Y, Schneider W, Luft FC, et al. Prolonged cold preservation augments vascular injury independent of renal transplant immunogenicity and function. Kidney Int 2001 Sep;60(3):1173-1181.
[23] Wilhelm SM, Simonson MS, Robinson AV, Stowe NT, Schulak JA. Cold ischemia induces endothelin gene upregulation in the preserved kidney. J Surg Res 1999 Jul;85(1):101-108.
[24] Ojo AO, Wolfe RA, Held PJ, Port FK, Schmouder RL. Delayed graft function: risk factors and implications for renal allograft survival. Transplantation 1997 Apr 15;63(7):968-974.

[25] Locke JE, Segev DL, Warren DS, Dominici F, Simpkins CE, Montgomery RA. Outcomes of kidneys from donors after cardiac death: implications for allocation and preservation. Am J Transplant 2007 Jul;7(7):1797-1807.
[26] Kayler LK, Srinivas TR, Schold JD. Influence of CIT-induced DGF on kidney transplant outcomes. Am J Transplant 2011 Dec;11(12):2657-2664.
[27] Dittrich S, Groneberg DA, von Loeper J, Lippek F, Hegemann O, Grosse-Siestrup C, et al. Influence of cold storage on renal ischemia reperfusion injury after non-heart-beating donor explantation. Nephron Exp Nephrol 2004;96(3):e97-102.
[28] Siedlecki A, Irish W, Brennan DC. Delayed graft function in the kidney transplant. Am J Transplant 2011 Nov;11(11):2279-2296.
[29] Opelz G, Dohler B. Multicenter analysis of kidney preservation. Transplantation 2007 Feb 15;83(3):247-253.
[30] Simpkins CE, Montgomery RA, Hawxby AM, Locke JE, Gentry SE, Warren DS, et al. Cold ischemia time and allograft outcomes in live donor renal transplantation: is live donor organ transport feasible? Am J Transplant 2007 Jan;7(1):99-107.
[31] Hernandez D, Estupinan S, Perez G, Rufino M, Gonzalez-Posada JM, Luis D, et al. Impact of cold ischemia time on renal allograft outcome using kidneys from young donors. Transpl Int 2008 Oct;21(10):955-962.
[32] Chatziantoniou C, Dussaule JC. Is kidney injury a reversible process? Curr Opin Nephrol Hypertens 2008 Jan;17(1):76-81.
[33] Barrientos A, Portoles J, Herrero JA, Torralbo A, Prats D, Gutierrez-Millet V, et al. Glomerular hyperfiltration as a nonimmunologic mechanism of progression of chronic renal rejection. Transplantation 1994 Mar 15;57(5):753-756.
[34] Giral-Classe M, Hourmant M, Cantarovich D, Dantal J, Blancho G, Daguin P, et al. Delayed graft function of more than six days strongly decreases long-term survival of transplanted kidneys. Kidney Int 1998 Sep;54(3):972-978.
[35] Parikh CR, Jani A, Mishra J, Ma Q, Kelly C, Barasch J, et al. Urine NGAL and IL-18 are predictive biomarkers for delayed graft function following kidney transplantation. Am J Transplant 2006 Jul;6(7):1639-1645.
[36] Hall IE, Yarlagadda SG, Coca SG, Wang Z, Doshi M, Devarajan P, et al. IL-18 and urinary NGAL predict dialysis and graft recovery after kidney transplantation. J Am Soc Nephrol 2010 Jan;21(1):189-197.
[37] Koyner JL, Vaidya VS, Bennett MR, Ma Q, Worcester E, Akhter SA, et al. Urinary biomarkers in the clinical prognosis and early detection of acute kidney injury. Clin J Am Soc Nephrol 2010 Dec;5(12):2154-2165.
[38] McLaren AJ, Jassem W, Gray DW, Fuggle SV, Welsh KI, Morris PJ. Delayed graft function: risk factors and the relative effects of early function and acute rejection on long-term survival in cadaveric renal transplantation. Clin Transplant 1999 Jun;13(3):266-272.
[39] Lebranchu Y, Halimi JM, Bock A, Chapman J, Dussol B, Fritsche L, et al. Delayed graft function: risk factors, consequences and parameters affecting outcome-results from MOST, A Multinational Observational Study. Transplant Proc 2005 Jan-Feb;37(1):345-347.

[40] Rosenthal JT, Danovitch GM, Wilkinson A, Ettenger RB. The high cost of delayed graft function in cadaveric renal transplantation. Transplantation 1991 May;51(5):1115-1118.

[41] Sanfilippo F, Vaughn WK, Spees EK, Lucas BA. The detrimental effects of delayed graft function in cadaver donor renal transplantation. Transplantation 1984 Dec;38(6):643-648.

[42] Mikhalski D, Wissing KM, Ghisdal L, Broeders N, Touly M, Hoang AD, et al. Cold ischemia is a major determinant of acute rejection and renal graft survival in the modern era of immunosuppression. Transplantation 2008 Apr 15;85(7 Suppl):S3-9.

[43] Nicholson ML, Metcalfe MS, White SA, Waller JR, Doughman TM, Horsburgh T, et al. A comparison of the results of renal transplantation from non-heart-beating, conventional cadaveric, and living donors. Kidney Int 2000 Dec;58(6):2585-2591.

[44] Gagandeep S, Matsuoka L, Mateo R, Cho YW, Genyk Y, Sher L, et al. Expanding the donor kidney pool: utility of renal allografts procured in a setting of uncontrolled cardiac death. Am J Transplant 2006 Jul;6(7):1682-1688.

[45] D'Alessandro AM, Fernandez LA, Chin LT, Shames BD, Turgeon NA, Scott DL, et al. Donation after cardiac death: the University of Wisconsin experience. Ann Transplant 2004;9(1):68-71.

[46] Whiting JF, Delmonico F, Morrissey P, Basadonna G, Johnson S, Lewis WD, et al. Clinical results of an organ procurement organization effort to increase utilization of donors after cardiac death. Transplantation 2006 May 27;81(10):1368-1371.

[47] Tojimbara T, Fuchinoue S, Iwadoh K, Koyama I, Sannomiya A, Kato Y, et al. Improved outcomes of renal transplantation from cardiac death donors: a 30-year single center experience. Am J Transplant 2007 Mar;7(3):609-617.

[48] Summers DM, Johnson RJ, Allen J, Fuggle SV, Collett D, Watson CJ, et al. Analysis of factors that affect outcome after transplantation of kidneys donated after cardiac death in the UK: a cohort study. Lancet 2010 Oct 16;376(9749):1303-1311.

[49] Sung RS, Guidinger MK, Christensen LL, Ashby VB, Merion RM, Leichtman AB, et al. Development and current status of ECD kidney transplantation. Clin Transpl 2005:37-55.

[50] Saidi RF, Elias N, Kawai T, Hertl M, Farrell ML, Goes N, et al. Outcome of kidney transplantation using expanded criteria donors and donation after cardiac death kidneys: realities and costs. Am J Transplant 2007 Dec;7(12):2769-2774.

[51] Hordijk W, Hoitsma AJ, van der Vliet JA, Hilbrands LB. Results of transplantation with kidneys from non-heart-beating donors. Transplant Proc 2001 Feb-Mar;33(1-2):1127-1128.

[52] Daemen JH, de Vries B, Oomen AP, DeMeester J, Kootstra G. Effect of machine perfusion preservation on delayed graft function in non-heart-beating donor kidneys--early results. Transpl Int 1997;10(4):317-322.

[53] Johnson RJ, Fuggle SV, O'Neill J, Start S, Bradley JA, Forsythe JL, et al. Factors influencing outcome after deceased heart beating donor kidney transplantation in the United Kingdom: an evidence base for a new national kidney allocation policy. Transplantation 2010 Feb 27;89(4):379-386.

[54] Barlow AD, Metcalfe MS, Johari Y, Elwell R, Veitch PS, Nicholson ML. Case-matched comparison of long-term results of non-heart beating and heart-beating donor renal transplants. Br J Surg 2009 Jun;96(6):685-691.
[55] Singh RP, Farney AC, Rogers J, Zuckerman J, Reeves-Daniel A, Hartmann E, et al. Kidney transplantation from donation after cardiac death donors: lack of impact of delayed graft function on post-transplant outcomes. Clin Transplant 2011 Mar-Apr;25(2):255-264.
[56] Snoeijs MG, Schaubel DE, Hene R, Hoitsma AJ, Idu MM, Ijzermans JN, et al. Kidneys from donors after cardiac death provide survival benefit. J Am Soc Nephrol 2010 Jun;21(6):1015-1021.
[57] Hoogland ER, Snoeijs MG, Winkens B, Christaans MH, van Heurn LW. Kidney Transplantation from Donors after Cardiac Death: Uncontrolled versus Controlled Donation. Am J Transplant 2011 Jul;11(7):1427-1434.
[58] Taylor CJ, Kosmoliaptsis V, Sharples LD, Prezzi D, Morgan CH, Key T, et al. Ten-year experience of selective omission of the pretransplant crossmatch test in deceased donor kidney transplantation. Transplantation 2010 Jan 27;89(2):185-193.
[59] Lapchinsky AG. Recent results of experimental transplantation of preserved limbs and kidneys and possible use of this technique in clinical practice. Ann N Y Acad Sci 1960 May 31;87:539-571.
[60] Carrel A, Lindbergh CA. The Culture of Whole Organs. Science 1935 Jun 21;81(2112):621-623.
[61] Calne RY, Pegg DE, Pryse-Davies J, Brown FL. Renal Preservation by Ice-Cooling: an Experimental Study Relating to Kidney Transplantation from Cadavers. Br Med J 1963 Sep 14;2(5358):651-655.
[62] Collins GM, Bravo-Shugarman M, Terasaki PI. Kidney preservation for transportation. Initial perfusion and 30 hours' ice storage. Lancet 1969 Dec 6;2(7632):1219-1222.
[63] Opelz G, Terasaki PI. Kidney preservation: perfusion versus cold storage-1975. Transplant Proc 1976 Mar;8(1):121-125.
[64] Collins GM, Halasz NA. Current aspects of renal preservation. Urology 1977 Jul;10(1 Suppl):22-32.
[65] Collins GM, Halasz NA. Simplified 72-hr kidney storage. Surg Forum 1974;25(0):275-277.
[66] Slapak M, Wilson A, Clyne C, Bagshaw H, Naik RB, Lee HA. Hyperosmolar citrate versus perfudex: a functional comparison in clinical kidney preservation. Transplant Proc 1979 Mar;11(1):478-481.
[67] Jablonski P, Howden B, Marshall V, Scott D. Evaluation of citrate flushing solution using the isolated perfused rat kidney. Transplantation 1980 Oct;30(4):239-243.
[68] Belzer FO, Glass NR, Sollinger HW, Hoffmann RM, Southard JH. A new perfusate for kidney preservation. Transplantation 1982 Mar;33(3):322-323.
[69] Hauet T, Han Z, Doucet C, Ramella-Virieux S, Hadj Aissa A, Carretier M, et al. A modified University of Wisconsin preservation solution with high-Na+ low-K+ content reduces reperfusion injury of the pig kidney graft. Transplantation 2003 Jul 15;76(1):18-27.

[70] Groenewoud AF, Isemer FE, Stadler J, Heideche CD, Florack G, Hoelscher M. A comparison of early function between kidney grafts protected with HTK solution versus Euro-Collins solution. Transplant Proc 1989 Feb;21(1 Pt 2):1243-1244.
[71] Minor T, Olschewski P, Tolba RH, Akbar S, Kocalkova M, Dombrowski F. Liver preservation with HTK: salutary effect of hypothermic aerobiosis by either gaseous oxygen or machine perfusion. Clin Transplant 2002 Jun;16(3):206-211.
[72] Fridell JA, Mangus RS, Tector AJ. Clinical experience with histidine-tryptophan-ketoglutarate solution in abdominal organ preservation: a review of recent literature. Clin Transplant 2009 Jun-Jul;23(3):305-312.
[73] Lynch RJ, Kubus J, Chenault RH, Pelletier SJ, Campbell DA, Englesbe MJ. Comparison of histidine-tryptophan-ketoglutarate and University of Wisconsin preservation in renal transplantation. Am J Transplant 2008 Mar;8(3):567-573.
[74] Stevens RB, Skorupa JY, Rigley TH, Yannam GR, Nielsen KJ, Schriner ME, et al. Increased primary non-function in transplanted deceased-donor kidneys flushed with histidine-tryptophan-ketoglutarate solution. Am J Transplant 2009 May;9(5):1055-1062.
[75] Boku N, Tanoue Y, Kajihara N, Eto M, Masuda M, Morita S. A comparative study of cardiac preservation with Celsior or University of Wisconsin solution with or without prior administration of cardioplegia. J Heart Lung Transplant 2006 Feb;25(2):219-225.
[76] Boudjema K, Grandadam S, Compagnon P, Salame E, Wolf P, Ducerf C, et al. Efficacy and safety of Celsior preservation fluid in liver transplantation: one-year follow up of a prospective, multicenter, non-randomized study. Clin Transplant 2011 Apr 21.
[77] Fridell JA, Mangus RS, Powelson JA. Organ preservation solutions for whole organ pancreas transplantation. Curr Opin Organ Transplant 2010 Dec 9.
[78] Nunes P, Mota A, Figueiredo A, Macario F, Rolo F, Dias V, et al. Efficacy of renal preservation: comparative study of Celsior and University of Wisconsin solutions. Transplant Proc 2007 Oct;39(8):2478-2479.
[79] O'Callaghan JM, Knight SR, Morgan RD, Morris PJ. Preservation solutions for static cold storage of kidney allografts: a systematic review and meta-analysis. Am J Transplant 2012 Apr;12(4):896-906.
[80] Vaziri N, Thuillier R, Favreau FD, Eugene M, Milin S, Chatauret NP, et al. Analysis of machine perfusion benefits in kidney grafts: a preclinical study. J Transl Med 2011 Jan 25;9:15.
[81] Belzer FO, Ashby BS, Dunphy JE. 24-Hour and 72-Hour Preservation of Canine Kidneys. Lancet 1967 Sep 9;2(7515):536-538.
[82] Belzer FO. Current methods of kidney storage. Cryobiology 1969 May-Jun;5(6):444-446.
[83] Moers C, Smits JM, Maathuis MH, Treckmann J, van Gelder F, Napieralski BP, et al. Machine perfusion or cold storage in deceased-donor kidney transplantation. N Engl J Med 2009 Jan 1;360(1):7-19.
[84] Moers C, Pirenne J, Paul A, Ploeg RJ, Machine Preservation Trial Study Group. Machine perfusion or cold storage in deceased-donor kidney transplantation. N Engl J Med 2012 Feb 23;366(8):770-771.

[85] Jochmans I, Moers C, Smits JM, Leuvenink HG, Treckmann J, Paul A, et al. Machine perfusion versus cold storage for the preservation of kidneys donated after cardiac death: a multicenter, randomized, controlled trial. Ann Surg 2010 Nov;252(5):756-764.
[86] Treckmann J, Moers C, Smits JM, Gallinat A, Maathuis MH, van Kasterop-Kutz M, et al. Machine perfusion versus cold storage for preservation of kidneys from expanded criteria donors after brain death. Transpl Int 2011 Jun;24(6):548-554.
[87] Watson CJ, Wells AC, Roberts RJ, Akoh JA, Friend PJ, Akyol M, et al. Cold machine perfusion versus static cold storage of kidneys donated after cardiac death: a UK multicenter randomized controlled trial. Am J Transplant 2010 Sep;10(9):1991-1999.
[88] Jochmans I, Moers C, Ploeg R, Pirenne J. To perfuse or not to perfuse kidneys donated after cardiac death. Am J Transplant 2011 Feb;11(2):409-410.
[89] Monbaliu D, Heedfeld V, Liu Q, Wylin T, van Pelt J, Vekemans K, et al. Hypothermic machine perfusion of the liver: is it more complex than for the kidney? Transplant Proc 2011 Nov;43(9):3445-3450.
[90] Bond M, Pitt M, Akoh J, Moxham T, Hoyle M, Anderson R. The effectiveness and cost-effectiveness of methods of storing donated kidneys from deceased donors: a systematic review and economic model. Health Technol Assess 2009 Aug;13(38):iii-iv, xi-xiv, 1-156.
[91] Valero R, Cabrer C, Oppenheimer F, Trias E, Sanchez-Ibanez J, De Cabo FM, et al. Normothermic recirculation reduces primary graft dysfunction of kidneys obtained from non-heart-beating donors. Transpl Int 2000;13(4):303-310.
[92] Gravel MT, Arenas JD, Chenault R,2nd, Magee JC, Rudich S, Maraschio M, et al. Kidney transplantation from organ donors following cardiopulmonary death using extracorporeal membrane oxygenation support. Ann Transplant 2004;9(1):57-58.
[93] Lee CY, Tsai MK, Ko WJ, Chang CJ, Hu RH, Chueh SC, et al. Expanding the donor pool: use of renal transplants from non-heart-beating donors supported with extracorporeal membrane oxygenation. Clin Transplant 2005 Jun;19(3):383-390.
[94] Reznik O, Bagnenko S, Skvortsov A, Ananyev A, Senchik K, Loginov I, et al. Rehabilitation of ischemically damaged human kidneys by normothermic extracorporal hemoperfusion in situ with oxygenation and leukocyte depletion. Transplant Proc 2010 Jun;42(5):1536-1538.
[95] Reznik O, Bagnenko S, Scvortsov A, Loginov I, Ananyev A, Senchik K, et al. The use of in-situ normothermic extracorporeal perfusion and leukocyte depletion for resuscitation of human donor kidneys. Perfusion 2010 Sep;25(5):343-348.
[96] Maessen JG, van der Vusse GJ, Vork M, Kootstra G. Intermediate normothermic perfusion during cold storage of ischemically injured kidneys. Transplant Proc 1989 Feb;21(1 Pt 2):1252-1253.
[97] Maessen JG, van der Vusse GJ, Vork M, Kootstra G. The beneficial effect of intermediate normothermic perfusion during cold storage of ischemically injured kidneys. A study of renal nucleotide homeostasis during hypothermia in the dog. Transplantation 1989 Mar;47(3):409-414.

[98] Brasile L, Stubenitsky BM, Booster MH, Arenada D, Haisch C, Kootstra G. Transfection and transgene expression in a human kidney during ex vivo warm perfusion. Transplant Proc 2002 Nov;34(7):2624.

[99] Brasile L, Stubenitsky BM, Booster MH, Arenada D, Haisch C, Kootstra G. Hypothermia--a limiting factor in using warm ischemically damaged kidneys. Am J Transplant 2001 Nov;1(4):316-320.

[100] Brasile L, Stubenitsky BM, Booster MH, Lindell S, Araneda D, Buck C, et al. Overcoming severe renal ischemia: the role of ex vivo warm perfusion. Transplantation 2002 Mar 27;73(6):897-901.

[101] Brasile L, Stubenitsky BM, Booster MH, Haisch C, Kootstra G. NOS: the underlying mechanism preserving vascular integrity and during ex vivo warm kidney perfusion. Am J Transplant 2003 Jun;3(6):674-679.

[102] Hosgood SA, Nicholson ML. First in Man Renal Transplantation After Ex Vivo Normothermic Perfusion. Transplantation 2011 Aug 11.

[103] Asher J, Wilson C, Gok M, Shenton BK, Stamp S, Wong YT, et al. Transplantation from non heart beating donors in Newcastle upon Tyne. Ann Transplant 2004;9(1):59-61.

[104] Gok MA, Pelzers M, Glatz JF, Shenton BK, Buckley PE, Peaston R, et al. Do tissue damage biomarkers used to assess machine-perfused NHBD kidneys predict long-term renal function post-transplant? Clin Chim Acta 2003 Dec;338(1-2):33-43.

[105] Gok MA, Pelsers M, Glatz JF, Shenton BK, Peaston R, Cornell C, et al. Use of two biomarkers of renal ischemia to assess machine-perfused non-heart-beating donor kidneys. Clin Chem 2003 Jan;49(1):172-175.

[106] Jochmans I, Pirenne J. Graft quality assessment in kidney transplantation: not an exact science yet! Curr Opin Organ Transplant 2011 Apr;16(2):174-179.

[107] Sonnenday CJ, Cooper M, Kraus E, Gage F, Handley C, Montgomery RA. The hazards of basing acceptance of cadaveric renal allografts on pulsatile perfusion parameters alone. Transplantation 2003 Jun 27;75(12):2029-2033.

[108] Guarrera JV, Goldstein MJ, Samstein B, Henry S, Reverte C, Arrington B, et al. 'When good kidneys pump badly': outcomes of deceased donor renal allografts with poor pulsatile perfusion characteristics. Transpl Int 2010 Apr 1;23(4):444-446.

[109] de Vries B, Snoeijs MG, von Bonsdorff L, Ernest van Heurn LW, Parkkinen J, Buurman WA. Redox-active iron released during machine perfusion predicts viability of ischemically injured deceased donor kidneys. Am J Transplant 2006 Nov;6(11):2686-2693.

[110] Ross H, Escott ML. Gaseous oxygen perfusion of the renal vessels as an adjunct in kidney preservation. Transplantation 1979 Nov;28(5):362-364.

[111] Fischer JH, Kulus D, Hansen-Schmidt I, Isselhard W. Adenine nucleotide levels of canine kidneys during hypothermic aerobic or anaerobic storage in Collins solution. Eur Surg Res 1981;13(2):178-188.

[112] Treckmann JW, Paul A, Saad S, Hoffmann J, Waldmann KH, Broelsch CE, et al. Primary organ function of warm ischaemically damaged porcine kidneys after retrograde oxygen persufflation. Nephrol Dial Transplant 2006 Jul;21(7):1803-1808.

[113] Treckmann J, Nagelschmidt M, Minor T, Saner F, Saad S, Paul A. Function and quality of kidneys after cold storage, machine perfusion, or retrograde oxygen persufflation: results from a porcine autotransplantation model. Cryobiology 2009 Aug;59(1):19-23.

[114] Edwards ML. Hyperbaric oxygen therapy. Part 1: history and principles. J Vet Emerg Crit Care (San Antonio) 2010 Jun;20(3):284-288.

[115] Edwards ML. Hyperbaric oxygen therapy. Part 2: application in disease. J Vet Emerg Crit Care (San Antonio) 2010 Jun;20(3):289-297.

[116] Muralidharan V, Christophi C. Hyperbaric oxygen therapy and liver transplantation. HPB (Oxford) 2007;9(3):174-182.

[117] Guibert EE, Petrenko AY, Balaban CL, Somov AY, Rodriguez JV, Fuller BJ. Organ Preservation: Current Concepts and New Strategies for the Next Decade. Transfus Med Hemother 2011;38(2):125-142.

[118] Pegg DE, Wusteman MC, Foreman J. Metabolism of normal and ischemically injured rabbit kidneys during perfusion for 48 hours at 10 C. Transplantation 1981 Nov;32(5):437-443.

[119] Stegemann J, Hirner A, Rauen U, Minor T. Gaseous oxygen persufflation or oxygenated machine perfusion with Custodiol-N for long-term preservation of ischemic rat livers? Cryobiology 2009 Feb;58(1):45-51.

[120] Minor T, Isselhard W, Yamamoto Y, Obara M, Saad S. The effects of allopurinol and SOD on lipid peroxidation and energy metabolism in the liver after ischemia in an aerobic/anaerobic persufflation. Surg Today 1993;23(8):728-732.

[121] Hosgood SA, Nicholson ML. The role of perfluorocarbon in organ preservation. Transplantation 2010 May 27;89(10):1169-1175.

[122] Clark LC,Jr, Gollan F. Survival of mammals breathing organic liquids equilibrated with oxygen at atmospheric pressure. Science 1966 Jun 24;152(730):1755-1756.

[123] Brandhorst H, Asif S, Andersson K, Theisinger B, Andersson HH, Felldin M, et al. A new oxygen carrier for improved long-term storage of human pancreata before islet isolation. Transplantation 2010 Jan 27;89(2):155-160.

[124] Maluf DG, Mas VR, Yanek K, Stone JJ, Weis R, Massey D, et al. Molecular markers in stored kidneys using perfluorocarbon-based preservation solution: preliminary results. Transplant Proc 2006 Jun;38(5):1243-1246.

[125] Marada T, Zacharovova K, Saudek F. Perfluorocarbon improves post-transplant survival and early kidney function following prolonged cold ischemia. Eur Surg Res 2010;44(3-4):170-178.

[126] Hosgood SA, Mohamed IH, Nicholson ML. The two layer method does not improve the preservation of porcine kidneys. Med Sci Monit 2011 Jan;17(1):BR27-33.

[127] Berkowitz HD, Mendham J, Miller LD. Importance of circulating microparticles for optimal renal perfusion. Surg Forum 1973;24:293-295.

[128] Berkowitz HD, McCombs P, Sheety S, Miller LD, Sloviter H. Fluorochemical perfusates for renal preservation. J Surg Res 1976 Jun;20(6):595-600.

[129] Honda K. Fundamental and clinical studies on intracadaveric organ perfusion with Fluosol-DA. Prog Clin Biol Res 1983;122:327-330.

[130] Thuillier R, Dutheil D, Trieu MT, Mallet V, Allain G, Rousselot M, et al. Supplementation With a New Therapeutic Oxygen Carrier Reduces Chronic Fibrosis and Organ Dysfunction in Kidney Static Preservation. Am J Transplant 2011 Sep;11(9):1845-1860.

[131] Johnson JL, Dolezal MC, Kerschen A, Matsunaga TO, Unger EC. In vitro comparison of dodecafluoropentane (DDFP), perfluorodecalin (PFD), and perfluoroctylbromide (PFOB) in the facilitation of oxygen exchange. Artif Cells Blood Substit Immobil Biotechnol 2009;37(4):156-162.

[132] Lundgren CE, Bergoe GW, Tyssebotn IM. Intravascular fluorocarbon-stabilized microbubbles protect against fatal anemia in rats. Artif Cells Blood Substit Immobil Biotechnol 2006;34(5):473-486.

[133] Daniels FH, McCabe RE,Jr, Leonard EF. The use of hemoglobin solutions in kidney perfusions. Crit Rev Biomed Eng 1984;9(4):315-345.

[134] Brasile L, DelVecchio P, Amyot K, Haisch C, Clarke J. Organ preservation without extreme hypothermia using an Oxygen supplemented perfusate. Artif Cells Blood Substit Immobil Biotechnol 1994;22(4):1463-1468.

[135] Humphreys MR, Ereth MH, Sebo TJ, Slezak JM, Dong Y, Blute ML, et al. Can the kidney function as a lung? Systemic oxygenation and renal preservation during retrograde perfusion of the ischaemic kidney in rabbits. BJU Int 2006 Sep;98(3):674-679.

[136] Gage F, Leeser DB, Porterfield NK, Graybill JC, Gillern S, Hawksworth JS, et al. Room temperature pulsatile perfusion of renal allografts with Lifor compared with hypothermic machine pump solution. Transplant Proc 2009 Nov;41(9):3571-3574.

[137] Regner KR, Nilakantan V, Ryan RP, Mortensen J, White SM, Shames BD, et al. Protective effect of Lifor solution in experimental renal ischemia-reperfusion injury. J Surg Res 2010 Dec;164(2):e291-7.

[138] Bonventre JV, Yang L. Cellular pathophysiology of ischemic acute kidney injury. J Clin Invest 2011 Nov 1;121(11):4210-4221.

[139] Bonventre JV. Pathophysiology of AKI: injury and normal and abnormal repair. Contrib Nephrol 2010;165:9-17.

[140] Hosgood SA, Bagul A, Kaushik M, Rimoldi J, Gadepalli RS, Nicholson ML. Application of nitric oxide and carbon monoxide in a model of renal preservation. Br J Surg 2008 Aug;95(8):1060-1067.

[141] Oruc O, Inci K, Aki FT, Zeybek D, Muftuoglu SF, Kilinc K, et al. Sildenafil attenuates renal ischemia reperfusion injury by decreasing leukocyte infiltration. Acta Histochem 2010 Jul;112(4):337-344.

[142] Nafar M, Sahraei Z, Salamzadeh J, Samavat S, Vaziri ND. Oxidative stress in kidney transplantation: causes, consequences, and potential treatment. Iran J Kidney Dis 2011 Nov;5(6):357-372.

[143] Savas M, Yeni E, Ciftci H, Yildiz F, Gulum M, Keser BS, et al. The antioxidant role of oral administration of garlic oil on renal ischemia-reperfusion injury. Ren Fail 2010 Jan;32(3):362-367.

[144] Chatterjee PK. Novel pharmacological approaches to the treatment of renal ischemia-reperfusion injury: a comprehensive review. Naunyn Schmiedebergs Arch Pharmacol 2007 Oct;376(1-2):1-43.

[145] Haug CE, Colvin RB, Delmonico FL, Auchincloss H,Jr, Tolkoff-Rubin N, Preffer FI, et al. A phase I trial of immunosuppression with anti-ICAM-1 (CD54) mAb in renal allograft recipients. Transplantation 1993 Apr;55(4):766-72; discussion 772-3.

[146] Harlan JM, Winn RK. Leukocyte-endothelial interactions: clinical trials of anti-adhesion therapy. Crit Care Med 2002 May;30(5 Suppl):S214-9.

[147] Edelstein CL, Ling H, Schrier RW. The nature of renal cell injury. Kidney Int 1997 May;51(5):1341-1351.

[148] Yates PJ, Hosgood SA, Nicholson ML. A biphasic response to nitric oxide donation in an ex vivo model of donation after cardiac death renal transplantation. J Surg Res 2012 Jun 15;175(2):316-321.

[149] Dal Secco D, Moreira AP, Freitas A, Silva JS, Rossi MA, Ferreira SH, et al. Nitric oxide inhibits neutrophil migration by a mechanism dependent on ICAM-1: role of soluble guanylate cyclase. Nitric Oxide 2006 Aug;15(1):77-86.

[150] Caumartin Y, Stephen J, Deng JP, Lian D, Lan Z, Liu W, et al. Carbon monoxide-releasing molecules protect against ischemia-reperfusion injury during kidney transplantation. Kidney Int 2011 May;79(10):1080-1089.

[151] Hanto DW, Maki T, Yoon MH, Csizmadia E, Chin BY, Gallo D, et al. Intraoperative administration of inhaled carbon monoxide reduces delayed graft function in kidney allografts in Swine. Am J Transplant 2010 Nov;10(11):2421-2430.

[152] Hosgood SA, Nicholson ML. Hydrogen sulphide ameliorates ischaemia-reperfusion injury in an experimental model of non-heart-beating donor kidney transplantation. Br J Surg 2010 Feb;97(2):202-209.

[153] Liu YH, Lu M, Bian JS. Hydrogen sulfide and renal ischemia. Expert Rev Clin Pharmacol 2011 Jan;4(1):49-61.

[154] Cassis P, Azzollini N, Solini S, Mister M, Aiello S, Cugini D, et al. Both darbepoetin alfa and carbamylated erythropoietin prevent kidney graft dysfunction due to ischemia/reperfusion in rats. Transplantation 2011 Aug 15;92(3):271-279.

[155] Hu L, Yang C, Zhao T, Xu M, Tang Q, Yang B, et al. Erythropoietin Ameliorates Renal Ischemia and Reperfusion Injury via Inhibiting Tubulointerstitial Inflammation. J Surg Res 2011 Jul 19.

[156] Martinez F, Kamar N, Pallet N, Lang P, Durrbach A, Lebranchu Y, et al. High dose epoetin beta in the first weeks following renal transplantation and delayed graft function: Results of the Neo-PDGF Study. Am J Transplant 2010 Jul;10(7):1695-1700.

[157] Aydin Z, Mallat MJ, Schaapherder AF, van Zonneveld AJ, van Kooten C, Rabelink TJ, et al. Randomized Trial of Short-Course High-Dose Erythropoietin in Donation After Cardiac Death Kidney Transplant Recipients. Am J Transplant 2012 Mar 19.

[158] Patel NS, Kerr-Peterson HL, Brines M, Collino M, Rogazzo M, Fantozzi R, et al. The delayed administration of pHBSP, a novel non-erythropoietic analogue of erythropoietin, attenuates acute kidney injury. Mol Med 2012 Mar 8.

[159] Eldaif SM, Deneve JA, Wang NP, Jiang R, Mosunjac M, Mutrie CJ, et al. Attenuation of renal ischemia-reperfusion injury by postconditioning involves adenosine receptor and protein kinase C activation. Transpl Int 2010 Feb;23(2):217-226.

[160] Szwarc I, Mourad G, Argiles A. Post-conditioning to reduce renal ischaemia/reperfusion injury. Nephrol Dial Transplant 2009 Jul;24(7):2288-9; author reply 2289-90.

[161] Basu S, Meisert I, Eggensperger E, Krieger E, Krenn CG. Time course and attenuation of ischaemia-reperfusion induced oxidative injury by propofol in human renal transplantation. Redox Rep 2007;12(4):195-202.

[162] Snoeijs MG, Vaahtera L, de Vries EE, Schurink GW, Haenen GR, Peutz-Kootstra CJ, et al. Addition of a water-soluble propofol formulation to preservation solution in experimental kidney transplantation. Transplantation 2011 Aug 15;92(3):296-302.

[163] Zhuo W, Liao L, Xu T, Wu W, Yang S, Tan J. Mesenchymal stem cells ameliorate ischemia-reperfusion-induced renal dysfunction by improving the antioxidant/oxidant balance in the ischemic kidney. Urol Int 2011;86(2):191-196.

[164] Hara Y, Stolk M, Ringe J, Dehne T, Ladhoff J, Kotsch K, et al. In vivo effect of bone marrow-derived mesenchymal stem cells in a rat kidney transplantation model with prolonged cold ischemia. Transpl Int 2011 Nov;24(11):1112-1123.

[165] Kwon O, Miller S, Li N, Khan A, Kadry Z, Uemura T. Bone marrow-derived endothelial progenitor cells and endothelial cells may contribute to endothelial repair in the kidney immediately after ischemia-reperfusion. J Histochem Cytochem 2010 Aug;58(8):687-694.

[166] Ciancio G, Burke GW, Gaynor JJ, Roth D, Kupin W, Rosen A, et al. A randomized trial of thymoglobulin vs. alemtuzumab (with lower dose maintenance immunosuppression) vs. daclizumab in renal transplantation at 24 months of follow-up. Clin Transplant 2008 Mar-Apr;22(2):200-210.

[167] Brennan DC, Daller JA, Lake KD, Cibrik D, Del Castillo D, Thymoglobulin Induction Study Group. Rabbit antithymocyte globulin versus basiliximab in renal transplantation. N Engl J Med 2006 Nov 9;355(19):1967-1977.

Chapter 11

Hypertension After Renal Transplantation

Mithat Tabaković, Nermin N. Salkić, Fahir Baraković and Senaid Trnačević

Additional information is available at the end of the chapter

http://dx.doi.org/10.5772/51012

1. Introduction

Hypertension after kidney transplantation is an important factor for both graft and patient survival. Arterial hypertension in renal graft recipient is defined as the blood pressure higher than 140/90 mmHg. According to the recent guidelines, the target blood pressure should be less than 138/85 mmHg.[1]

Blood pressure in renal graft recipient is one of the most important factors with negative impact on the survival of kidney graft. Correlation between blood pressure and long-term graft survival is extremely significant.[2] The introduction of the calcineurin inhibitors into the post transplant immunosupressive protocols has increased the prevalence of hypertension after kidney transplantation.

2. Epidemiology

Cardiovascular disease is the most frequent cause of morbidity and mortality after renal transplantation and remains a significant barrier to improve long-term outcomes.Although transplantation improves life expectancy compared with dialysis, survival remains well below general population estimates. Approximately 50% of patients die with a functioning transplant, with approximately 50% of these deaths from cardiovascular disease or stroke.[3] Cardiovascular death rates underestimate the full impact of this disease process given the large number of nonfatal events, including acute myocardial infarction, cardiac arrhythmias, heart failure, and stroke, that affect quality of life.

Transplant recipients are at an increased cardiovascular risk secondary to a variety of modifiable and non modifiable factors, which should be early recognized, continuously monitored and, if possible, thoroughly treated. Blood pressure (BP) represents a non-immunological risk factor that should be readily amenable to intervention. Nevertheless, control rates are disturbingly poor and arterial hypertension is observed in the majority of this patient population. The blood pressure frequently rises after kidney transplantation, as hypertension develops in up to 60 to 80 or more percent of renal allograft recipients.[4-6] Also, it is not unusual have poorly controlled blood pressure among kidney transplant recipients. In a single center study, for example, only 5 percent of kidney transplant patients were normotensive as defined by blood pressures less than 130/80 mmHg as measured by ambulatory blood pressure monitoring. [6]

3. Pathophysiology and causes

There are different factors that cause the appearance of hypertension: renal artery stenosis, immunosuppressive medications especially calcineurin inhibitors (cyclosporine and tacrolimus), corticosteroids, graft dysfunction, chronic allograft nephropathy (CAN), recurrent or "de novo" disease as well as genetic predisposition of donor and recipent.

Most transplant recipients have suffered from long-lasting chronic kidney disease (CKD) and have been treated with hemodialysis or peritoneal dialysis for a certain period. These patients exhibit structural and functional vascular abnormalities, as reflected by the high prevalence of elevated systolic BP and increased pulse pressure. BP in these patients is usually difficult to manage and often volume or salt-dependent. Older age, diabetes mellitus and a high cardiovascular disease burden are common comorbidities.

An association between hypertension and deterioration of renal function does not prove a causal relationship. Hypertension after transplantation might simply be the result of a deterioration in graft function rather than vice versa. Retrospective studies demonstrating an association between hypertension after transplantation and graft survival, cannot differentiate between cause and effect.[2, 7]

The first evidence that hypertension per se may lead to graft damage was the observation that not only hypertension after transplantation, but also hypertension before transplantation is associated with later CAN. Hypertension before transplantation increased the risk for later CAN by a factor of 3.4, the magnitude which was only surpassed by late (>60 days after transplantation) acute rejection episodes, which increased the risk for CAN by 5.5.[8]

Studies in animals support the concept of hypertension-induced graft damage. In two different hypertensive animal models (clipped native kidney plus allograft [9] or transplantation into spontaneous hypertensive rats [10]) it was shown that hypertension may aggravate graft damage.

Another elegantly designed study on rat allograft models explored the mechanisms by which hypertension contribute to CAN. [11] Rats were either left normotensive or were made hypertensive by treatment with deoxycorticosterone acetate (DOCA) and salt. Proteinuria was measured monthly, grafts were harvested at 3 and 6 months for semi-quantitative real time PCR for smooth muscle cell-growth factors PDGF and TGF-β and for immunohistology. Systolic blood pressure was markedly elevated in rats receiving DOCA/salt. Proteinuria was elevated in untreated allografts compared to isografts and was further raised in hypertensive animals. Expression of mRNA for PDGF was higher in allografts than in isografts and was highest in hypertensive animals. Similarly, significantly more tubular cells expressing the 'proliferating cell nuclear antigen' as well as more extracellular matrix deposition were observed in hypertensive animals compared to untreated allografts. In addition, increased expression of MHC I and II was observed in hypertensive animals by both immunohistology and RT–PCR. Thus, hypertension may influence the immunogenicity of the graft.

These data indicate that hypertension of the recipient acts together with alloantigen-dependent factors on the expression of growth factors in the graft thought to be responsible for the morphological changes observed in CAN, particularly the vascular changes with proliferation of smooth muscle cells leading to neointimal proliferation.[12] Hypertension may initiate inflammatory pathways or act synergistically with alloantigen-dependent factors on graft injury.

3.1. Role of immunosupressive drugs in development of hypertension

Immunosuppressive drugs have an important role in the development of hypertension in renal transplant patient. The majority of patients that use cyclosporine do have hypertension that usually normalizes after discontinuation of the incriminated immunosuppressant. Patients that have been using cyclosporine for more than a year develop a need for antihypertensive drug(s) in 20-100% of cases.[13] Most often, it is only a slightly elevated blood pressure that can be successfully controlled with antihypertensives. However, children can develop a serious hypertension combined with neurological complications including "grand mal" convulsions after transplantation, due to high doses of cyclosporine and vasoconstriction.[14]

Before cyclosporine A was introduced in 1983, 50% of the patients with transplanted kidney developed hypertension. After calcineurin inhibitors (cyclosporine and tacrolimus) were introduced the incidence of hypertension surged up to 70-90%.[15] The usage of cyclosporine and tacrolimus is associated with reduced production of nitrogen oxide and increased production of endothelin as well as reduced endothel function. These factors lead to the reduction of vasodilatation on one hand and the increase of vasoconstriction on the other hand, which consequently lead to hypertension. Cyclosporine nephrotoxicity and resulting chronic nephrosclerosis, thrombotic microangiopathy are probably caused by increased sympathic activity, and reduced renal prostaglandin synthesis as well as stimulation of renin-angiotensin-aldosterone (RAAS) systems. [16]

Many authors agree that the influence of cyclosporine and tacrolimus on incidence of post-transplant hypertension is evident. However, the probability for developing a post-transplant hypertension in patients on tacrolimus, is at least 5% lower than in those on cyclosporine therapy. However, the others argue that tacrolimus in higher doses is no different from cyclosporine in terms of risk for development of post-transplant hypertension. [17]

Calcineurin inhibitor (CNI) free immunosuppression has, therefore, been advocated due to the favorable cardio-metabolic profile. In patients receiving belatacept-based immunosuppressive regimens and the mammalian target of Rapamycin (mTOR) inhibitor sirolimus both systolic and diastolic blood pressure were lower compared with patients on CNI.[18]

Cyclosporine-induced hypertension was more of a problem in the early years of its widespread use in which target levels and treatment doses were significantly higher than today. However, in the modern era of individualized immunosuppression and after the publication of the results of the Efficacy Limiting Toxicity Elimination (ELITE)-Symphony study [19, 20] CNI minimization but not complete avoidance is being supported as the best available treatment strategy. Furthermore, findings that chronic humoral rejection may be a major cause of chronic allograft changes and late allograft failure annihilate the common perception that CNIs are responsible for interstitial fibrosis and tubular atrophy.[21] Thus, CNI-free combinations are reserved only for selected patients and CNIs are considered to be essential for the management of renal transplant recipients.

Corticosteroids as integral part of basic immunosuppressive protocols also have an important role as one of the possible causes for post-transplant hypertension. Volume retention caused by corticosteroids partially explains its hypertensive properties. It is proven that the decrease of corticosteroid dose leads to a significant decrease of post-transplant hypertension, as well as reduced body mass index that is considered to be one of the causes for the appearance of post-transplant hypertension.[22] Corticosteroids can deteriorate hypertension with their hemodynamic and hormone properties reflecting through salt and water retention. The usual steroid dose, 10 mg per day or less, however, does not present a significant cause of hypertension.[23]

The well known side-effects of corticosteroids have motivated interest in steroid-free immunosuppression for as long as these agents are available. Steroid withdrawal is possible in many transplant recipients with comparable patient and graft survival.[24, 25] Unfortunately, rejection rates are higher and allograft fibrosis seems to be more common. Still, there may be a advantageous trade-off in terms of reduction of cardiovascular risk factors including hypertension, diabetes and dyslipidaemia.[26] Corticosteroids may contribute more to hypertension early after transplantation or during pulse rejection therapy due to higher doses administered.[27] Glucocorticosteroid-mediated hypertension seems to result from increased peripheral vascular resistance through direct action on the vascular smooth muscle cells and not through the activation of the mineralcorticoid receptor.[28]

3.2. Role of allograft nephropathy in development of hypertension

It is accepted for a fact that chronic graft nephropathy is one of the main causes of hypertension after kidney transplantation.[29] Hypertension is quite often the first clinical sign of chronic graft rejection. A great number of authors highlight the association between chronic graft nephropathy and hypertension more than the degree of tissue match (HLA), suggesting that hypertension is merely one of the causes of chronic graft nephropathy rather than its consequence.[8]

Hypertension is an independent risk factor for the graft dysfunction with the normal creatinine level, as well as with the patients that have been previously treated for acute rejection. The most frequent consequence of hypertension is hypertrophy of the left chamber, angina pectoris, myocardial infarction, stroke, heart weakness, arrhythmia, and sudden death.[15] With the appropriate treatment it is possible to induce regression of the left ventricle hypertrophy and reduce the risk of cardiovascular diseases. [30]

3.3. Donor and recipient related factors and the development of hypertension

Small increases in BP in donors after transplantation do occur and effects are more noticeable in donors with lower nephron mass.[31] However, apart from fetal programming, nephron mass declines continuously with age and prevalence of nephrosclerosis increases linearly and independently from other risk factors from 2.7% for patients aged 18-29 years to 73% for those aged 70-77 years.[32] Older kidney donors (>55 years) have slightly less than half the number of functioning glomeruli compared with younger ones according to a recent report.[33]

Apart from ongoing injury, congenital endowment and donor's age appear to be critical determinants of transplant nephron mass. Therefore, it is not surprising that donor age and graft size are related to the development of posttransplant hypertension. Recipients of older deceased kidney donors are more likely to be hypertensive, whereas patients with low kidney transplant to recipient weight ratios are in need of more intense antihypertensive regimens.[34, 35]

Kidney recipients that have received kidney from donors with positive family history for hypertension have the higher possibility of developing artery hypertension than the recipients who have received the kidney from donors without family history. However, patients having primary hypertension as the cause of terminal renal insufficiency, become normotensive after bilateral nephrectomy and successful kidney transplantation from normotensive donor.[36]

Recipient’s native kidneys and pre-transplant hypertension are described as independent factor associated with post-transplant hypertension. They can cause hypertension in graft recipient via renin-angiotensin system.[29] Also, blood pressure in the recipient's transplant can be influenced by re-emergence of primary disease, “de novo” glomerulonephritis and obstructive uropathy.

3.4. Posttransplant hypertension due to renal transplant artery stenosis

Incidence of renal artery stenosis falls within the range of 2-6% and it is comparably much lower than 80% incidence of developing post-transplant hypertension.[37] The donors younger than 5 years, termino-terminal anastomosis with internal iliac artery as well as the implantation of right kidney are associated with frequent renovascular complications. In a retrospective study of 29 recipients with stenosis and a case-control group of 58 patients, an increased risk of stenosis was significantly associated with CMV infection and delayed function.[38] In contrast to termino-terminal anastomosis with the internal iliac artery, termino-terminal anastomosis with the external iliac artery, in children, decreases renal artery stenosis incidence.

Posttransplant hypertension due to renal transplant artery stenosis is important to identify because it is a correctable form of hypertension. Although it can present at any time, renal artery stenosis usually becomes evident between three months and two years posttransplant.[39]

Clinical suspicion for renal artery stenosis should be raised in situations when audible sound can be recorded during the graft auscultation or in the case of abrupt deterioration of graft function after administration of angiotensin-converting enzyme inhibitor. Hypertension caused by renal artery stenosis is frequently associated with the occurrence of diuretic resistant oedema without significant proteinuria, and with the reduced graft function. It is often associated with polycythaemia.

Stenosis can occur on the anastomosis, but also proximal or distal from anastomosis. Typical time of occurrence is 6-24 months after transplantation. Factors that can cause the renal artery stenosis are: artery injury during explantation and implantation, intimal injury during cannulation or weak technique of vascular suture.[40]

The prevalence of anastomotic renal transplant artery stenosis is difficult to assess. This is due in part to discrepancies in the definition of hemodynamically significant lesions and the use of different diagnostic modalities. It has been suggested that functionally significant stenosis occurs in up to 12 percent of transplant recipients with hypertension, with a range of incidence from 1 to 23 percent.[38]

As with other causes of bilateral renal artery stenosis or unilateral stenosis in a solitary kidney, the administration of an angiotensin converting enzyme (ACE) inhibitor or angiotensin II receptor blocker (ARB) to a patient with transplant renal artery stenosis can lead to a reversible decline in glomerular filtration rate. [39, 41] Thus, an elevation in plasma creatinine concentration in this setting is suggestive but not diagnostic of renovascular disease in the graft. Persistent uncontrolled hypertension, flash pulmonary edema, and an acute elevation in blood pressure are other common features of this disorder.[42]

Although various different imaging techniques may be utilized to diagnose renal artery stenosis, arteriography is the preferred modality. However, since arteriography is invasive, magnetic resonance arteriography or CT angiography are increasingly utilized techniques to screen and/or diagnose transplant recipients for the presence of renovascular disease.[39, 43]

The options available to correct stenosis of the renal artery include angioplasty (with or without stenting) and surgery.

3.5. Consequences of posttransplant hypertension

Hypertension is one of the main risk factors for cardiovascular diseases and reduction of transplant and patient survival. Over the past ten years, the survival of kidney grafts and patients have been recording a significant improvement.

There is little doubt that uncontrolled posttransplant hypertension contributes considerably to graft failure and affects patient survival negatively. The Collaborative Transplant Study (CTS) group first demonstrated a strong and graded relationship between posttransplant BP and renal allograft failure [2], results that have also been validated in subsequent studies.[44] Furthermore, persistently poor controlled posttransplant hypertension (defined as SBP above 140 mm Hg) was found to be associated with poor outcomes, namely worse graft survival and increased cardiovascular mortality.[45]

The study of 29.000 kidney recipients confirms that the increase of systolic and diastolic pressure leads to the higher risk of graft failure. Chronic kidney failure is significantly associated with high blood pressure. It is proven that hypertension is an independent risk factor in kidney graft failure. It has been reported that in hypertensive recipients with systolic blood pressure higher than 150mmHg after the first year from transplantation, there is up to 15% better graft survival in four-years period, with prescribed antihypertensive therapy. [46]

4. Treatment of posttransplant hypertension

4.1. General considerations and proncíples

The target blood pressure is based in part upon the presence or absence of proteinuria and/or additional comorbid conditions, such as diabetes mellitus and/or atherosclerotic cardiovascular disease.[1, 5] The K/DOQI guidelines recommend that the target blood pressure should be less than 130/80 mmHg.[1] For those with significant proteinuria (greater than a spot urine total protein to creatinine ratio of 500 to 1000 mg/g), the K/DOQI work group suggests that a lower systolic blood pressure goal should be considered. The European best practice guidelines recommend a blood pressure goal of less than 125/75 mmHg for proteinuric patients. [47]

The recommended BP targets in renal transplant recipients do not differ from the BP targets of nontransplanted patients at high cardiovascular risk, such as diabetic patients and patients with CKD or established cardiovascular disease. It is important to note that the recommendation to lower systolic BP below 130 mmHg in high-risk hypertensive individuals of the (nontransplanted) general population is not even supported by consistent trial evidence [48] but also, a series of recent publications report no significant benefit or even potential clinical harm by targeting lower BP levels in those patients.

Posttransplant hypertension should be treated to protect against cardiovascular disease and against possible hypertensive injury to the graft. It has been suggested that long-term renal allograft survival may be negatively influenced by posttransplant hypertension. [7, 49]

There are also clinical data showing benefits with blood pressure control. This was best shown in a study of nearly 25,000 first deceased donor kidney recipients.[45] Among patients with systolic blood pressures >140 mmHg at one year post-transplant, improved long-term allograft outcome was observed among patients with systolic pressures controlled to less than 140 mmHg at three years versus those with sustained increases in systolic pressure.

The goal of treatment is to protect graft function and reduce the risk of cardiovascular complications. By applying general life style modifications such as weight control, limited salt and fat intake, moderate physical activity and smoking cessation it is possible to achieve better graft function.[50]

No antihypertensive drug class is contraindicated in the renal transplant recipient and the selection of a specific agent depends mainly on the presence or absence of other comorbidities.[1, 51] The reluctance in the use renin-angiotensine-aldosterone system (RAAS) blockers and the ability of calcium channel blockers (CCBs) to counteract the systemic and renal vasoconstrictive effects of CNIs has influenced the choice of antihypertensive therapy.[52] CCBs are currently considered the therapeutic standard for the treatment of posttransplant hypertension. A recent meta-analysis of a total of 60 randomized controlled trials enrolling nearly 4000 kidney transplant recipients showed that CCBs were the preferred first-line agents.[53] Yet, in the majority of renal transplant recipients, multiple drugs must be given to effectively treat hypertension. As attaining BP targets is more important than selection of individual agents, every drug class may be appropriate after considering the individual contraindications and the patient's risk profile.[54, 55]

It is necessary to determine the causes of post-transplant hypertension and then establish appropriate therapy. Hypertensive patients not taking cyclosporine or tacrolimus should be started on antihypertensive medications. Calcium channel blockers, ACE inhibitors, and beta-blockers all may be effective in this setting. A diuretic may also be necessary in patients with allograft dysfunction in whom volume expansion often contributes to the rise in blood pressure.

In patient on calcineurin inhibitor, an attempt should be made to reduce the calcineurin inhibitor dose in hypertensive patients receiving one of these agents. If the patient remains hypertensive, therapy with a calcium channel blocker or a diuretic (with concurrent salt restriction) should be begun. Other antihypertensive drugs can be added if the blood pressure is not controlled with a calcium channel blocker.

Patients with resistant hypertension should undergo renal arteriography to exclude renal artery stenosis unless there are findings (such as renal insufficiency and an active urine sediment) suggesting possible recurrence of the primary disease. Angioplasty (with or without stenting) or surgery is indicated if a significant stenosis is found. In the absence of renovascular disease, recurrent disease, or rejection, consideration should be given to removal of the native kidneys if there is no other way to control the hypertension.[56, 57]

4.2. Calcium channel blockers

Many physicians prefer a calcium channel blocker because in addition to proven antihypertensive efficacy, it minimizes cyclosporine-induced renal vasoconstriction.[15, 58] The influence on renal hemodynamics positively affects the reduction of fluids and also the acting of calcineurin inhibitors. Clinical studies show that the usage of calcium antagonists with calcineurin inhibitors is connected with the reduction of delayed graft function, with lower number of acute rejection episodes and improvement of long-term graft survival.[59]

A large number of studies have evaluated the efficacy of calcium channel blockers in kidney transplant patients. A 2009 systematic review of 29 studies with 2262 patients that compared calcium channel blockers to placebo or no treatment as well as seven studies with 405 patients that compared calcium channel blockers with ACE inhibitors found that calcium channel blockers were the most effective antihypertensive agent.[53] This systematic review included studies in which patients were not taking a calcineurin inhibitor.

CCBs and ACE inhibitors equally lower the blood pressure. However, in parallel head-to-head two year study which compared nifedipine and lisinopril, it was demonstrated that calcium antagonists improved renal function in 20% more patients than those taking lisinopril.[46]

Calcium channel blockers may have significant drug interactions with cyclosporine, tacrolimus, sirolimus or everolimus (Table 1).[60] Verapamil, diltiazem, nicardipine, and amlodipine (to a minor extent), but not nifedipine or isradipine, slow cyclosporine/tacrolimus metabolism and elevate the plasma cyclosporine concentration. [60, 61] Some physicians have recommended the use of nifedipine to prevent this interaction, while others prefer verapamil or diltiazem since the inhibition of cyclosporine/tacrolimus metabolism permits the use of lower cyclosporine doses.

4.3. Beta blockers

Some authors argue that beta blockers should be first line of treatment in patients with posttransplant hypertension and co-existing heart disease.[62] Beta blockers may increase the triglyceride level, and decrease HDL cholesterol level and in already established dislipidemia in immunosupriminary patients may lead to the additional increase in lipid levels.[63] Beta blockers also contribute to the development of diabetes.

Nevertheless, in patients with heart disease and myocardial inarction they should be part of usual treatment. Left ventricle hypertrophy is an independent factor of mortality in 60 % of the patients with terminal kidney insufficiency while hypertension is a decisive factor in hypertrophy pathogenesis of the left chamber. [64]

4.4. ACE inhibitors and angiotenzin II receptor blockers

The role of ACE inhibitors/angiotensin II receptor blockers in the transplant patient is incompletely defined. These drugs effectively lower the blood pressure and experiments in

Drug class	Indication/benefits	Side-effects/contraindications
a-Blockers	Prostate hypertrophy	Orthostatic hypotension
b-Blockers	Refractory hypertension Hyperkalemia Chronic graft dysfunction Heart failure Coronary artery disease Atrial fibrillation	Hypokalemia Metabolic syndrome Glucose intolerance AV-block grade 2 or 3 Asthma/severe COPD Peripheral artery disease
Calcium channel blockers	Coronary artery disease Supraventricular tachycardia (non-DHPs) Peripheral artery disease	Edema Interactions with CNIs (non-DHPs) Proteinuria
Centrally acting agents	Useful in patients with CKD and after kidney transplantation (increased sympathetic tone)	Bradycardia if used with b- blockers
Diuretics	Heart failure Volume overload	Gout/hyperuricemia Hyponatremia
RAAS blockers	Left ventricular hypertrophy Systolic heart failure Proteinuria	Hyperkalemia Significant transplant artery stenosis Pregnancy
Vasodilators	Refractory hypertension	Orthostatic hypotension Fluid sequestration if used without diuretics (minoxidil)

AV atrioventricular; CKD-chronic kidney disease; CNI-calcineurin inhibitor; COPD-chronic obstructive pulmonary disease; DHP-dihydropyridine; GFR-glomerular filtration rate; LVH-left ventricular hypertrophy; RAAS-renin–angiotensin–aldosterone system.

Table 1. Potential indications/benefits and side-effect/contraindications of various antihypertensive classes in treatment of hypertension after renal transplantation

animals suggest that they may partially protect against cyclosporine nephrotoxicity when compared to similar blood pressure control with hydrochlorothiazide, reserpine, minoxidil, hydralazine, or furosemide. [65, 66]

ACE inhibitors slow down chronic insufficiency of native kidney, and are used for a very long time as an alternative in hypertension treatment.[67, 68] The protective functioning effects of ACE inhibitor are founded on the decrease of both intraglomerular pressure and proteinuria. It is important to point out that angiotensin-converting enzyme inhibitors and angiotensin II receptor blockers inhibit the activation of transforming growth factor –β (TGF), which is included in pathogenesis of chronic kidney failure. The ability of angiotensin-converting enzyme inhibitor to slow down the development of chronic kidney failure is proven on animal experiments and it is documented in the recent report.[69]

However, there are several potential risks with ACE inhibitors/angiotensin II receptor blockers in calcineurin-inhibitor treated patients. The combination of ACE inhibition and cyclosporine-induced vascular disease can induce a modest decline in glomerular filtration rate via the same mechanism described above for renal artery stenosis [68].[70] Early after transplantation (within three to six months post-transplantation), the increase in serum creatinine concentration may confound the ability to accurately detect acute rejection.

Cyclosporine/tacrolimus tends to raise the plasma potassium concentration, primarily by decreasing urinary potassium excretion. This effect can be exacerbated by an ACE inhibitor, which reduces angiotensin II production and subsequent aldosterone secretion. Thus, ACE inhibitors should be avoided in patients who already have a plasma potassium concentration above 5.0 meq/L.

ACE inhibitors can induce anemia in transplant recipients, lowering the hematocrit by as much as 5 to 10 percent [69] via an effect that may be enhanced by cyclosporine.[71] Why this occurs is incompletely understood but a similar phenomenon probably accounts for the efficacy of ACE inhibition in posttransplant erythrocytosis.

To assess the safety and efficacy of ACE inhibitors and angiotensin II receptor blockers (ARBs) in kidney transplant recipients, a large number of retrospective and prospective studies have been performed. The magnitude of these effects was evaluated in a 2009 systematic review of 10 studies with 445 patients that compared angiotensin converting enzyme inhibitors to placebo or no treatment and of 7 studies with 405 patients that compared angiotensin converting enzyme inhibitors to calcium channel blockers.[53] Compared with calcium channel blockers, angiotensin converting enzyme inhibitors were associated with a decrease in GFR, proteinuria level, and hemoglobin value and an increased incidence of hyperkalemia.

No definitive conclusions with respect to GFR and allograft loss could be reached when angiotensin converting enzyme inhibitors were compared with placebo or no treatment. Several retrospective studies in patients with chronic allograft nephropathy have reported benefits with these agents in terms of slowing the progression of renal failure and possibly mortality.

4.5. Conclusion

In conclusion, a great number of patients after renal replacement treatment have poorly controlled blood pressure. Numerous studies bring evidence that poorly controlled hypertension poses a significant threat to both patient and graft which is why blood pressure control may be as equally important as tailoring the individualized immunosupressive regime.

Author details

Mithat Tabaković*, Nermin N. Salkić, Fahir Baraković and Senaid Trnačević
University Clinical Center Tuzla, Internal Medicine Hospital, Tuzla, Bosnia and Herzegovina

* Corresponding Author

5. References

[1] K/DOQI clinical practice guidelines on hypertension and antihypertensive agents in chronic kidney disease. American journal of kidney diseases: the official journal of the National Kidney Foundation. 2004;43:S1-290.

[2] Opelz G, Wujciak T, Ritz E. Association of chronic kidney graft failure with recipient blood pressure. Collaborative Transplant Study. Kidney international. 1998;53:217-22.

[3] Ojo AO, Hanson JA, Wolfe RA, Leichtman AB, Agodoa LY, Port FK. Long-term survival in renal transplant recipients with graft function. Kidney international. 2000;57:307-13.

[4] Kasiske BL, Anjum S, Shah R, Skogen J, Kandaswamy C, Danielson B, et al. Hypertension after kidney transplantation. American journal of kidney diseases: the official journal of the National Kidney Foundation. 2004;43:1071-81.

[5] Mangray M, Vella JP. Hypertension after kidney transplant. American journal of kidney diseases: the official journal of the National Kidney Foundation. 2011;57:331-41.

[6] Paoletti E, Gherzi M, Amidone M, Massarino F, Cannella G. Association of arterial hypertension with renal target organ damage in kidney transplant recipients: the predictive role of ambulatory blood pressure monitoring. Transplantation. 2009;87:1864-9.

[7] Cheigh JS, Haschemeyer RH, Wang JC, Riggio RR, Tapia L, Stenzel KH, et al. Hypertension in kidney transplant recipients. Effect on long-term renal allograft survival. American journal of hypertension. 1989;2:341-8.

[8] Frei U, Schindler R, Wieters D, Grouven U, Brunkhorst R, Koch KM. Pre-transplant hypertension: a major risk factor for chronic progressive renal allograft dysfunction? Nephrology, dialysis, transplantation: official publication of the European Dialysis and Transplant Association - European Renal Association. 1995;10:1206-11.

[9] Kusaka M, Ziai F, Hancock WW, Tilney NL, Mackenzie HS. Systemic hypertension accelerates chronic rejection of renal allografts in the rat. Transplantation proceedings. 1999;31:869.

[10] Szabo A, Patschan O, Kuttler B, Muller V, Philipp T, Rettig R, et al. Hypertension accelerates the pace of chronic graft dysfunction in the rat. Transplant international: official journal of the European Society for Organ Transplantation. 1998;11 Suppl 1:S10-4.

[11] Schindler R, Tanriver Y, Tullius S, Neuhaus P, Frei U. Chronic allograft nephropathy in the rat is aggravated by hypertension and improved by ACE-inhibition (abstract). European Society of Organ Transplantation. Oslo, 1999.

[12] Schindler R, Tanriver Y, Frei U. Hypertension and allograft nephropathy--cause, consequence, or both? Nephrology, dialysis, transplantation: official publication of the European Dialysis and Transplant Association - European Renal Association. 2000;15:8-10.

[13] Schorn T, Frei U, Brackmann H, Lorenz M, Vogt P, Wiese B, et al. Cyclosporine-associated posttransplant hypertension incidence and effect on renal transplant function. Transplantation proceedings. 1988;20:610-4.

[14] Joss DV, Barrett AJ, Kendra JR, Lucas CF, Desai S. Hypertension and convulsions in children receiving cyclosporin A. Lancet. 1982;1:906.

[15] First MR, Neylan JF, Rocher LL, Tejani A. Hypertension after renal transplantation. Journal of the American Society of Nephrology: JASN. 1994;4:S30-6.

[16] Cosio FG, Larson TS. Cardiovascular disease after transplantation: do we know all of the variables? American journal of transplantation: official journal of the American

Society of Transplantation and the American Society of Transplant Surgeons. 2003;3:915-6.
[17] Pirsch JD, Miller J, Deierhoi MH, Vincenti F, Filo RS. A comparison of tacrolimus (FK506) and cyclosporine for immunosuppression after cadaveric renal transplantation. FK506 Kidney Transplant Study Group. Transplantation. 1997;63:977-83.
[18] Steigerwalt SP, Brar N, Dhungel A, Butcher D, Steigerwalt S, El-Ghouroury M, et al. Improved 24-hour blood pressure control with sirolimus versus calcineurin inhibitor based immunosuppression in renal transplant recipients. Transplantation proceedings. 2009;41:4184-7.
[19] Ekberg H, Bernasconi C, Tedesco-Silva H, Vitko S, Hugo C, Demirbas A, et al. Calcineurin inhibitor minimization in the Symphony study: observational results 3 years after transplantation. American journal of transplantation: official journal of the American Society of Transplantation and the American Society of Transplant Surgeons. 2009;9:1876-85.
[20] Ekberg H, Tedesco-Silva H, Demirbas A, Vitko S, Nashan B, Gurkan A, et al. Reduced exposure to calcineurin inhibitors in renal transplantation. The New England journal of medicine. 2007;357:2562-75.
[21] Einecke G, Reeve J, Sis B, Mengel M, Hidalgo L, Famulski KS, et al. A molecular classifier for predicting future graft loss in late kidney transplant biopsies. The Journal of clinical investigation. 2010;120:1862-72.
[22] Taler SJ, Textor SC, Canzanello VJ, Schwartz L, Porayko M, Wiesner RH, et al. Role of steroid dose in hypertension early after liver transplantation with tacrolimus (FK506) and cyclosporine. Transplantation. 1996;62:1588-92.
[23] Nagasako SS, Koch Nogueira PC, Machado PG, Medina Pestana JO. Arterial hypertension following renal transplantation in children-a short-term study. Pediatr Nephrol. 2003;18:1270-4.
[24] Luan FL, Steffick DE, Gadegbeku C, Norman SP, Wolfe R, Ojo AO. Graft and patient survival in kidney transplant recipients selected for de novo steroid-free maintenance immunosuppression. American journal of transplantation: official journal of the American Society of Transplantation and the American Society of Transplant Surgeons. 2009;9:160-8.
[25] Luan FL, Steffick DE, Ojo AO. Steroid-free maintenance immunosuppression in kidney transplantation: is it time to consider it as a standard therapy? Kidney international. 2009;76:825-30.
[26] Knight SR, Morris PJ. Steroid avoidance or withdrawal after renal transplantation increases the risk of acute rejection but decreases cardiovascular risk. A meta-analysis. Transplantation. 2010;89:1-14.
[27] Veenstra DL, Best JH, Hornberger J, Sullivan SD, Hricik DE. Incidence and long-term cost of steroid-related side effects after renal transplantation. American journal of kidney diseases: the official journal of the National Kidney Foundation. 1999;33:829-39.
[28] Goodwin JE, Zhang J, Geller DS. A critical role for vascular smooth muscle in acute glucocorticoid-induced hypertension. Journal of the American Society of Nephrology: JASN. 2008;19:1291-9.

[29] Ponticelli C, Montagnino G, Aroldi A, Angelini C, Braga M, Tarantino A. Hypertension after renal transplantation. American journal of kidney diseases: the official journal of the National Kidney Foundation. 1993;21:73-8.
[30] Schmieder RE, Martus P, Klingbeil A. Reversal of left ventricular hypertrophy in essential hypertension. A meta-analysis of randomized double-blind studies. JAMA: the journal of the American Medical Association. 1996;275:1507-13.
[31] brahim HN, Foley R, Tan L, Rogers T, Bailey RF, Guo H, et al. Long-term consequences of kidney donation. The New England journal of medicine. 2009;360:459-69.
[32] Rule AD, Amer H, Cornell LD, Taler SJ, Cosio FG, Kremers WK, et al. The association between age and nephrosclerosis on renal biopsy among healthy adults. Annals of internal medicine. 2010;152:561-7.
[33] Tan JC, Busque S, Workeneh B, Ho B, Derby G, Blouch KL, et al. Effects of aging on glomerular function and number in living kidney donors. Kidney international. 2010;78:686-92.
[34] Cosio FG, Henry M, Pesavento TE, Ferguson RM, Kim S, Lemeshow S. The relationship between donor age and cadaveric renal allograft survival is modified by the recipient's blood pressure. American journal of transplantation: official journal of the American Society of Transplantation and the American Society of Transplant Surgeons. 2003;3:340-7.
[35] Giral M, Foucher Y, Karam G, Labrune Y, Kessler M, de Ligny BH, et al. Kidney and recipient weight incompatibility reduces long-term graft survival. Journal of the American Society of Nephrology: JASN. 2010;21:1022-9.
[36] Mailloux LU, Levey AS. Hypertension in patients with chronic renal disease. American ournal of kidney diseases: the official journal of the National Kidney Foundation. 1998;32:S120-41.
[37] Merkus JW, Huysmans FT, Hoitsma AJ, Buskens FG, Skotnicki SH, Koene RA. Renal allograft artery stenosis: results of medical treatment and intervention. A retrospective analysis. Transplant international: official journal of the European Society for Organ Transplantation. 1993;6:111-5.
[38] Audard V, Matignon M, Hemery F, Snanoudj R, Desgranges P, Anglade MC, et al. Risk factors and long-term outcome of transplant renal artery stenosis in adult recipients after treatment by percutaneous transluminal angioplasty. American journal of transplantation: official journal of the American Society of Transplantation and the American Society of Transplant Surgeons. 2006;6:95-9.
[39] Bruno S, Remuzzi G, Ruggenenti P. Transplant renal artery stenosis. Journal of the American Society of Nephrology: JASN. 2004;15:134-41.
[40] Sutherland RS, Spees EK, Jones JW, Fink DW. Renal artery stenosis after renal transplantation: the impact of the hypogastric artery anastomosis. The Journal of urology. 1993;149:980-5.
[41] Hricik DE, Browning PJ, Kopelman R, Goorno WE, Madias NE, Dzau VJ. Captopril-induced functional renal insufficiency in patients with bilateral renal-artery stenoses or renal-artery stenosis in a solitary kidney. The New England journal of medicine. 1983;308:373-6.
[42] Voiculescu A, Schmitz M, Hollenbeck M, Braasch S, Luther B, Sandmann W, et al. Management of arterial stenosis affecting kidney graft perfusion: a single-centre study

in 53 patients. American journal of transplantation: official journal of the American Society of Transplantation and the American Society of Transplant Surgeons. 2005;5:1731-8.

[43] Humar A, Matas AJ. Surgical complications after kidney transplantation. Seminars in dialysis. 2005;18:505-10.

[44] Mange KC, Cizman B, Joffe M, Feldman HI. Arterial hypertension and renal allograft survival. JAMA: the journal of the American Medical Association. 2000;283:633-8.

[45] Opelz G, Dohler B. Improved long-term outcomes after renal transplantation associated with blood pressure control. American journal of transplantation: official journal of the American Society of Transplantation and the American Society of Transplant Surgeons. 2005;5:2725-31.

[46] Midtvedt K, Hartmann A. Hypertension after kidney transplantation: are treatment guidelines emerging? Nephrology, dialysis, transplantation: official publication of the European Dialysis and Transplant Association - European Renal Association. 2002;17:1166-9.

[47] European best practice guidelines for renal transplantation. Section IV: Long-term management of the transplant recipient. IV.5.2. Cardiovascular risks. Arterial hypertension. Nephrology, dialysis, transplantation: official publication of the European Dialysis and Transplant Association - European Renal Association. 2002;17 Suppl 4:25-6.

[48] Zanchetti A, Grassi G, Mancia G. When should antihypertensive drug treatment be initiated and to what levels should systolic blood pressure be lowered? A critical reappraisal. Journal of hypertension. 2009;27:923-34.

[49] Sanders CE, Jr., Curtis JJ. Role of hypertension in chronic renal allograft dysfunction. Kidney international Supplement. 1995;52:S43-7.

[50] Barnas U, Schmidt A, Haas M, Oberbauer R, Mayer G. The effects of prolonged angiotensin-converting enzyme inhibition on excretory kidney function and proteinuria in renal allograft recipients with chronic progressive transplant failure. Nephrology, dialysis, transplantation: official publication of the European Dialysis and Transplant Association - European Renal Association. 1996;11:1822-4.

[51] Adams PL. Long-term patient survival: strategies to improve overall health. American journal of kidney diseases: the official journal of the National Kidney Foundation. 2006;47:S65-85.

[52] Baroletti SA, Gabardi S, Magee CC, Milford EL. Calcium channel blockers as the treatment of choice for hypertension in renal transplant recipients: fact or fiction. Pharmacotherapy. 2003;23:788-801.

[53] Cross NB, Webster AC, Masson P, O'Connell P J, Craig JC. Antihypertensives for kidney transplant recipients: systematic review and meta-analysis of randomized controlled trials. Transplantation. 2009;88:7-18.

[54] Chapman N, Chen CY, Fujita T, Hobbs FD, Kim SJ, Staessen JA, et al. Time to re-appraise the role of alpha-1 adrenoceptor antagonists in the management of hypertension? Journal of hypertension. 2010;28:1796-803.

[55] Hausberg M, Tokmak F, Pavenstadt H, Kramer BK, Rump LC. Effects of moxonidine on sympathetic nerve activity in patients with end-stage renal disease. Journal of hypertension. 2010;28:1920-7.

[56] Curtis JJ, Luke RG, Diethelm AG, Whelchel JD, Jones P. Benefits of removal of native kidneys in hypertension after renal transplantation. Lancet. 1985;2:739-42.
[57] Fricke L, Doehn C, Steinhoff J, Sack K, Jocham D, Fornara P. Treatment of posttransplant hypertension by laparoscopic bilateral nephrectomy? Transplantation. 1998;65:1182-7.
[58] Textor SC, Canzanello VJ, Taler SJ, Wilson DJ, Schwartz LL, Augustine JE, et al. Cyclosporine-induced hypertension after transplantation. Mayo Clinic proceedings Mayo Clinic. 1994;69:1182-93.
[59] Ladefoged SD, Andersen CB. Calcium channel blockers in kidney transplantation. Clinical transplantation. 1994;8:128-33.
[60] Kovarik JM, Beyer D, Bizot MN, Jiang Q, Allison MJ, Schmouder RL. Pharmacokinetic interaction between verapamil and everolimus in healthy subjects. British journal of clinical pharmacology. 2005;60:434-7.
[61] Lake KD. Management of drug interactions with cyclosporine. Pharmacotherapy. 1991;11:110S-8S.
[62] Olyaei AJ, deMattos AM, Bennett WM. A practical guide to the management of hypertension in renal transplant recipients. Drugs. 1999;58:1011-27.
[63] Donahoo WT, Kosmiski LA, Eckel RH. Drugs causing dyslipoproteinemia. Endocrinology and metabolism clinics of North America. 1998;27:677-97.
[64] Foley RN, Parfrey PS, Harnett JD, Kent GM, Martin CJ, Murray DC, et al. Clinical and echocardiographic disease in patients starting end-stage renal disease therapy. Kidney international. 1995;47:186-92.
[65] Lafayette RA, Mayer G, Meyer TW. The effects of blood pressure reduction on cyclosporine nephrotoxicity in the rat. Journal of the American Society of Nephrology: JASN. 1993;3:1892-9.
[66] Pichler RH, Franceschini N, Young BA, Hugo C, Andoh TF, Burdmann EA, et al. Pathogenesis of cyclosporine nephropathy: roles of angiotensin II and osteopontin. Journal of the American Society of Nephrology: JASN. 1995;6:1186-96.
[67] Maschio G, Oldrizzi L, Rugiu C. [Risk factors for the progression of chronic kidney failure]. Annali italiani di medicina interna: organo ufficiale della Societa italiana di medicina interna. 1993;8:35-7.
[68] Ruggenenti P, Perna A, Gherardi G, Gaspari F, Benini R, Remuzzi G. Renal function and requirement for dialysis in chronic nephropathy patients on long-term ramipril: REIN follow-up trial. Gruppo Italiano di Studi Epidemiologici in Nefrologia (GISEN). Ramipril Efficacy in Nephropathy. Lancet. 1998;352:1252-6.
[69] Noris M, Mister M, Pezzotta A, Azzollini N, Cassis P, Benigni A, et al. ACE inhibition limits chronic injury of kidney transplant even with treatment started when lesions are established. Kidney international. 2003;64:2253-61.
[70] Curtis JJ, Laskow DA, Jones PA, Julian BA, Gaston RS, Luke RG. Captopril-induced fall in glomerular filtration rate in cyclosporine-treated hypertensive patients. Journal of the American Society of Nephrology: JASN. 1993;3:1570-4.
[71] Gaston RS, Julian BA, Curtis JJ. Posttransplant erythrocytosis: an enigma revisited. American journal of kidney diseases: the official journal of the National Kidney Foundation. 1994;24:1-11

Chapter 12

Transplant Renal Artery Stenosis

Taqi Toufeeq Khan and Mirza Anzar Baig

Additional information is available at the end of the chapter

http://dx.doi.org/10.5772/50396

1. Introduction

Transplant renal artery stenosis (TRAS) is an increasingly recognized, potentially reversible complication of kidney transplantation. It has become an important curable cause of hypertension, graft dysfunction and graft loss in kidney recipients. The incidence varies from 1% to 23%[1] and can be attributed to several factors, first, the absence of the definition of hemodynamically significant TRAS, hence, the reported stenosis ranges widely from 50% to 90% [2-5]. Second, the ready availability of noninvasive screening modalities, such as color Doppler ultrasonography (DUS) and magnetic resonance angiography (MRA), may have led to an increase in the number of suspected cases and third, the intensity with which diagnosis and screening is pursued [1]. The vast majority of cases present between 3 months to 2 years after transplantation but can also present earlier or later [6]. The usual presentation is worsening or new onset hypertension and /or graft dysfunction in the absence of rejection, drug toxicity, ureteric obstruction and infection. Several etiologic mechanisms have been proposed for TRAS, acute rejection [7], suture technique, atherosclerotic arterial disease in the donor or recipient, arterial trauma during organ procurement or transplant, cytomegalovirus (CMV) [8, 9], deceased donor transplants, prolonged cold ischemia and arterial kinking because of a longer renal artery [1,11]. Angiography remains the gold standard for diagnosis and planning appropriate therapy [1]. Percutaneous transluminal balloon angioplasty (PTA) is the preferred initial mode of therapy since it is minimally invasive, safe and effective, with success rates reported between 20% and 88%[1, 12,]. Post PTA recurrence prompted the primary placement of endovascular stents to maintain long term patency [13]. Surgical repair of TRAS is technically challenging due to the dense scar tissue around the allograft, it can result in graft loss and may be indicated in cases where PTA has either failed or is not an option [6]. The hypothesis of downstream effects of renal ischemia and hypoperfusion are introduced for the first time in an attempt to explain its association with ureteric stenosis [14].

2. Etiology

There are 3 main lesions seen in TRAS: the common variety is at or close to the anastomosis, another is a localized lesion, which can be proximal or distal to the anastomosis and lastly, diffuse or multiple stenoses.

2.1. Surgical technique and perfusion

The early presentation of TRAS is suggestive of a technical reason, late presentations especially after many years suggests progression of recipient atherosclerosis. The most common cause of stenosis is related to poor technique and usually located at the site of anastomosis, especially in end to end anastomoses [8, 12] when arteries with unequal diameters are approximated. Other technical reasons that may result in TRAS are: the damage to the intima caused by application of vascular clamps, the healing of which would result in stenosis, the degree of stenosis depending on the degree of initial intimal damage.

Torsion of the allograft at the time of final placement [11] at the time of closure of the incision can lead to kinking that can cause turbulent flow and simulate TRAS [1]. In cases where the renal artery is longer than the vein, kinking and knuckling of the artery is unavoidable because the vein is shorter and prevents a smooth contour. This is especially true in deceased donor right kidney allograft that is without the contiguous inferior vena cava needed for renal vein augmentation to match the length of the right renal artery [11]. This problem is compounded if the renal artery has early bifurcation and cannot be shortened to match the vein because multiple arterial anastomoses would then be required (Fig 1).

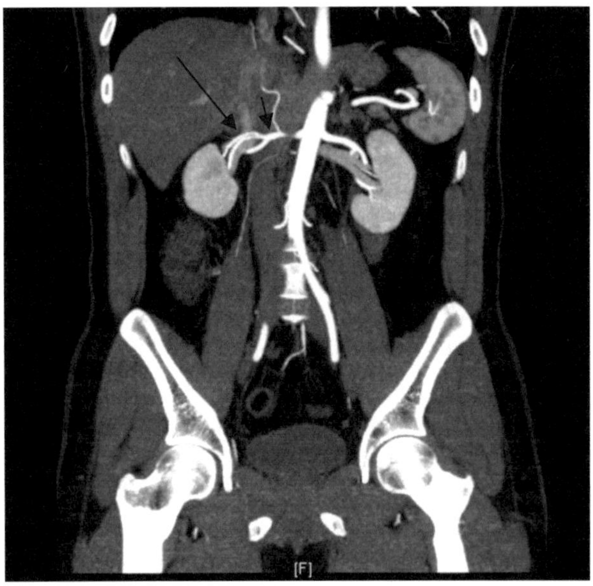

Figure 1. Early bifurcation of the right renal artery . One stump of the renal artery is possible only when it is divided proximal to its bifurcation (short arrow) , rendering it twice the length of the vein (long arrow) that can cause kinking.

Another aspect of technique involves damage to the renal artery at the time of allograft recovery. Rough handling and stretching of the artery can result in intimal injury and dissection, and arteries always need to be handled with great care because success of the entire transplant depends on this arterial inflow. TRAS is allegedly more common in deceased donor transplantation, because of an inherent longer cold ischemia associated with the procedure[12], and not intimal injury. The reason intimal injury is unlikely is because the cannula used for cold perfusion is placed in the aorta, at a distance from the renal arteries, and the renal artery orifices remain untouched. Theoretically at least, intimal injury is more likely in live donor allograft perfusion because the perfusion cannulae are placed directly within the renal artery lumen and have the potential for injury, especially in smaller arteries where an intravenous plastic cannula may be required, and the tip of this plastic cannula can injure the intima if care is not exercised.

2.2. Acute cellular rejection (ACR)

Wong et al found a significantly higher incidence of ACR in their TRAS group compared to controls (0.67 vs 0.35 episodes per patient) with significantly poorer patient and graft survival [7]. Acute rejection was also found to occur more frequently in patients with TRAS (48%) compared to the non TRAS group (27%), although the difference was insignificant [9]. In another paper, 7 of 17 patients with acute rejection also developed TRAS [12]. We also reported our only case of TRAS in a deceased donor recipient, who presented with worsening of hypertension and graft dysfunction, 4 weeks after an episode of ACR [15]. Perfusion injury to the renal artery in this donor was unlikely because the perfusion cannula was placed in the aorta, at a distance from the origin of the renal arteries. Twenty percent of pediatric enbloc and 7% of adult transplants developed TRAS in a study from Spain but the authors found no association between ACR and TRAS in their cohort of 367 pediatric enbloc and adult single kidney transplants over a 13-year period. Interestingly, they found nearly 46% of TRAS lesions proximal to the anastomosis resulting from recipient atherosclerosis [16]. The hypothesis that immune mediated intimal injury was the major factor in the development of TRAS [7] has never been proven and there is no strong definitive evidence that acute rejection causes TRAS. There appears to be only is a weak association or perhaps a coincidental finding.

2.3. CMV infection

Pouria et al found CMV infection significantly more in patients with TRAS than controls (36 vs 12) and claim that CMV contributes to the development of a stenosis [8]. In another paper, the same group reported an increased incidence of ACR in their TRAS cases but deny the CMV association with steroid therapy for ACR [7]. Their hypothesis is that CMV induced arterial injury in immune suppressed patients is via local infection and the mitogenic actions of viral gene products within the arterial wall [8]. It is hypothesized that healing that follows this intimal damage causes fibrosis and leads to stenosis of the artery. CMV was also associated with TRAS in a French study, and in their multivariate analysis, only CMV and delayed graft function were significantly and independently associated with TRAS and poor long term outcome [9].

2.4. Progression of recipient atherosclerosis

As more older and diabetic patients become kidney recipients, there is increased risk of peripheral vascular disease and reduced blood flow to the lower limb. These are patients who should be examined for a bruit because of proximal stenoses in the common iliac artery or the aorta. In a Spanish study, Marques et al found 46% of stenoses were caused by recipient atherosclerosis that caused symptoms of TRAS and these stenotic lesions were proximal to the anastomoses [16]. These lesions can limit arterial flow to the allograft and behave like TRAS (pseudo TRAS) and may simultaneously also have signs and symptoms of lower limb ischemia [17, 18]. Progression of atherosclerosis in these cases can result in stenosis, either at the anastomosis or more diffusely. Stenoses that cause symptoms later or many years after transplant is suggestive of recipient atherosclerotic disease that may involve either the renal artery, or more proximally, the external iliac, common iliac or the infrarenal aorta.

2.5. Calcineurin toxicity

Nodular hyaline deposits in the media of afferent arterioles (arteriolar hyalinosis) are commonly considered irreversible changes, and also regarded as a hallmark of CNI nephrotoxicity. These are characterized by the replacement of necrotic smooth muscle cells by focal or circular lumpy protein (hyaline) deposits at the periphery of the wall of afferent arterioles. Eventually, these nodular hyaline deposits become sufficiently large to cause narrowing of the vascular lumen resulting in stenosis that can cause hypoperfusion, ischemia and TRAS like symptoms [19].

3. Pathogenesis

The most common site for a TRAS lesion is close to the arterial anastomosis, but these may also be located at a distance from it. The number of stenoses depends on the etiology, they can be single or several, affecting different sites along the artery which is suggestive of varied times and causes or it may uniformly involve the whole vessel. The anastomotic stenosis are generally related to technique, may also be related to trauma to arteries during recovery of the allograft or the application of clamps at the time of anastomosis. Poor surgical technique can also result in narrowing of the neo ostium especially when end to end union is attempted, especially where there is disparity in the diameter of opposing lumens. These would present early after surgery because the reason is mechanical [6].

Intimal injury caused by rough handling and stretching of the artery can be either small intimal flaps or dissections that would heal as a scar or hyperplasia, resulting in narrowing. Late stenoses, those which present several years after transplantation are suggestive of progression of atherosclerosis and can involve the allograft artery or its proximal inflow [5]. Diffuse stenoses discovered late can be the result of immune mediated endothelial damage because the histology resembles vascular rejection. There is no clear evidence that rejection is the primary insult that over time results in a stenotic lesion.

Prolonged cold ischemia in deceased donor transplantation may cause arterial injury that heals with fibrosis and causes narrowing, TRAS is less common in live donor transplantation because the cold ischemia is much shorter.

Mechanical narrowing of the renal artery by kinking produces the same effect as a stenosis by reducing inflow and causing ischemia. This is observed when the artery is longer than the vein, usually in right kidneys. In right kidneys from deceased donors, the absence of a contiguous inferior vena cava prevents augmentation of the vein to match the longer renal artery and causes kinking if the discrepancy is not corrected. The kinking may be difficult to correct without further surgery, it is thus imperative that attention be paid to any discrepancy in vascular lengths.

4. Pathophysiology

Hypertension caused by TRAS is the clinical equivalent of the experiments carried out by Goldblatt in the 1930s [18]. He took the approach of experimentally compromising renal arterial blood flow by placing a clamp on the main renal artery. He got the idea from pathologists that intrarenal sclerosis of arteries and arterioles were commonly found at autopsy in patients dying with hypertension. Recognizing that no experimental procedure existed for creating the vascular pathology seen in human hypertensive kidneys, he reasoned that if impaired renal blood flow was the fundamental cause, this could be mimicked by constricting the main renal artery.

Silver clips were set for varying degrees of constriction and placed on the renal artery of dogs. Goldblatt observed that minimal occlusion of the main renal artery was sufficient to induce a rise in blood pressure within 24 to 72 hours. In control experiments constriction of the splenic or femoral arteries did not result in elevated blood pressure. Once hypertension was established, removal of the clip resulted in return of blood pressure to normal levels, a finding suggesting that the ischemic kidney maintained the elevated blood pressure. In some experiments, instead of removing the clip, the clipped kidney was removed. This resulted in a return of blood pressure to normal levels. Subsequently placing a clip on the main renal artery of the remaining kidney resulted in reelevation of blood pressure. In Goldblatt's early studies, hypertension in most animals lasted from 4 to 6 weeks and then blood pressures returned to normal levels, even though the clamps were still in place. Goldblatt noticed that the return to normal blood pressure was associated with conspicuous development of collateral arterial circulation to the kidney, particularly through the renal capsule. In subsequent experiments he decapsulated the kidney and enclosed it in a membrane to prevent revascularization. When the renal artery of such animals was constricted, hypertension occurred and persisted.

Goldblatts one kidney, one clip (1K1C) model is where a clip is applied to one renal artery and the contralateral kidney is removed. The transplanted kidney, unlike the clipped kidney is denervated and ischemia fails to elicit sympathetic activation. In the ischemic 1K1C model, this single kidney responds with activation of renin angiotensin system, sodium retention and increase in the extracelluar volume. The increased volume improves renal perfusion which inhibits the RAS. In this new milieu, hypertension is sustained by the expanded volume and renin levels remain normal or low.

In animal experiments, a decrease in kidney perfusion is observed only after the renal artery lumen is narrowed by more than 50% [20]. Similar findings are reported in humans during angiography, the renal vascular resistance increases to levels which impair perfusion only after arterial lumen is narrowed by 50% [21]. When the renal perfusion pressure drops by at least 15mmHg as a result of TRAS, severe hypertension and renal failure ensue, becoming irreversible if left untreated.

Glomerular filtration rate (GFR) is generally not affected, even though the perfusion pressure is low because intracapillary pressure is sustained by increasing the postglomerular resistance which increases the filtration fraction. There is a critical period during which revascularization can be successful, however, if the ischemia becomes chronic, restoring renal blood flow at this time usually will not result in improvement because of the chronic changes. When revascularization is performed before these changes, the postglomerular resistance is reduced with prompt diuresis and improvement in hypertension [22]. This has clinical implications, because prolonged renal ischemia causes irreversible changes, every effort must be made to restore kidney perfusion in a timely manner after diagnosis to prevent such permanent damage and renal failure. An indication of these permanent changes may be reflected by the intrarenal resistive indices (RIs) on DUS, and RIs over 0.8 reflect such structural changes that will prevent any functional recovery following revascularization. A clinical study was undertaken in transplant recipients by Radermacher et al to assess whether RIs over 0.8 reflected structural changes and predicted early graft loss and death [23]. They showed that significantly more patients with RIs over 0.8 had lower creatinine clearance, required dialysis and died, than patients with RIs less than 0.8 ($P<0.001$ for all comparisons) . This effectively means that if any transplant recipient with TRAS has RIs over 0.8, the chances of revascularization are not enough to warrant invasive treatment. Initially in TRAS, the intrarenal RIs are less than 0.55, however, if untreated, the associated hypertension results in arteriolosclerosis, fibrosis and kidney atrophy with an increase in RIs. Presence of RIs between 0.55 and 0.8 suggests that permanent structural changes have not occurred and that revascularization can be successful.

5. Clinical presentation

Worsening or de novo hypertension is the usual initial presentation, in some cases, there may be an increased requirement of anti hypertensive medication. Renal hypoperfusion activates the renin angiotensin system (RAS) with resulting fluid retention, which with hypertension can cause edema, congestive cardiac failure or recurrent pulmonary edema. Patients can also remain asymptomatic except for hypertension. Injudicious diuretic therapy or addition of angiotensin converting enzyme inhibitors or angiotensin receptor blockers to the anti hypertensive regime can cause acute deterioration in renal function or renal failure.

A bruit may be heard over the graft in some cases, although not specific for TRAS because the stenosis can involve any artery proximal to the anastomosis. Renal dysfunction in the absence of rejection, ureteric obstruction and infection is not observed until a critical stenosis is reached, and there is much debate about this critical degree of stenosis or when does a stenosis become 'significant'. Objectively, stenosis of the transplant renal artery only achieves significance once there is evidence of renal impairment, because it indicates a level of renal hypoperfusion or ischemia that is unable to sustain adequate renal function.

6. Differential diagnosis

Any condition that causes hypertension and graft dysfunction must be included in the list of differential diagnosis. During the early period following transplantation, calcineurin inhibitor (CNI) levels are highest, and toxicity can induce reversible hemodynamic changes that mimic those observed in TRAS. This is the result of an increase in resistance at the site of afferent arteriole that causes glomerular hypoperfusion, increased FF, sodium and water retention and hypertension. Chronic CNI toxicity will produce irreversible vascular changes with graft failure [24]. TRAS must be differentiated from proximal aortic or iliac stenosis associated with recipient atherosclerosis, that may have progressed as a consequence of treatment with CNIs and steroids. In these cases, a bruit may be audible below the umbilicus. Other considerations are hypertension as a result of native atrophic kidneys and as a consequence of chronic rejection.

6.1. Diagnosis – Laboratory tests

Plasma renin. Lower levels may be observed in TRAS because the fluid retention and volume expansion that causes hypertension may not fully activate the RAS.

Increased levels may be secondary to diuretic therapy or in some cases of acute rejection.

Serum potassium may be elevated with high CNI levels.

6.2. Isotope scanning

Isotope renal scanning had good sensitivity (75%) but the poor specificity (67%) made it unpopular [25]. Scintigraphy using Captopril [26] was useful in evaluating segmental arteries but Losartan scintigraphy [27] was considered an improvement, but is rarely used now.

6.3. DUS

This is an excellent modality for diagnosis and follow-up for TRAS. Its many advantages are that it is non-invasive, inexpensive, has good sensitivity (87-94%) and specificity (86-100%), can be performed at the bedside, can evaluate hemodynamic significance, grading and localization of stenoses and assess revascularization. The information derived from this depends heavily on the experience and skill of the person operating the machine. Two types of data are necessary for evaluation of a stenosis, the peak systolic velocity (PSV) at the site of stenosis, and the intra renal RIs. At times, PSV may not be obtainable by DUS but scans carried out during microbubble infusion can quantify total and regional renal blood flow [28].

6.4. Extra renal doppler

This is a scan of the renal artery from the anastomosis to the hilum of the kidney and PSV is measured along its entire course. At the site of a stenosis, there is an increase in PSV of >2m/sec. The advantages are a high accuracy in ascertaining the severity of stenosis with the ability to localize the site of stenosis. The main disadvantage is that it is operator dependent, it is also time consuming because it requires an angle of interrogation parallel to the course of the artery.

6.5. Intra renal doppler

This analyzes the Doppler signal in the intrarenal arteries distal to the stenosis. The normal intrarenal spectral waveform has a sharp systolic rise, a gradual reduction in velocity of flow in late systole, and, low velocity forward flow throughout diastole (Fig 2).

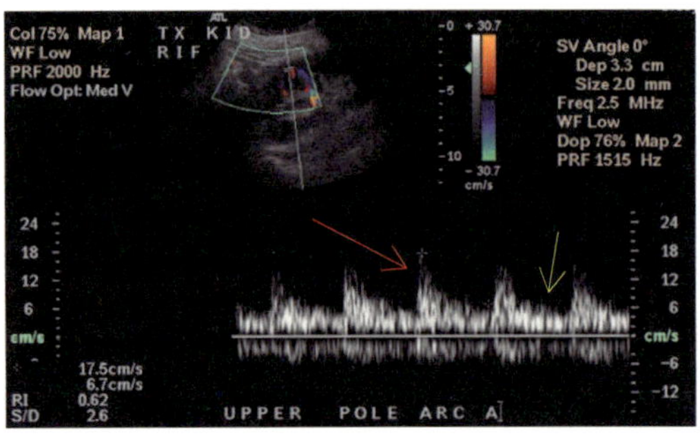

Figure 2. Normal intrarenal waveform, note the sharp systolic upstroke (red arrow), a gradual reduction in velocity and low velocity flow during diastole (yellow arrow).

The parvus tardus waveform is considered diagnostic of a proximal stenosis, and is a small amplitude waveform with a prolonged systolic rise or prolongation of the acceleration time (Fig 3) [29].

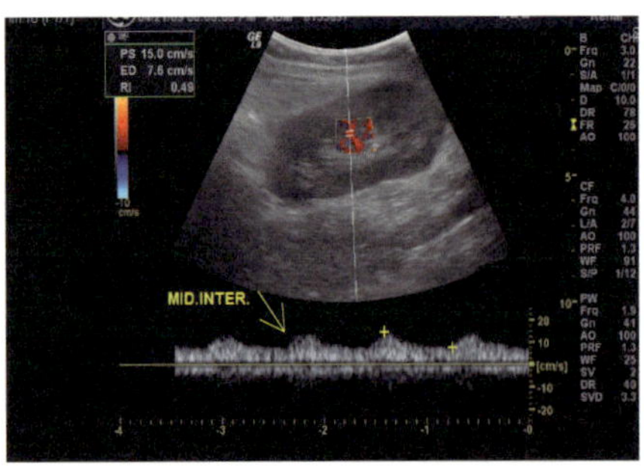

Figure 3. Intrarenal parvus tardus waveform, note the low amplitude and slow systolic rise waveform (yellow arrow) with RI of 0.49.

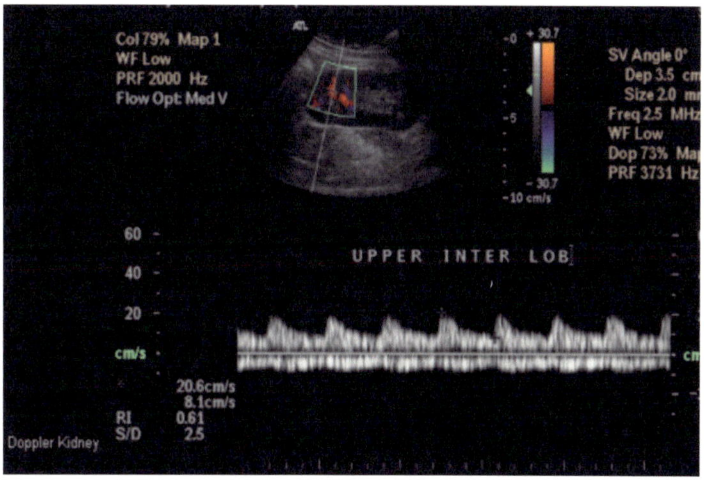

Figure 4. Post revascularization intrarenal Doppler. Normal waveform is seen confirming successful restoration of blood flow.

It must be remembered that this waveform can be produced by a stenosis at any point proximal to the artery studied. This Doppler scan is not as operator dependent as the extra renal Doppler and also cannot localize the site of stenosis.

In cases of TRAS, RIs in the intrarenal arteries are reduced because it is distal to the stenosis and subject to reduced blood flow. An RI of <0.55 is considered diagnostic of TRAS alongwith the parvus tardus waveform, both reflecting reduced blood flow [30].

6.6. Spiral computerized tomography

Provides three- dimensional imaging of the vascular anatomy and the images are superior to conventional angiography. It requires less contrast medium and does not require arterial access. Unlike angiography, it cannot be used for angioplasty.

6.7. MRA

This imaging modality has a sensitivity of 67-100% and specificity of 75-100%, but is expensive with limited availability. There is no radiation involved and the contrast used in not nephrotoxic [31].

6.8. Angiography

This is the gold standard for diagnosis of TRAS and provides a road map that is helpful in planning treatment. Besides confirming the diagnosis and localizing the site of stenosis, it provides immediate access for PTA and placement of a stent and the outcome can be confirmed right away with another angiography (Fig 4, 5). Carbon dioxide can be used as negative contrast in cases with renal impairment to provide images comparable to standard angiography [32].

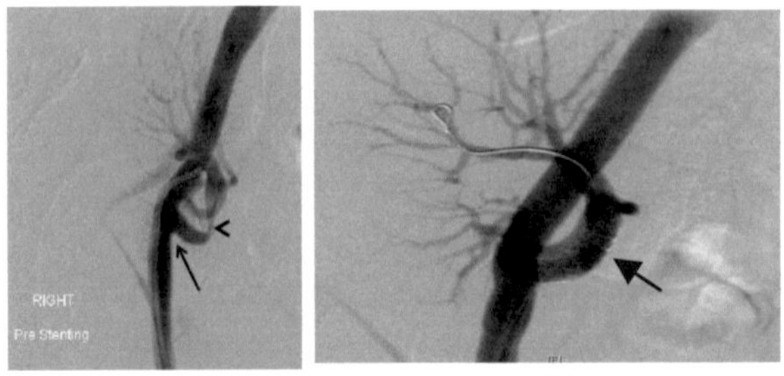

(a) (b)

Figure 5. (a)Angiography showing allograft renal artery stenosis (arrowhead) away from site of anastomosis (arrow). (b)Post stenting angiography showing the stent in place (arrow).

7. Treatment

7.1. Conservative treatment

This is indicated when renal function is at baseline values and intrarenal RIs are >0.55 on Doppler. This suggests that renal blood flow is adequate and the stenosis is not hemodynamically significant. In such patients, the treatment of hypertension should include low dose angiotensin converting enzyme inhibitors (ACEi) and serum potassium and creatinine checked in 7-10 days. A 30% increase in serum creatinine from the baseline in cases of TRAS indicates decreased intravascular volume, low albumin or decreased cardiac output. An increase in serum potassium should be treated with exchange resins. Long term treatment should be considered if low dose ACEi are tolerated and replaced with longer acting agents. This will also help in reducing cardiovascular complications. TRAS should be monitored by Doppler at least every 6 months for evidence of progression of the stenosis by comparing the new RI and PSV values with previous ones.

7.2. Angioplasty and stenting

Before the onset of renal impairment, it can be implied that the amount of blood flow possible through the stenosis is enough to maintain normal renal function. When the stenosis becomes hemodynamically significant with evidence of renal hypoperfusion, an angiogram should be carried out to confirm the diagnosis, followed by an angioplasty to dilate the stenosis and stenting, an option that is gaining popularity. PTA is the preferred initial mode of therapy for TRAS. It is minimally invasive and safe with a reported success rate of 70-90% [33]. The variable success rate for PTA may be related to the location and length of the stenosis, and the best results have been reported when the lesions are short, linear and not at the site of anastomosis [1]. When used in anastomotic lesions, PTA alone has a low success rate with an increased risk of complications, but better results are reported when PTA is combined with stenting [34]. In cases where the artery is kinked, PTA is ineffective because the kink is related to the disparity in length of artery and vein and the kink will return once the balloon is withdrawn. After PTA alone, the short term recurrence rate of up to 30% is a major disadvantage, this risk of recurrence can however be significantly reduced when PTA and stenting are carried out during the same procedure [35]. The low recurrence rates with primary stenting has prompted radiologists to consider stenting during the first PTA. Hung Su reported on 9 cases of TRAS treated with primary stenting after PTA without any evidence of any recurrence after a 4 year follow-up [13]. A novel development to reduce stent occlusion was the introduction of stents that release agents like rapamycin and enoxaparin locally to inhibit intimal hyperplasia [36].

8. Surgery

Indications for surgery include stenoses at the anastomotic site, kinks, severe stenosis inaccessible to PTA, failed PTA and recurrent lesions. Access to the renal arteries can be technically challenging because of scar tissue and adhesions, and serious complications can develop, including graft loss [6]. The success and minimal invasiveness of PTA and stenting has relegated surgery to the position of a salvage procedure when no other options are available. Surgical reconstruction of the transplant renal artery using preserved, blood type-matched, cadaveric donor iliac artery grafts appears promising. In a study from Wisconsin, patients treated with surgical reconstruction, hemodynamically significant TRAS lesions were noted at or within 1 to 2 mm of the anastomosis in 13 patients, in the middle of the renal artery in 4, and secondary to a kink in 2 patients. Surgical treatment was undertaken in seven patients following unsuccessful PTA. Two patients also had aneurysms of the iliac artery. Reconstruction using cadaveric iliac artery was successful in 19 of 21 (90%) patients, and only 1 these patients (4.8%) failed due to recurrence, with a median follow-up of 42 months. Graft loss secondary to TRAS occurred in only two patients. The authors claim not to have seen any long-term complications related to cadaveric iliac artery grafts [37].

9. Defining significant stenosis

After being diagnosed with TRAS on DUS, it is important to know which patients need regular monitoring and which patients require an angiogram and treatment? The lack of such a definition of significant TRAS needs to be addressed and should include both refractory hypertension and importantly, graft dysfunction (in the absence of rejection, obstruction and infection). If TRAS is causing significant ischemia and hypoperfusion, it should cause graft dysfunction. Calculating the degree of stenosis as a percentage is subjective and prone to inaccuracies and reminiscent of the classification of Mirizzi syndrome that was based on the percentage of bile duct diameter affected by stenosis [38]. The increased availability of DUS has increased the diagnosis of TRAS by 12.4% but by only 2.4% in patients already suspected of having TRAS based on the presence of refractory hypertension and renal impairment, highlighting the importance of clinical diagnosis [7]. This increase in suspected cases include those in whom the stenosis is not significant, because their renal function is normal and need only regular monitoring and follow-up like all transplant recipients. The question that needs an answer is, would an angiogram be carried out on a recipient with refractory hypertension or Doppler findings of TRAS without graft dysfunction? The advent of renal impairment on top of refractory hypertension indicates that the present renal blood flow is not enough to maintain normal renal function and should be labeled as significant. When this point is reached, serious consideration should be given to invasive diagnosis and appropriate treatment. We feel that graft dysfunction should be considered mandatory for the diagnosis of TRAS.

An interesting issue not discussed in the literature is regarding the other effects of ischemia resulting from TRAS? This ischemia, we feel, is the crux of the matter, greater the hypoperfusion, less the blood flow to the kidney. The only proximal blood supply of the ureter is derived from the renal artery in the hilum, which is usually distal to the TRAS lesion. It can be hypothesized that this ischemia will affect that part of the ureter that is furthest from the hilum. It is somewhat surprising that no downstream complications (appropriately termed) of allograft ischemia have been reported except from our center [14].

10. Conclusions

Worsening hypertension is suggestive of TRAS, significant stenosis and ischemia result in graft dysfunction. Early diagnosis is crucial because prompt treatment can restore perfusion, prevent graft loss and cardiovascular complications. DUS is easily available and is accurate, with documentation of PSVs, RIs and parvus tardus waveforms. It can confirm revascularization and monitor renal perfusion as part of follow-up. PTA and primary stenting remain the treatment of choice, while the failures and recurrences can be treated surgically. Incidence of long standing TRAS must be reduced because it causes irreversible structural changes reflected by intrarenal RIs of >0.8, when successful revascularization is unlikely.

Author details

Taqi Toufeeq Khan and Mirza Anzar Baig
Section of renal Transplant Surgery,
Department of Nephrology and Transplantation, Riyadh Military Hospital, Saudi Arabia

Acknowledgement

Figures 2-5 with permission from CHIRURGICA, Edizioni Minerva medica-Torino.

11. References

[1] Fervenza FC, Lafayette RA, Alfrey EJ, Petersen J. Renal artery stenosis in kidney transplantation. Am J Kid Dis 1998;31:142-148.
[2] Faenza A, Spolaora R, Poggioli G, Selleri et al. Renal artery stenosis after renal transplantation. Kidney Int Suppl 1983;14:S54-S59.
[3] Lo CY, Cheng IK, Tso WK, Mak KO. Percutaneous transluminal angioplasty for transplant renal artery stenosis. Trans Proc 1996;28:1468-1469.

[4] Lacombe M. arterial stenosis complicating renal allotransplantation in man. A study of 38 cases. Ann Surg 1975;181:283-288.
[5] Becker BN, Odorico JS, Becker YT, Leversen G et al. Peripheral vascular disease and renal transplant artery stenosis: reappraisal of transplant renovascular disease. Clin Transplant 1999;13:349-355.
[6] Roberts JP, Ascher NL, Fryd DS, Hunter DW et al. Transplant renal artery stenosis. Transplantation 1989;48:580-583.
[7] Wong W, Fynn SP, Higgins RM, Walters H et al. Transplant renal artery stenosis in 77 patients- does it have an immunological cause? Transplantation 1996;61:215-219.
[8] Pouria S, State OI, Wong W, Hendry BM. CMV infection is associated with transplant renal artery stenosis. QJM 1998;91:185-189.
[9] Audarda V, Matignona M, Hemeryb F, Snanoudjc R et al. Risk Factors and Long-Term Outcome of Transplant Renal Artery Stenosis in Adult Recipients After Treatment by Percutaneous Transluminal Angioplasty. Am J Transpl 2006;6:95-99.
[10] Gray DWR. Graft renal artery stenosis in the transplanted kidney. Transplant Rev 1994; 8:15–21.
[11] Khan T, Baig MA, Zahid R, Mousa D. Right renal vein augmentation in deceased donor kidney transplantation: importance of the contiguous inferior vena cava. Urotoday Int J 2010;3(6): doi:10.3834/uij.1944-784.2010.12.08.
[12] Patel NH, Jindal RM, Wilkin T, et al. Renal artery stenosis in renal artery allografts: Retrospective study of predisposing factors and outcomes after percutaneous transluminal angioplasty. Radiology 2001;219:663–667.
[13] Khan T, Baig MA. Distal ureteric obstruction resulting from transplant renal artery stenosis: A case report. Urotoday Int J 2011 April;4(2):art 21. doi:10.3834/uij.1944-5784.2011.04.03.
[14] Khan T, Baig MA. Primary endoluminal stenting for transplant renal artery stenosis: A case report. CHIRURGIA 2011;24:1-2.
[15] Bruno S, Remuzzi G, Ruggenenti P. Transplant renal artery stenosis. J AM Soc Nephrol 2004;15:134-141.
[16] Marques M, Prats D, Fructuoso AS, Naranjo P et al. incidence of renal artery stenosis in pediatric enbloc and adult single kiney transplants. Transplantation 2001;71:164-166.
[17] Aslam S, Salifu MO, Ghali H, Markell MS et al. common iliac artery stenosis presenting as renal allograft dysfunction in two diabetic recipients. Transplantation 2001;71:814-817.
[18] Goldblatt H, Lynch J, Hanzal RF, Summerville WW. Studies on experimental hypertension: 1. the production of persistent elevation of systolic blood pressure by means of renal ischemia. J Exp Med 1934;59:347-379.
[19] Mihatsch MJ, Kyo M, Morozumi K, Yamaguchi Y et al. the side effects of cyclosporine-A and tacrolimus. Clin Nephrol 1998;46:356-363.
[20] Imanishi M, Akabane S, Takamiya M, Kawamura M et al. Critical degree of renal arterial ischemia that causes hypertension in dogs. Angiology 1992;43:833-842.
[21] Bruno S, Ferrari S, Remuzzi G, Ruggenenti P. Doppler ultrasound in post transplant renal artery stenosis: a reliable tool for assessing effectiveness of revascularization.? Transplantation 2003;76:147-153.

[22] Liard JF, Peters G. Mechanism of fall of blood pressure after unclamping in rats with Goldblatt hypertension. Experientia 1980;26:743-745.
[23] Radermacher J, Mengel M, Ellis S, Stuht S et al. The renal artery resistance index and renal allograft survival. N Engl J Med 2003; 349:115-124.
[24] Sawaya B, Provenzano R, Kupin L, Venkat KK. Cyclosporine induced renal microangiopathy. Am J Kid Dis 1988;12:534-537.
[25] Erley CM, Duda SH, Wakat J-P, Sokler M et al. Non invasive procedures for diagnosis of renovascular hypertension in renal transplant recipients: A prospective analysis. Transplantation 1992; 54:863-867.
[26] Mousa D, Hamilton D, Hassan A, Al-Sulaiman M et al. The diagnosis of segmental transplant renal artery stenosis by Captopril renography. J Nucl Med 1999;24:504-505.
[27] Fuster D, Marco MP, Setoain FJ, Oppenheimer F et al. A case of renal artery stenosis after transplantation: can Losartan be more accurate than Captopril renography? Clin Nucl Med 1998;23:731-734.
[28] Wei K, Le E, Bin JP, Coggins M et al. Quantification of renal blood flow with contrast enhanced ultrasound. J Am Coll Cardiol 2001;37:1135-1140.
[29] Stavros AT, Parker SH, Yakes WF et al. Segmental stenoses of the renal artery: pattern recognition of tardus and parvus abnormalities with duplex sonography. Radiology 1992;184:487-492.
[30] Ardalan MR, Tarzamani MK, Shoja MM. A correlation between direct and indirect Doppler ultrasonographic measures in transplant renal artery stenosis. Transplant Proc 2007;39:1436-1438.
[31] Vasbinder GBC, Nelemans PJ, Kessels AGH, Kroon AA et al. Diagnostic tests for renal artery stenosis in patients suspected of having renovascular hypertension. Ann Int Med 2001;135:401-411.
[32] Moresco KP, Patel NH, Namyslowski J, Shah H et al. Carbon dioxide angiography of the transplanted kidney: technical considerations and imaging findings. Am J Roentgenol 1998;9:1271-1276.
[33] Greenstein S, Verstanding A, McLean G, Dafoe DC et al. Percutaneous transluminal angioplasty. Transplantation 1987;43:29-32.
[34] Chiu TY, Leu HB, Wu TC, Chen JW et al. Endovascular stenting treatment for drug refractory hypertension due to ostial stenosis of transplant renal artery. J Chin med Assoc 2004;67:189-192.
[35] Leerrtouwer TC, Gussenhoven EJ, Bosch JL, van Jaarsveld BC et al. Stent placement for renal artery stenosis: where do we stand? A meta analysis. Radiology 2000;216:78-85.
[36] Keisz RS, Buszman P, Martin JL, Deutsch E et al. Local delivery of enoxaparin to decrease re stenosis after stenting: results of initial mulitcenter trial: Polish-American local Lovenox NIR assessment study (The Polonia study). Circulation 2001;103:26-31.
[37] Shames BD, Odorico JS, D;Allessandro AM, Pirsch JD et al. Surgical repair of transplant renal artery stenosis with preserved cadaveric iliac artery grafts. Ann Surg 2003;237:116-122.
[38] Toufeeq Khan TF, Sherazi ZA, Muniandy S, Hayat FZ. Mirizzi syndrome: a simplified surgical approach and classification. Sing Med J 1999;40:1781-173.

Surgical Advances in Laparoscopic Donor Nephrectomy

Cheguevara Afaneh, Meredith J. Aull, Joseph J. Del Pizzo and Sandip Kapur

Additional information is available at the end of the chapter

http://dx.doi.org/10.5772/53945

1. Introduction

1.1. Historical overview

Since it was first described in the 1990s, conventional laparoscopic donor nephrectomy has been the standard of care at most major transplant centers. Clayman et al. described the first successful conventional laparoscopic nephrectomy in 1991 for intrinsic renal disease [1]. Several years later, a conventional laparoscopic donor nephrectomy procedure was successfully performed in a large animal model [2], while Ratner and colleagues described the first successful conventional laparoscopic live donor nephrectomy one year later [3]. Donor were discharged home within two days and most returned to work within two weeks postoperatively. Moreover, recipient outcomes were significantly better than deceased donor allografts.

Over the next decade following the advent of conventional laparoscopic donor nephrectomy, the number of kidney transplants performed in the United States nearly doubled. The ability to perform the procedure using the conventional laparoscopic approach certainly influenced the willingness of donors to donate [4]. Moreover, the ease of donation has lead to more unexpected results, including altruistic donors, innovative protocols for ABO incompatibility and positive crossmatches, as well as kidney paired donation [5-7].

Laparoendoscopic single site surgery represents the next step in the evolution of conventional laparoscopic surgery. It is performed through a single small skin incision, often partially concealed at the umbilicus. Recently, several institutions, including our own, have reported on this technique for live donor nephrectomy [8-10]. Cosmesis, as well as possibly decreased postoperative pain and port-site related complications, are among the possible benefits compared to the conventional laparoscopic approach. Recipients have experienced similar postoperative results as those receiving allografts using the conventional laparoscopic procurement technique [11, 12].

2. Preoperative evaluation

2.1. Initial evaluation

All potential donors undergo a complete surgical, medical, and psychological evaluation in accordance with the clinical practice guidelines established by the American Society for Transplantation and the Consensus Statement on the Live Organ Donor [13, 14]. A discussion of the medical work-up is discussed elsewhere in this textbook. After a thorough medical and psychological evaluation, the patient is referred to the surgeon for preoperative consideration of anatomy and functional status of the donor kidneys.

2.2. Surgical preoperative considerations

2.2.1. Anatomy and functionality

The use of preoperative imaging is a vital component of proper surgical planning. This allows determination of potential donor kidney size, function, and anatomy. This allows for determination of the safest and most feasible surgical approach. Potential donors typically undergo spiral computed tomography (CT) scans with intravenous contrast administration with vascular reconstructions to properly assess the renal hilum prior to surgery [15]. Magnetic resonance angiography is an alternative to spiral CT for evaluation of potential kidneys. Renal scintigraphy usually obtained when there is a >1 cm size discrepancy between kidneys.

2.2.2. Laterality

Choosing the side of the nephrectomy should be given careful considering. The right kidney presents a technical challenge. Procurement of the right kidney using the endoscopic GIA stapling device to divide the anatomically shorter right renal vein results in losing anywhere from 1 cm to 1.5 cm from the total length [16]. This leads to a relatively short renal vein that complicates the recipient procedure and has been associated with acute renal vein thrombosis and early graft loss [17]. Short renal vasculature is no longer avoidable given surgical innovations. Left kidneys are preferentially chosen if the renal vasculature and function are comparable. Multiple left renal arteries or anomalous left renal veins are not absolute contraindications to procuring the left kidney [17]. The feasibility of procuring the right kidney has been clearly described from hand-assisted laparoscopy to the conventional laparoscopic approach to even using the laparoendoscopic single site approach [11, 18, 19].

2.2.3. Contraindications

The contraindications to laparoendoscopic single site surgery are the same as those for any laparoscopic abdominal procedure. Certainly, previous abdominal surgery further complicates any laparoscopic procedure; it does not confer an absolute contraindication. In fact, the rate of conversion of laparoendoscopic single site surgery remains relatively low (<5%) as has been our experience [12].

3. Operative technique

3.1. Positioning

Patients are placed in a modified flank position, and a 5 centimeter vertical periumbilical incision is made with the abdominal skin on stretch. After creation of a vertical midline anterior rectus fasciotomy, the abdomen is entered. The Gel Point device (Applied Medical, Rancho Santa Margarita, CA) as seen in figure 1 with three trocars already in place is inserted into the abdomen and pneumoperitoneum is established. Two 5-mm trocars and one 15-mm trocar are used. A bariatric 10-mm rigid laparoscope is used through the 15mm port with a right angle attachment for the light cord to maximize space for triangulation. Standard, non articulating laparoscopic instruments are used in the majority of the procedure. For right sided kidneys, a fourth trocar is placed through the Gelpoint device and a Diamond-Flex retractor (***Genzyme*** Surgical Products, Tucker, GA) is used for exposure after mobilization of the right lobe of the liver by division of the triangular and coronary ligaments.

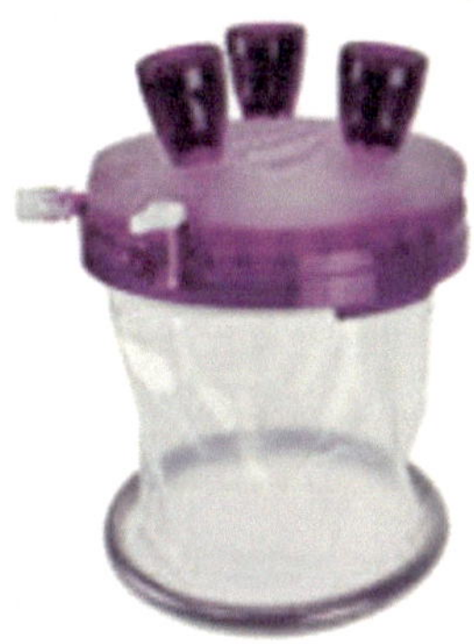

Figure 1. Gelport™ device. Three trocars are in place traversing the gel cap.

3.2. Procurement technique

3.2.1. Left kidney

When procuring the left kidney using the laparoendoscopic single site procurement technique, the descending colon, pancreas and spleen are mobilized generously en bloc without the need for continuous retraction. The ureter and gonadal vein are identified and lifted off of the psoas muscle together, maintaining periureteral attachments and dissected towards the hilum. The lumbar vein, if present, is divided between titanium clips. The renal vein is skeletonized and the adrenal vein is divided between titanium clips, and the adrenal gland is released from the upper pole. The renal artery is dissected down to its aortic origin, and the interaortocaval region is skeletonized. Lastly, the posterior attachments were dissected free from the kidney. A 12-mm trocar replaces one of the 5-mm trocars in anticipation of using the EndoGIA vascular stapling device (United States Surgical, Norwalk CT).

Once the recipient team is ready, the ureter and gonadal vein are divided together at the pelvic brim. The renal artery and then vein are divided using the vascular stapling device. An Endocatch bag is introduced, and the allograft is gently entrapped and extracted by removing the Gel cap. If necessary, the fascial incision is extended 1-2 cm to facilitate removal of the graft, taking care to leave the overlying skin intact without further extension of the incision. Fascia and skin are closed in the standard fashion after ensuring adequate hemostasis. No articulating or specialized laparoscopic instruments are needed and no extraumbilical incisions need to be made. The incision is well-concealed in the umbilicus using this technique (Figure 2).

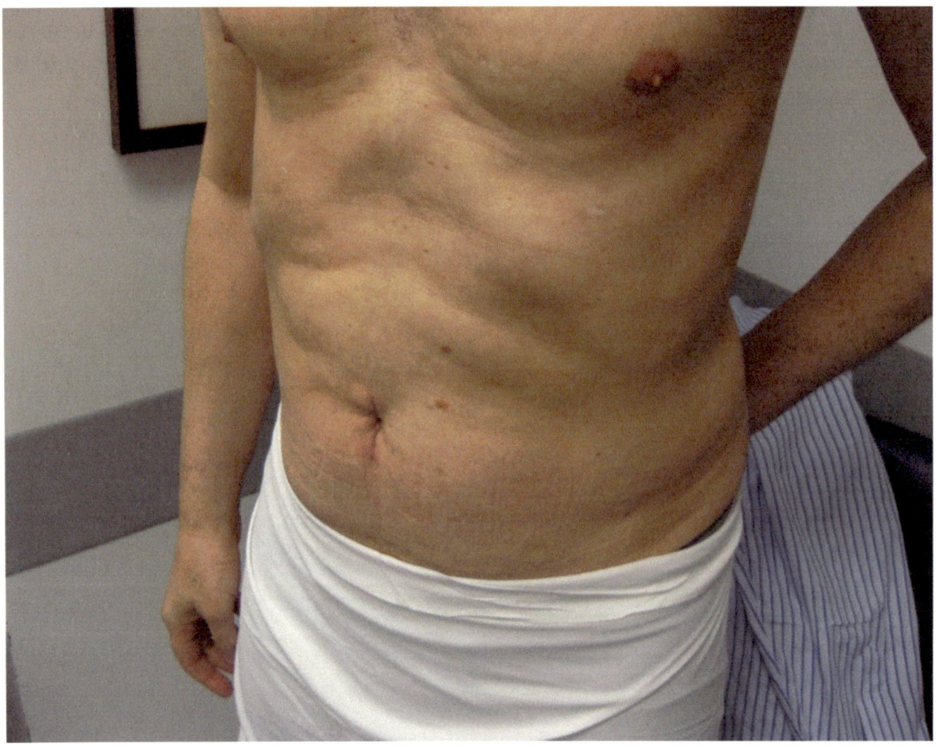

Figure 2. Postoperative incision. In this figure, the patient is 8 weeks postoperatively from a laparoendoscopic single site left donor nephrectomy.

3.2.2. *Right kidney*

The initial three trocars are placed as described above for left kidneys; however, the right kidney procurement technique requires a fourth trocar for retraction of the liver. Using mostly one handed dissection, the duodenum is kocherized bluntly to expose the inferior vena cava (IVC). The hepatic flexure is gently lifted and the plane between Gerota's fascia and the mesocolon is identified. The colon is bluntly dissected and mobilized in a medial and caudal direction, down to the iliac vasculature. The ureter and gonadal vein are identified and lifted off of the psoas muscle together, maintaining periureteral attachments and dissected towards the hilum. At this point, a fourth trocar (5mm) is placed through the Gelport™ device for retraction of the right lobe of the liver (Figure 3).

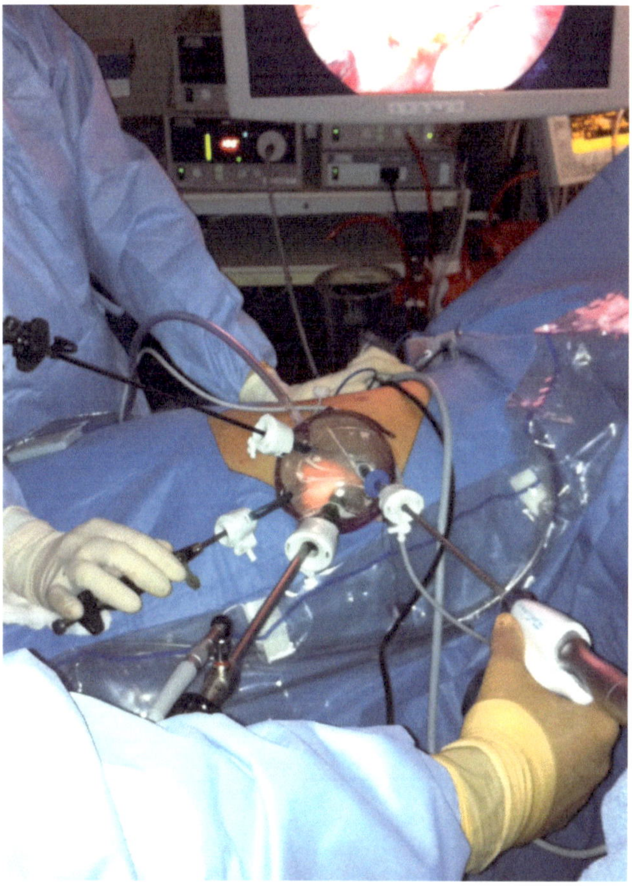

Figure 3. Port placement for right sided kidney. In this figure, the four trocars are present traversing the Gelport™ device.

The renal vein is skeletonized down to the level of the IVC. The renal artery is dissected medial to the lateral edge of the IVC to maximize length, and the interaortocaval region is skeletonized. The adrenal gland is dissected free from the medial upper pole of the kidney using a harmonic scalpel. Lastly, the posterior and lateral attachments are divided. A 12-mm trocar replaces one of the 5-mm trocars in anticipation of using the EndoGIA vascular stapler (United States Surgical, Norwalk CT).

Once the recipient team is ready, the ureter is divided at the pelvic brim. The kidney is then retracted laterally. Using an EndoGIA vascular stapler, the renal artery is divided first, followed by the vein, with the vein being divided flush with the IVC to maximize length. An Endocatch bag is introduced, and the allograft is gently entrapped and extracted.

3.2.3. Obese donors

Obese donors represent a technically more challenging population. The technique mirrors that of the normal BMI donors; however there are several important technical aspects to consider [20]. First, mobilization of adjacent organs may be more difficult. Given the amount of intra-abdominal fat, visualization may be more difficult. As a result, there may be increased difficulty in identifying key landmarks. Male donors have additional visceral adipose tissue which may make it more difficult to retract [21]. The amount of perirenal fat must be taken into consideration when planning safe extraction of the allograft from an obese patient to avoid a renal laceration [20]. The incision remains well-concealed, even this population (Figure 4A&B).

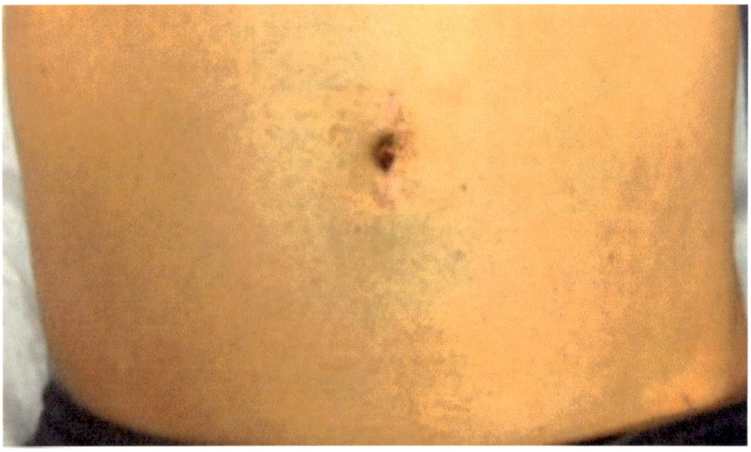

A.

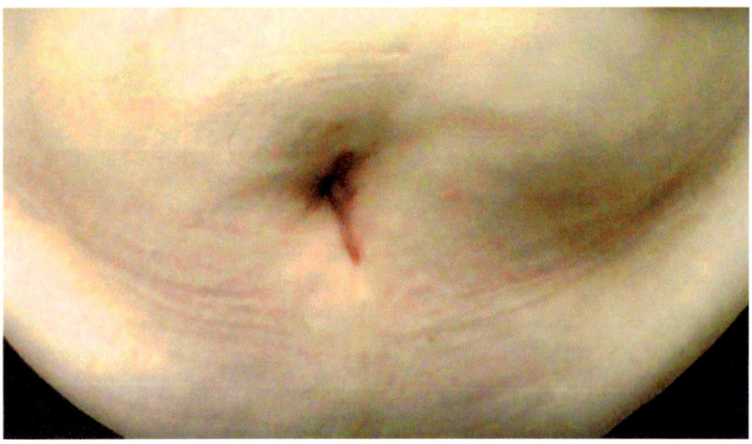

B.

Figure 4. Obese versus normal BMI. The images depict donors approximately 2 weeks following laparoendoscopic single site donor nephrectomy. Panel A is a non-obese donor and panel B is an obese donor.

4. Donor considerations

4.1. Morbidity

The donor nephrectomy is a unique procedure, as it entails operating on a healthy individual, as opposed to surgery for specific disease processes. To justify the procedure, the potential complications must be minimized as donor safety should be the priority.

Initial studies evaluating donor safety compared the open to the conventional laparoscopic approach. Various studies and reviews have demonstrated a complication rate ranging from 0% to 38% using the open procurement approach and 0% to 30% with the conventional laparoscopic approach [22, 23]. More recent studies have reported complications of less than 10% in conventional laparoscopic donor nephrectomy [24, 25]. In a single surgeon series of 750 laparoscopic donor nephrectomies, Harper et al. used the modified Clavien-Dindo system and reported an overall complication rate of 5.5% [24]. The majority of complications were classified as minor, with most (66%) being grade 1. Moreover, there were only four cases converted to an open procedure (0.4%). These values are similar to our experience as our complication rate for conventional laparoscopic donor nephrectomy was approximately 7%. Moreover, only one patient in that cohort required conversion to an open procedure (0.15%) [25].

Given the relatively novel nature of the laparoendoscopic single site procurement technique, donor morbidity must remain minimal. We reported a similar complication rate (approximately 7%) large series of laparoendoscopic single site donor nephrectomies, comparable to our conventional laparoscopic procurement technique [12, 25]. Other smaller, single center series have demonstrated similar outcomes comparing laparoendoscopic single site donor nephrectomies to conventional laparoscopic donor nephrectomies [26, 27]. Kurien and colleagues reported the first randomized controlled trial of 50 patients comparing conventional laparoscopic donor nephrectomies versus laparoendoscopic single-site donor nephrectomies [28]. They reported an intraoperative and postoperative complication rate of 16% in the laparoendoscopic single-site donor group, which was similar to the conventional laparoscopic donor nephrectomy group.

Certain complications are more specific to the laterality of the donor kidney. For example, in right sided donors, liver lacerations and injuries to the retro-aortic renal arteries are more common. On the other hand, intraoperative complications related to splenic lacerations during mobilization of the splenic flexure of the colon or injuries to the supra-adrenal branches of the left renal vein are more common in left sided donors [29].

4.2. Technical considerations

The use of laparoendoscopic single site surgery in living donor kidney procurement offers a new set of challenges to the laparoscopic surgeon. Technical limitations including a reduced working space and lack of instrument triangulation make it a technically challenging procedure. These limitations are more pronounced in the obese patient, where difficulties in exposure and visualization already exist, including additional visceral adipose tissue that is more difficult to retract. Overweight male donors were even found to have higher rates of conversion to open procedures compared to overweight female donors, possibly related to the visceral fat distribution [21].

Procuring the right kidney poses additional threats as previous studies have demonstrated an increased risk of renal vein thrombosis [17, 18]. Our initial experience with hand-assisted laparoscopy saw a renal vein thrombosis rate of less than 3% [30]. In fact, we had not had any cases of renal vein thrombosis with the conventional laparoscopic procurement technique, or even more recently, with the laparoendoscopic single site donor nephrectomy technique [19, 30]. An important technical consideration is firing the stapling device flush against the IVC, while laterally retracting the kidney to maximize renal vein length to avoid this complication.

Various studies have compared outcomes of transplantation of kidneys with a single artery versus those with multiple arteries (Figure 5). Most of these studies have demonstrated similar survival and graft function between the two groups [31-33]. However, other studies have shown that kidneys harvested with multiple arteries are technically difficult leading to increased complications, such as vascular thrombosis, increased bleeding during nephrectomy, and increased operating times [34]. Our experience using the laparoendoscopic single site donor nephrectomy technique to procure kidneys with multiple vessels has been similar to those with single renal arteries and veins (approximate complication rate of 6%).

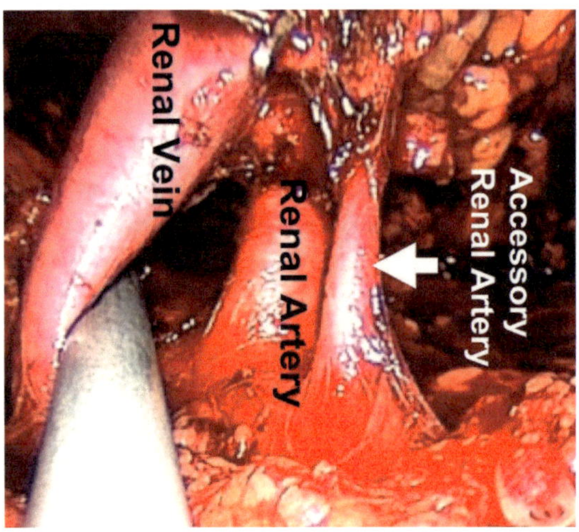

Figure 5. Multiple renal arteries. The image depicts a kidney with multiple renal arteries.

4.3. Donor satisfaction

The true benefits of laparoendoscopic single site donor nephrectomy remain to be seen. Canes et al. compared 17 laparoendoscopic single site donor nephrectomies to a matched pair of 17 conventional laparoscopic donor nephrectomies and found no difference in standard perioperative parameters [27]. They did however identify superior patient scar satisfaction, decreased oral analgesic use, and improved convalescence in the laparoendoscopic single site cohort. Kurien and colleagues demonstrated no difference in convalescence parameters in their randomized controlled trial comparing 25 laparoendoscopic single site donor nephrectomies to 25 conventional laparoscopic donor nephrectomies [28]. The laparoendoscopic cohort did have less pain requirements and a one-half day improvement in hospital stay; however, the warm ischemia time was slightly increased in that cohort. In an analysis of our series of our first 100 laparoendoscopic single site donor nephrectomies, the laparoendoscopic group had a slight, but significant improvement in convalescence compared to a group of 100 matched conventional laparoscopic donor nephrectomies [12]. However, the laparoendoscopic group had significantly longer operative times by almost 30 minutes on average.

5. Recipient outcomes

5.1. Allograft function

The benefit of live donor nephrectomy, compared to receiving an allograft from a deceased donor, is the prompt functionality of the allograft with more durable function. Comparisons of early and late allograft function in the recipient of open versus conventional laparoscopic donor nephrectomy have already been shown in several studies, including two randomized controlled trials [35, 36]. Similarly, all recent studies comparing allografts procured with the laparoendoscopic single site technique have shown similar early allograft function compared to allografts via conventional laparoscopic approaches [10-12, 28]. Moreover, these results have also been seen with right sided allografts, despite the shorter vasculature when compared to either right or left allografts [19, 30]. In addition, allografts from obese donors have seen similar early allograft function as allografts from non-obese donor irrespective of procurement technique [20]. In all of these studies, the incidence of delayed graft function remained low (<5%).

5.2. Survival

Graft survival following conventional laparoscopic donor nephrectomy has been excellent. Given the infancy of the laparoendoscopic single site procurement technique, long-term or even intermediate-term follow-up remains limited. However, short-term follow-up suggests patient survival remains excellent at 1 year (100%) as well as overall graft survival at 1 year (98%) [11]. Kurien et al. demonstrated similar 1 year outcomes, including both patient and graft survival of 100% [28]. At the present, short-term outcomes appear similar to conventional laparoscopic procurement techniques.

6. Conclusion

The single incision approach represents a technological advancement in renal allograft organ recovery. Perhaps with time, this could represent a paradigm shift that will require evolution of instrumentation, technique, and training models, just as conventional laparoscopic donor nephrectomies did over a decade and a half ago. At this time, the benefits of single incision technique appears limited to superior cosmesis and a small improvement in convalescence. With time, however, the laparoendoscopic single site donor nephrectomy technique may further decrease the barriers to live organ donation and transplantation.

Author details

Cheguevara Afaneh, Meredith J. Aull, Joseph J. Del Pizzo and Sandip Kapur
Department of Surgery, Division of Transplant Surgery, New York-Presbyterian Hospital- Weill Cornell Medical College, New York, NY, USA

Joseph J. Del Pizzo
Department of Urology, New York-Presbyterian Hospital- Weill Cornell Medical College, New York, NY, USA

7. References

[1] Clayman, R.V.; Kavoussi, L.R.; Soper, N.J., et al.. Laparoscopic nephrectomy. *N Engl J Med*,Vol.324, No.19, (May 1991), pp. 1370-1371.
[2] Gill, I.S.; Carbone, J.M.; Clayman, R.V., et al. Laparoscopic live-donor nephrectomy. *J Endourol*, Vol.8, No.2, (April 1994), pp. 143-148.
[3] Ratner, L.E.; Cisek, L.J.; Moore, R.G., et al. Laparoscopic live donor nephrectomy. *Transplantation*, Vol.60, No.9, (November 1995), pp. 1047-1049.
[4] Ratner, L.E.; Hiller, J.; Sroka, M., et al. Laparoscopic live donor nephrectomy removes discentives to live donation. *Transplant Proc*, Vol.29, No.8, (December 1997), pp. 3402-3403.
[5] Montgomery, R.; Simpkins, C.E.; Segev, D.L. New options for patients with donor incompatibilities. *Transplantation*, Vol.82, No.2, (July 2006), pp. 164-165.
[6] Montgomery, R.A.; Zachary, A.A.; Ratner, L.E., et al. Clinical results from transplanting incompatible live kidney donor/recipient pairs using kidney paired donation. *JAMA*, Vol. 294, No.13, (October 2005), pp. 1655-1663.
[7] Leeser, D.B.; Aull, M.J.; Afaneh, C., et al. Living donor kidney paired donation transplantation: A single center experience. *Clin Transplant* 2012; 26(3):E213–E222.
[8] Canes, D.; Desai, M.M.; Aron, M., et al. Transumbilical single-port surgery: Evolution and current status. *Eur Urol*, Vol.54, No.5, (November 2008), pp. 1020-1029.
[9] Gill, I.S.; Canes, D.; Aron, M., et al. Single port transumbilical (E-NOTES) donor nephrectomy. *J Urol*, Vol.180, No.2, (August 2008), pp. 637-641.
[10] Gimenez, E.; Leeser, D.; Wysock, J., et al. Laparoendoscopic single site live donor nephrectomy: Initial experience. *J Urol*, Vol.184, No.5, (November 2010), pp. 2049-2053.
[11] Afaneh, C.; Aull, M.J.; Gimenez, E., et al. Comparison of laparoendoscopic single-site donor nrephrectomy and conventional laparoscopic donor nephrectomy: donor and recipient outcomes. *Urology*, Vol.78, No.6, (December 2011), pp. 1332-1337.

[12] Wang, G.J.; Afaneh, C.; Aull, M., et al. Laparoendoscopic single site live donor nephrectomy: single institution report of initial 100 cases. *J Urol*, Vol.186, No.6, (December 2011), pp. 2333-2337.
[13] Abecassis, M.; Adams, M.; Adams, P., et al. For the Live Organ Donor Consensus Group: Consensus statement on the live organ donor. *JAMA*, Vol.284, No.22, (December 2000), pp. 2919-2926.
[14] Kasiske, B.L.; Ravenscraft, M.; Ramos, E.L., et al. The evaluation of living renal transplant donors: clinical practice guidelines. Ad Hoc Clinical Practice Guidelines Subcommittee of the Patient Care and Education Committee of the American Society of Transplant Physicians. *J Am Soc Nephrol*, Vol.7, No.11, (November 1996), pp. 2288-2313.
[15] Smith, P.A.; Ratner, L.E.; Lynch, F.C., et al. Role of CT angiography in the preoperative evaluation for laparoscopic nephrectomy. *Radiographics*, Vol.18, No.3, (May-June 1998), pp. 589.
[16] Ratner, L.E.; Kavoussi, L.; Chavin, K., et al. Laparoscopic live donor nephrectomy: technical consideration and vascular length. *Transplantation*, Vol.65, No.12, (June 1998), pp. 1657-1658.
[17] Mandal, A.K.; Cohen, C.; Montgomery, R.A., et al. Should the indications for laparoscopic live donor nephrectomy of the right kidney be the same as for the open procedure? Anomalous left renal vasculature is not a contraindication to laparoscopic left donor nephrectomy. *Transplantation*, 2001;71(5):660-4.
[18] Buell, J.F.; Hanaway, M.J.; Potter, S.R., et al. Surgical techniques in right laparoscopic donor nephrectomy. *J Am Coll Surg*, 2002;195(1):131-7.
[19] Afaneh, C.; Ramasamy, R.; Leeser, D.B., et al. Is right-sided laparoendoscopic single-site donor nephrectomy feasible? *Urology*, Vol.77, No.6, (June 2011), pp. 1365-1369.
[20] Afaneh, C.; Sheth, S.; Aull, M.J., et al. Laparoendoscopic single-site nephrectomy in obese living renal donors. *J Endourol*, Vol.26, No.2, (February 2012), pp. 140-146.
[21] Kok, N.F.; Izzermans, J.N.; Schouten, O., et al. Laparoscopic donor nephrectomy in obese donors: easier to implement in overweight women? *Transpl Int*, Vol.20, No.11, (November 2007), pp. 956-961.
[22] Merlin, T.L.; Scott, D.F.; Rao, M.M, et al. The safety and efficacy of laparoscopic live donor nephrectomy: a systematic review. *Transplantation*, Vol.70, No.12, (December 2000), pp. 1659-1666.
[23] Tooher, R.I.; Rao, M.M.; Scott, D.F., et al. A systematic review of laparoscopic live-donor nephrectomy. *Transplantation*, Vol.78, No.3, (August 2004), pp. 404-414.
[24] Harper, J.D.; Breda, A.; Leppert, J.T., et al. Experience with 750 consecutive laparoscopic donor nephrectomies—is it time to use a standardized classification of complications? *J Urol*, Vol.183, No.5, (May 2010), pp. 1941-1946.
[25] Ramasamy, R.; Afaneh, C.; Katz, M., et al. Comparison of complications of laparoscopic versus laparoendoscopic single site donor nephrectomy using the modified Clavien grading system. *J Urol*, Urol. 2011;186(4):1386-90.
[26] Andonian, S.; Rais-Bahrami, S.; Atalla, M.A., et al. Laparoendoscopic single-site Pfannenstiel versus standard laparoscopic donor nephrectomy. *J Endourol*, Vol.24, No.3, (March 2010), pp. 429-432.

[27] Canes, D.; Berger, A.; Aron, M., et al. Laparo-endoscopic single site (LESS) versus standard laparoscopic left donor nephrectomy: matched-pair comparison. *Eur Urol*, Vol.57, No.1, (January 2010), pp. 95-101.
[28] Kurien, A.; Rajapurker, S.; Sinha, L., et al. First prize: Standard laparoscopic donor nephrectomy versus laparoendoscopic single-site donor nephrectomy: a randomized comparative study. *J Endourol*, Vol.25, No.3, (March 2011), pp. 365-370.
[29] Minnee, R.C.; Bemelmen, W.A.; Maartense, S., et al. Left or right kidney in hand-assisted donor nephrectomy? A randomized controlled trial. *Transplantation*, Vol.85, No.2, (January 2008), pp. 203-208.
[30] Afaneh, C.; Aull, M.J.; Schubl, S., et al. The evolution of laparoscopic right donor nephrectomy: Progression to single site surgery. *J Transplant Technol Res*, Vol.1, Issue.2, No.103, (November 2011), pp. 1-7.
[31] Desai, M.R.; Ganuple, A.P.; Gupta, R., et al. Outcome of renal transplantation with multiple versus single renal arteries after laparoscopic live donor nephrectomy: A comparative study. *Urology*, Vol.69, No.5, (May 2007), pp. 824-827.
[32] Hsu, T.H.; Su, L.M.; Ratner, L.E.; Trock, B.J.; Kavoussi, L.R. Impact of renal artery multiplicity on outcomes of renal donors and recipients in laparoscopic donor nephrectomy. *Urology*, Vol.61, No.2, (February 2003), pp. 323-327.
[33] Saidi, R.; Kawai, T.; Kennealey, P., et al. Living donor kidney transplantation with multiple arteries: recent increase in modern era of laparoscopic donor nephrectomy, *Arch Surg*, Vol.144, No.5, (May 2009), pp. 472-475.
[34] Carter, J.T.; Freise, C.E.; McTaggart, R.A., et al. Laparoscopic procurement of kidneys with multiple renal arteries is associated with increased ureteral complications in the recipient. *Am J Transplant*, Vol.5, No.6, (June 2005), pp.1312-1318.
[35] Kok, N.F.; Lind, M.Y.; Hansson, B.M., et al. Comparison of laparoscopic and mini incision open donor nephrectomy: single blind randomized controlled trial. *BMJ*, Vol.333, No.7561, (July 2006), pp. 221.
[36] Simforoosh, N.; Basiri, A.; Tabibi, A., et al. Comparison of laparoscopic and open donor nephrectomy: a randomized controlled trial. *BJU Int*, Vol.95, No.6, (April 2005), pp. 851-855.

Chapter 14

Higher Volume and Better Outcomes Relationship in Kidney Transplant

Wui-Chiang Lee, Shu-Yun Tsao and Che-Chuan Loong

Additional information is available at the end of the chapter

http://dx.doi.org/10.5772/50385

1. Introduction

End-stage renal disease (ESRD) is a serious public health and medical problem in the world. The incidence and prevalence rates grow up in many countries (Figure 1). According to the recent United States Renal Data System (USRDS) report, the incidence of ESRD increases from 346 per million people in 2004 to 371 per million people in 2009 in the United States.(1) ESRD also has financial impacts on the health care delivery and insurance systems. For instance, in Taiwan, 68,000 chronic renal failure patients constitute 0.3% of national population, but they cost nearly 10% of health insurance resource in 2010.(2) In United States, total Medicare spending with ESRD cost 29 billion dollars in 2009.(3) Some developing countries and theirs patients with ESRD are unable to afford the tremendous cost of dialysis and kidney transplant. This leads to extremely public health and medical problem due to no substitute therapy can be provided owing to economic reason.(4)

2. Kidney transplant and donor shortage

Since Joseph Edward Murray successfully achieved the first kidney transplant surgery in 1954, kidney transplant has become one of the standard therapies for patients with ESRD. Hemodialysis, peritoneal dialysis and kidney transplant are regarded as replacement therapies for patients with ESRDs. Kidney transplant is widely believed to be the best option among all therapies.(5) Patients who receive kidney transplant are more likely to have higher satisfaction rate, better quality of life, and lower long-term utilization and cost than those who receive dialysis therapy.(5, 6) Although the death rate of patients within two weeks after receiving renal transplant surgery is 2.8 fold higher than those with hemodialysis therapy, the overall death rate 68% is lower than dialysis.(7)

The annual cost of dialysis is around $35,000 to $80,000 USD. The cost of kidney transplant is similar to dialysis in the first year, but the medical cost after surgery is lower than that receiving dialysis.(8-16) As a result, many countries promote kidney transplantation given the medical and financial benefits. Nevertheless, the amount of donated kidneys cannot satisfy the rapidly increasing need. The waiting times for kidney transplant surgery are from 3 to 6 years, and even longer in several countries such as United Kingdoms, Brazil, and Taiwan.(17-20) Therefore, many countries encourage expanded criteria donor (ECD) and donor after cardiac death (DCD). These two polices can increase amount of transplant surgery and reach good transplant results under well-planned and cooperative organizations.(21)

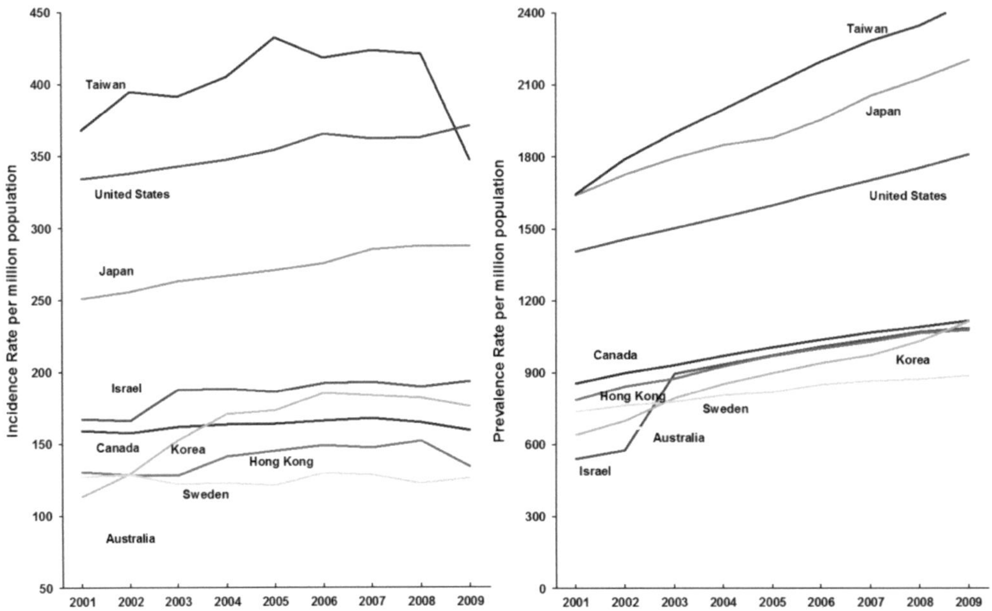

Figure 1. the incidence and prevalence of people with end-stage renal disease in different countries (retrieved parts of the statistics from the 2011 Annual Data Report, United States Renal Data System, http://www.usrds.org/2011/pdf/v2_ch012_11.pdf)

3. Organ procurement and allocation

The allocation and utilization of donated organs is as important as procurement. In developed countries, such as United States and United Kingdom that have executed organ transplant surgeries for decades, they have had well-established organ procurement organizations for procuring donors, organ harvest, and transplant. Whenever an organ donor is obtained, the transplant center distributes them according to the blood type, tissue matching result, disease severity, age, location, waiting time, and the shortest ischemic time to achieve the optimal transplant result. Health authorities will also request these centers must follow their patients to evaluate whether pre-set goals are achieved, such as efficiency of promotion, ratio of using expanded criteria donor, survival rate, and growth of transplant rate. The aim of disclosure of processing and outcome information of transplant to the public is not only providing necessary information to all patients, but also acting as performance parameters of all transplant centers.

However, such an organ procurement and allocation system is still at the beginning stage in many countries. Hospitals or the health care systems have to establish their own waiting and priority list. Usually there are few communications and cooperation across transplant centers, thus the limited donated organs cannot be fully utilized and allocated to the most needed recipients. To improve the efficiency of utilization and fairness of allocation, many countries such as Taiwan and Brazil have established a coordinating organization. They procure organ donation and set up the waiting list and the priority of organ utilization based on medical and ethical considerations. Patients with ESRDs have equal opportunity to share the limited organs as long as they fit the matching criteria. Previous studies showed that the number of kidney transplant increased significantly after establishment of the central coordinating organizations.(19)

4. Volume-outcome relationships in high-risk surgeries

Many studies have demonstrated that patients who receive surgery at higher-volume hospitals are more likely to have better outcomes.(22-30) The evidence for a positive relationship between provider volume and subsequent clinical outcomes for inpatients is substantial and compelling since its introduction in the literature mainly by Luft (31) and Flood (32, 33) in the 1980s. During the past 30 years, especially after 1995, a large body of studies has focused on measuring and explaining the relationship between inpatient outcomes and volume of services provided by hospitals and physicians. For certain diseases and procedures, a "higher volume and better outcomes" relationship has been recognized in several large-scale reviews.(30, 34) The Institute of Medicine released its synthesis of the evidence that 77% of peer-reviewed studies found significant inverse relationships between hospital volume and mortality (34); and another systematic review by Dudley et al (30, 34) reported similar findings. Extremely strong volume-outcome relationships have been chiefly identified for rare and high-risk procedures, including coronary artery bypass graft surgery,(35-40) pediatric cardiac surgery,(41-43) unruptured abdominal aortic aneurysm repair,(39, 44, 45) total hip replacement, (30, 34, 46, 47) and very high risk cancer surgeries such as for the pancreas,(48-52) esophagus,(50, 53, 54) and liver cancers.(53)

5. Causes for volume-outcome relationships

Although the association between the volume of inpatient services and outcomes of health care is substantial for many studies, the direction of causality has not been well defined. Three principal hypotheses have been advanced to explain this relationship:

First, the "practice makes perfect" hypothesis. Many studies support the "practice makes perfect" hypothesis, in that higher-volume providers develop more effective skills and treatments that result in better outcomes.(31, 55) According to this hypothesis, there is a learning effect among providers; that is, higher-volume providers develop more effective skills and treatments which result in better outcomes.(32, 33) It is plausible that regular experience is crucial to keep up skills and the lower-volume providers have poorer outcomes because they have lost a necessary edge.(56, 57) However, several studies that track changes in individual hospital volume over time found that fluctuating numbers of cases within the same hospital have no or minimal effects on outcomes.(36, 58) This implies that volume-outcome associations may reflect fixed differences in the overall quality of care between high and low-volume providers, rather than the hypothesis of "practice makes perfect" alone.(59)

Second, the "selective referral" hypothesis. Luft et al (60) argued that volume could be higher in hospitals with better outcomes because patients seek care at facilities with reputations for better performance. It is possible that for elective procedures providers who are well known might receive more referrals or self-referrals from patients themselves.(57) However, this is implausible in the case of emergency procedures where the opportunity for selective referral is low. Furthermore, given the fact that physicians do not usually use outcome information to make referrals,(61, 62) nor do patients flock to hospitals based on their outcome information,(63) selective referral alone cannot explain the whole story well. Luft et al (31) adopted a simultaneous-equation model to test the relative importance of the two explanations, and suggested that both hypotheses are valid and that the relative importance of the practice or referral explanation varies by diagnosis or procedure.

Third, the "outcome-related processes of care" hypothesis. An alternative hypothesis is that there is no direct causal relationship between volume and inpatient outcomes, and their correlation is due to other more specific intervening factors; that is, volume may be probably a proxy measure for other factors that affect care.(59) High-volume providers may have the economies of scale to improve their structural characteristics, such as recruiting experienced medical staff and investing in required equipment and information systems. These structural advantages may enable high-volume providers most likely to perform better processes of care, such as well-designed care plans, streamlined procedures, and higher adherence to evidence-based guidelines that improve clinical outcomes.(64-66) These findings are consistent with the framework of "Structure-Process-Outcome" hypothesized by Donabedian, that structure of care influences process which in turn influences outcomes.(67)

6. Volume-outcome relationship in kidney transplant

The outcome of kidney transplant is determined by a recipient's health status, surgical techniques, competency of the surgeons and staff, multidisciplinary care, infection control, and the ability to manage graft rejection after surgery. Kidney transplantation has achieved significant improvement for the past two decades. According to the USRDS 2010 annual report, one year survival of kidney transplant is about 98.7% for living donors, 96.7% for deceased donors, and 95.4% for synchronous pancreas and kidney transplant.(68)

Accumulating evidences have demonstrated the positive relationship between surgical volume and patient outcome in transplantation. The incidence and prevalence rates of ESRD are high in the United States and many European countries. The number of kidney transplant surgeries and the volume-outcome studies are also high in these countries. Axelrod et al. found that transplant outcomes are better at the higher volume centers.(24)

The unadjusted rate of renal graft loss within 1 year was significantly lower at high volume than low volume transplant centers. After adjustment, kidney transplant at low and very low volume centers was associated with a higher incidence of graft loss when compared with high volume centers. However, they did not identify clear minimal threshold volume for kidney transplantation. Edwards et al. (22) also found that as a group, liver-transplantation centers in the United States that perform 20 or fewer transplantations per year have mortality rates that are significantly higher than those at centers that perform more than 20 transplantations per year. They argued that information regarding the outcome of liver transplantation at transplantation centers should be made widely available to the public in a timely manner. Kim et al. (25) also found significant center-specific variation in the success of renal transplantation in Canada. There was significant center-specific variation in recipient and transplant characteristics (e.g. age, diabetes mellitus, donor source and center volume) as well as covariate-adjusted facility-specific outcome rates. There was a 3- to 4-fold difference in hazard rates of renal transplant outcomes among the 20 centers studied in Canada. Centers performing less than 200 transplants over the study period were associated with lower graft and patient survival. Using the North American Pediatric Transplant Cooperative Study database, Schurman et al. (23) found outcomes between groups existed, including the increasing rates of cadaver donor graft thrombosis and acute tubular necrosis with decreasing pediatric renal transplant center volume. Decreasing graft survival for decreasing center size groups was noted at 3 months after transplant. Superior graft survival in the high-volume centers noted at 3 months after transplant appears predominantly the result of lower rates of cadaver donor graft thrombosis and acute tubular necrosis.

For those with high incidence and prevalence rates of ESRD but low donation rates, such as Japan, Taiwan, Hong Kong, many hospitals and surgeons in these countries compete for limited number of renal transplant surgeries. The outcome and efficiency of transplant surgeries varied substantially among hospitals of different surgical volumes. One recent study based on a nationally representative data base in Taiwan revealed that kidney transplants performed at high-volume hospitals were more likely to result in fewer surgical complications, lower mortality, and higher survival for patients and transplanted grafts than those performed at low-volume hospitals.(69) Even though the mean age of the kidney recipients was older and the initial graft rejection rate was higher for patients at high surgical volume hospitals than at lower volume hospitals, the survival rates for recipients and grafts were significantly better at high- than low-volume hospitals. The mean transplant surgery cost was also lower at high- than low-volume hospitals. This study highlights the fact that nearly 77% of the surgeries were performed at six high-volume hospitals, which provided better quality of care than the low-volume counterparts. If all kidney transplants were performed at these high-volume hospitals, more patients and transplanted grafts would be saved and costs could be contained.

High volume hospitals are inevitably more likely to receive risky cases which in turn influence the outcomes of transplantation. This is to some extents the social responsibility of these high-volume and center-of-excellence hospitals. These hospitals can make efforts to minimize the influences of increasing risky cases. First of all, the differences in performance of surgeons and the surgical team will be more significant in high-risk than the average-risk cases. Transplant centers with the state-of-art techniques and well-trained surgical teams are more likely to increase the success rates of kidney transplant of risky cases than their counterparts. High volume of transplant cases means that the hospitals have enough capacity and capability to treat all kinds of patients. Secondly, the high-volume hospitals will not always treat risky cases as long as the establishment of the organ procurement and transplantation network. The allocation of the donated kidneys follows the pre-set standard of procedure including disease severity and many other factors such as tissue matching results, age, location, waiting time, and the shortest ischemic time.

7. The volume-based policies in risky surgeries and transplant

Evidence of the volume-outcome relationship has important and practical policy implications. Although volume has not been widely accepted as a quality indicator, it is a structural characteristic that is easy to calculate and that is often associated with quality in the literature. (70) If the "higher-volume and better-outcome" association exists and is strong in magnitude, it would support the concentration of some specific medical interventions in regional, high-volume centers in an attempt to increase patient safety and reduce mortality.(30, 71) Several other reasons to proceed with volume-based regionalization are: first, it is one of the few strategies that is feasible before the introduction of more reliable quality indicators; second, on average, it is more likely to result in better outcomes for patients; and third, it also creates an incentive for hospitals to collect and report the data needed to measure quality more accurately.(72)

The volume-based selective referral or regionalization policies have been implemented for certain risky surgeries as well as in organ transplantation in the United States.(73, 74) Several states in the United States have used certificate-of-need (CON) programs to review proposals for new construction and expanded services in an effort to control costs and to improve quality of care. These programs tend to regionalize cases in high-volume hospitals only.(75) Some studies found that the CON and regionalization of some high-risk procedures improves the quality of care in certain surgeries such as heart transplantation,(76) pancreas cancer,(77) and CABG.(78) Moreover, several independent organizations have begun providing the population with information about volumes at hospitals in their areas. Moreover, purchasers have the power to influence referral patterns by contracting with health plans even without direct support from the medical community. (79) Several large employers and health care purchasers in the US have combined to leverage improvements in health care quality such as the *Leapfrog Group*.(28) The purchasers set annual volume standards for some high-risk procedures and encourage patients to utilize hospitals that perform a high volume of these procedures.(80)

There is no rigid volume threshold for kidney transplantation after reviewing the literature available. However, kidney transplantation is usually conducted at limited number of transplant centers in the United States, Canada, and European countries. A number of studies have demonstrated the importance of the "center effect" as a prognostic factor in kidney transplantation.(26, 81-89) The variability in one year graft survival amongst US transplant centers has been shown to range from 30% to 40%. This effect has persisted despite advances in transplantation, which have led to improvements in short- and long-term graft and patient outcomes.(89, 90) No volume-based policy can be identified for countries with low donation rates.

Given the different socioeconomic status, culture, health care delivery and reimbursement systems, several factors shall be considered when health care authorities or hospitals plan to adopt the volume-based policies for high-risk surgeries. First of all, concentrating kidney transplant in a few high-volume hospitals could not only potentially decrease the quality of care because of work overload, but also reduce the proficiency of the remaining hospitals and their physicians in delivering kidney transplantation.(91, 92) Two controlled studies of perinatal regionalization showed no significant improvement in mortality.(93) One recent study by Hamilton et al.(58) found that the regionalization of major surgical procedures in Canada had minimal impact on death and readmission rates but showed a significant decline in the length of stay. Additionally, a volume-based referral program does not generate information about the causes of differences in quality among hospitals of varying volumes. It will also not help providers to determine how to improve quality of care except by boosting volume.

The second concern is for patient accessibility. There is clearly a tradeoff if time to treatment is increased by referring patients to high-volume centers or operators. Regionalization and selective referral could result inevitably in adverse outcomes by limiting patient choice and access to care, increasing unreasonable transfer and travel burdens and reducing the availability of surgical services in many locations, particularly in rural areas remote from the high-volume centers.(94, 95) The volume-based referral policy also may have unintended consequences for patients at lower-volume hospitals who have conditions that are not on the selective referral list. (79)

Third, patients might not benefit equally from regionalization or selective referrals. Nallamothu et al.(92) found that the beneficial effects of high-volume hospitals are only concentrated in a subgroup of patients with moderate to high risks of death. The experiences from the centralization of trauma centers further confirm that the higher-volume and better outcome benefits are only evident in high-risk patients.(95, 96) Thus, Nallamothu et al. suggest a transfer policy targeted at patients with moderate or higher risk.(71)

Finally, volume-based referral strategies would have substantial implications for hospitals, payers, and the society. First, regionalization and selective referral could create an unfair impact on the economic viability of small- to moderate-sized providers of lower-volume services.(97) Losing service volume could threaten the financial viability of local hospitals and their ability to recruit and retain physicians. (94) Second, reduced competition among providers may result in increased prices in many areas. Third, volume-based referral should not be expected to greatly reduce direct health care costs since the current evidence does not indicate that higher-volume hospitals achieve shorter lengths of hospital admissions.(74) Finally, the volume standards would inevitably create financial incentives for providers to increase the number of procedures, whether they are medically indicated or not.(98, 99).

8. Policy implications and suggestions

The relationship between hospitals' volume of kidney transplant surgery and patients' outcomes has been a quite debated issue. Although many studies have demonstrated that patients who receive surgery at higher-volume hospitals are more likely to have better outcomes, the volume-based healthcare policies shall be tailored according the prevalence of ESRD patients, the number of organ donors, the availability of high-quality transplant providers, the healthcare delivery and reimbursement systems, and the culture and social norms in each country. There is no one magic bullet to solve all problems in every country.

For many developed countries with abundant medical resources, well-experienced providers, and high organ donation rates, the release of transplant outcome information of each transplant center may be more important than using the volume of surgery as a proxy indicator. Therefore, the healthcare authorities had better establishing solid organ procurement and allocation systems so that the limited organs can be utilized in an efficient way.

On the other hand, the need and number of kidney transplant surgeries are also growing rapidly in many countries where organ donation has not been a social norm. When many hospitals and surgeons compete for the limited sources of donors, the medical societies and healthcare policy makers worth to concern the differences in quality and efficiency of kidney transplants between high- and low-volume hospitals . We suggest that policy makers consider the following volume-based strategies to improve the quality of kidney transplants. First, the healthcare authority can consider adopting a 'center of excellence policy", that is, regionalizing kidney transplant surgeries to hospitals that have performed kidney transplant surgeries above a certain volume threshold. This volume threshold can be decided by healthcare authorities, transplant expert groups, hospitals, and patient representatives. However, this policy shall take into consideration of the country's size, distribution of medical resources, and convenience of transportation. Second, the 'center of excellence' hospital should be accountable for regional kidney transplant quality and outcomes. All high-risk patients shall be referred to high-volume hospitals for intensive care. If kidney transplants for high-risk patients are allowed to be performed at low-volume hospitals, they shall be supervised by the 'center of excellence' hospitals. Third, the health care authorities can use a 'certificate of need' policy to review proposals for new construction and expand services in an effort to control costs and to improve kidney transplant quality.

9. Conclusions

When surgical quality information for kidney transplantation has not been systemically collected or disclosed to the public, hospital's volume of kidney transplants has served a convenient proxy quality indicator for patients and donors. In summary of all evidences available, patients who receive kidney transplant at high-volume hospitals are more likely to have better outcomes than at low-volume ones. This positive relationship has also been documented in many other high-risk surgeries. For areas with low organ donation rates and low volume of kidney transplant surgeries, volume-based strategies can be considered to ensure the quality of kidney transplant surgeries and to facilitate the highest utilization of limited kidney donors. Any regionalization or selective referral policy needs to be tailored based on the healthcare delivery and reimbursement systems, availability of medical resources, and culture background of the country. Hospital kidney transplant volume is just a proxy indicator on the population basis. The ultimate goal is that recipients and donors can access to comprehensive and transparent quality information of kidney transplant.

Author details

Wui-Chiang Lee
Department of Medical Affairs and Planning, Taipei Veterans General Hospital, Taipei, Taiwan (R.O.C)
Taiwan Joint Commission on Hospital Accreditation, Taiwan (R.O.C)
National Yang-Ming University School of Medicine, Taiwan (R.O.C)

Shu-Yun Tsao
Department of Surgery, Taipei Veterans General Hospital, Taiwan (R.O.C)

Che-Chuan Loong
National Yang-Ming University School of Medicine, Taiwan (R.O.C)
Division of Transplantation Surgery, Department of Surgery, Taipei Veterans General Hospital, Taiwan (R.O.C)

10. References

[1] Annual Data Report. United State Renal Data System; 2011 Chapter 12, International Comparison. Available from: http://www.usrds.org/2011/pdf/v2_ch012_11.pdf.
[2] Medical Utilization of Major Illness/Injury [database on the internet]. Bureau of National Health Insurance, Republic of China; 2010-[cited 2012 May 20].Available from http://www.nhi.gov.tw/webdata/webdata.aspx?menu=17&menu_id=661&WD_ID=689 &webdata_id=4004
[3] Annual Data Report [database on the internet]. United State Renal Data System; 2011-[cited 2012 May 20]. Chapter 11, Costs of ESRD. Available from: http://www.usrds.org/2011/pdf/v2_ch011_11.pdf
[4] Shrivastava A, Singh P, Bhandari M, Kumar A. Economics of Organ Transplantation in India. Transplantation Proceedings 1998;30:3121-2.
[5] Manninen DL, Evans RW, Dugan MK, Rader B. The costs and outcome of kidney transplant graft failure. Transplantation proceedings. 1991;23(1 Pt 2):1312-4.

[6] Niu SF, Li IC. Quality of life of patients having renal replacement therapy. J advanced nursing. 2005;51(1):15-21.

[7] Wolfe RA, Ashby VB, Milford EL, Ojo AO, Ettenger RE, Agodoa LYC, Held PJ, et al. Comparison of Mortality in all patient on dialysis,patients on dialysis awaiting transplantation,and recipents of a first cadaveric transplant. N Engl J Med . 1999;341:1725-30.

[8] Biesen WV, Lameire N, Peeters P, Vanholder R. Belgium's mixed private/public health care system and its impact on the cost of end-stage renal disease. Int J Health Care Finance Econ. 2007;7:133-48.

[9] Kleophas W, Reichel H. International study of health care organization and financing: development of renal replacement therapy in Germany. Int J Health Care Finance Econ. 2007;7:185-200.

[10] Pontoriero G, Pozzoni P, Vocchio LD, Locatelli F. International Study of Health Care Organization and Financing for renal replacement therapy in Italy: an evolving reality. Int J Health Care Finance Econ. 2007;2-3:201-15.

[11] Manns BJ, Mendelssohn DC, Taub KJ. The economics of end-stage renal disease care in Canada: incentives and impact on delivery of care. Int J Health Care Finance Econ. 2007;7:149-69.

[12] Hirth RA. The organization and financing of kidney dialysis and transplant care in the United States of America. Int J Health Care Finance Econ. 2007;7(4):301-18.

[13] Harris A. The organization and funding of the treatment of end-stage renal disease in Australia. Int J Health Care Finance Econ. 2007;7:113-32.

[14] Fukuhara S, Yamazaki C, Hayashino Y, Higashi T, Eichleay MA, Akiba T, et al. The organization and financing of end-stage renal disease treatment in Japan. Int J Health Care Finance Econ. 2007;7(2):217-31.

[15] Durand-Zaleski I, Combe C, Lang P. International Study of Health Care Organization and Financing for end-stage renal disease in France Int J Health Care Finance Econ. 2007;7(2-3):171-83.

[16] Ashton T, Marshall MR. The organization and financing of dialysis and kidney transplantation services in New Zealand. Int J Health Care Finance Econ. 2007;7(4):233-52.

[17] Organ Donation [database on the internet]. NHSBT; 2012-[cited 2012 May 20]. Waiting time to transplant. Available from http://www.organdonation.nhs.uk/ukt/about_transplants/waiting_time_to_transplant/waiting_time_to_transplant.asp

[18] Organ Procurement and Transplantation Network [database on the internet].US department HHS;2012- [cited 2012 May 11] . Waiting Time by Kidney PRA. Available from http://optn.transplant.hrsa.gov/latestData/rptStrat.asp

[19] Medina-Pestana JO. Organization of a High-Volume Kidney Transplant Program- "Assembly Line" Approach. Transplantation. 2006;81:1510-20.

[20] Vathsala A, Chow KT. Renal Transplantation in Singapore Ann Acad Med Singapore. 2009;38:291-9.

[21] James F.Whiting FD, Paul Morrissey, Giacomo Basadonna, Scott Johnson, Richard Rohrer, Kevin O'Connor,et al. Clinical Result of an Organ Procurement Organization Effort to Increase Utilization of Donors after Cardiac Death. Transplantation. 2006;81:1368-71.
[22] Edwards EB, Roberts JP, McBride MA, Schulak JA, Hunsicker LG. The effect of the volume of procedures at transplantation centers on mortality after liver transplantation. N Engl J Med. 1999;341(27):2049-53.
[23] Schurman SJ, Stablein DM, Perlman SA, Warady BA. Center volume effects in pediatric renal transplantation. A report of the North American Pediatric Renal Transplant Cooperative Study. Pediatric nephrology (Berlin, Germany). 1999;13(5):373-8.
[24] Axelrod DA, Guidinger MK, McCullough KP, Leichtman AB, Punch JD, Merion RM. Association of center volume with outcome after liver and kidney transplantation. Am J Transplant. 2004;4(6):920-7.
[25] Kim SJ, Schaubel DE, Jeffery JR, Fenton SS. Centre-specific variation in renal transplant outcomes in Canada. Nephrol Dial Transplant. 2004;19(7):1856-61.
[26] Lin HM, Kauffman HM, McBride MA, Davies DB, Rosendale JD, Smith CM, et al. Center-specific graft and patient survival rates: 1997 United Network for Organ Sharing (UNOS) report. JAMA. 1998;280(13):1153-60. Epub 1998/10/20.
[27] Hannan EL, Racz M, Ryan TJ, McCallister BD, Johnson LW, Arani DT, et al. Coronary angioplasty volume-outcome relationships for hospitals and cardiologists. JAMA. 1997;277(11):892-8.
[28] Birkmeyer JD, Siewers AE, Finlayson EV, Stukel TA, Lucas FL, Batista I, et al. Hospital volume and surgical mortality in the United States. N Engl J Med. 2002;346(15):1128-37.
[29] Vakili BA, Kaplan R, Brown DL. Volume-outcome relation for physicians and hospitals performing angioplasty for acute myocardial infarction in New York state. Circulation. 2001;104(18):2171-6.
[30] Dudley RA, Johansen KL, Brand R, Rennie DJ, Milstein A. Selective referral to high-volume hospitals: estimating potentially avoidable deaths. JAMA. 2000;283(9):1159-66.
[31] Luft HS, Hunt SS, Maerki SC. The volume-outcome relationship: practice-makes-perfect or selective-referral patterns? Health Serv Res. 1987;22(2):157-82.
[32] Flood AB, Scott WR, Ewy W. Does practice make perfect? Part II: The relation between volume and outcomes and other hospital characteristics. Med Care. 1984;22(2):115-25.
[33] Flood AB, Scott WR, Ewy W. Does practice make perfect? Part I: The relation between hospital volume and outcomes for selected diagnostic categories. Med Care. 1984;22(2):98-114.
[34] Halm EA, Lees C, Chassin MR. How is volume related to quality of care? A systematic review of the research literature. In: Hewitt M, ed. Interpreting the volume-outcome relationship in the context of health care quality. Washington, DC: Institute of Medicine; 2000.
[35] Showstack JA, Rosenfeld KE, Garnick DW, Luft HS, Schaffarzick RW, Fowles J. Association of volume with outcome of coronary artery bypass graft surgery. Scheduled vs nonscheduled operations. JAMA. 1987;257(6):785-9.

[36] Farley DE, Ozminkowski RJ. Volume-outcome relationships and in-hospital mortality: the effect of changes in volume over time. Med Care. 1992;30(1):77-94.
[37] Grumbach K, Anderson GM, Luft HS, Roos LL, Brook R. Regionalization of cardiac surgery in the United States and Canada. Geographic access, choice, and outcomes. JAMA. 1995;274(16):1282-8.
[38] Hannan EL, Siu AL, Kumar D, Kilburn H, Jr., Chassin MR. The decline in coronary artery bypass graft surgery mortality in New York State. The role of surgeon volume. JAMA. 1995;273(3):209-13.
[39] Hannan EL, O'Donnell JF, Kilburn H, Jr., Bernard HR, Yazici A. Investigation of the relationship between volume and mortality for surgical procedures performed in New York State hospitals. JAMA. 1989;262(4):503-10.
[40] Hannan EL, Kilburn H, Jr., Bernard H, O'Donnell JF, Lukacik G, Shields EP. Coronary artery bypass surgery: the relationship between inhospital mortality rate and surgical volume after controlling for clinical risk factors. Med Care. 1991;29(11):1094-107.
[41] Chang RK, Klitzner TS. Can regionalization decrease the number of deaths for children who undergo cardiac surgery? A theoretical analysis. Pediatrics. 2002;109(2):173-81.
[42] Hannan EL, Popp AJ, Tranmer B, Fuestel P, Waldman J, Shah D. Relationship between provider volume and mortality for carotid endarterectomies in New York state. Stroke. 1998;29(11):2292-7.
[43] Sollano JA, Gelijns AC, Moskowitz AJ, Heitjan DF, Cullinane S, Saha T, et al. Volume-outcome relationships in cardiovascular operations: New York State, 1990-1995. J Thorac Cardiovasc Surg. 1999;117(3):419-28.
[44] Dimick JB, Pronovost PJ, Cowan JA, Ailawadi G, Upchurch GR, Jr. The volume-outcome effect for abdominal aortic surgery: differences in case-mix or complications? Arch Surg. 2002;137(7):828-32.
[45] Pronovost PJ, Jenckes MW, Dorman T, Garrett E, Breslow MJ, Rosenfeld BA, et al. Organizational characteristics of intensive care units related to outcomes of abdominal aortic surgery. JAMA. 1999;281(14):1310-7.
[46] Solomon DH, Losina E, Baron JA, Fossel AH, Guadagnoli E, Lingard EA, et al. Contribution of hospital characteristics to the volume-outcome relationship: Dislocation and infection following total hip replacement surgery. Arthritis Rheum. 2002;46(9):2436-44.
[47] Matsen FA, 3rd. The relationship of surgical volume to quality of care: scientific considerations and policy implications. J Bone Joint Surg Am. 2002;84-A(8):1482-3.
[48] Birkmeyer JD, Finlayson SR, Tosteson AN, Sharp SM, Warshaw AL, Fisher ES. Effect of hospital volume on in-hospital mortality with pancreaticoduodenectomy. Surgery. 1999;125(3):250-6.
[49] Gordon TA, Burleyson GP, Tielsch JM, Cameron JL. The effects of regionalization on cost and outcome for one general high-risk surgical procedure. Ann Surg. 1995;221(1):43-9.
[50] Gordon TA, Bowman HM, Bass EB, Lillemoe KD, Yeo CJ, Heitmiller RF, et al. Complex gastrointestinal surgery: impact of provider experience on clinical and economic outcomes. J Am Coll Surg. 1999;189(1):46-56.

[51] Simunovic M, To T, Theriault M, Langer B. Relation between hospital surgical volume and outcome for pancreatic resection for neoplasm in a publicly funded health care system. Cmaj. 1999;160(5):643-8.
[52] Sosa JA, Bowman HM, Gordon TA, Bass EB, Yeo CJ, Lillemoe KD, et al. Importance of hospital volume in the overall management of pancreatic cancer. Ann Surg. 1998;228(3):429-38.
[53] Begg CB, Cramer LD, Hoskins WJ, Brennan MF. Impact of hospital volume on operative mortality for major cancer surgery. JAMA. 1998;280(20):1747-51.
[54] Patti MG, Corvera CU, Glasgow RE, Way LW. A hospital's annual rate of esophagectomy influences the operative mortality rate. J Gastrointest Surg. 1998;2(2):186-92.
[55] Luft HS, Bunker JP, Enthoven AC. Should operations be regionalized? The empirical relation between surgical volume and mortality. N Engl J Med. 1979;301(25):1364-9.
[56] Khuri SF, Daley J, Henderson W, Hur K, Demakis J, Aust JB, et al. The Department of Veterans Affairs' NSQIP: the first national, validated, outcome-based, risk-adjusted, and peer-controlled program for the measurement and enhancement of the quality of surgical care. National VA Surgical Quality Improvement Program. Ann Surg. 1998;228(4):491-507.
[57] Hlatky MA, Dudley RA. Operator volume and clinical outcomes of primary coronary angioplasty for patients with acute myocardial infarction. Circulation. 2001;104(18):2155-7.
[58] Hamilton SM, Johnston WC, Voaklander DC. Outcomes after the regionalization of major surgical procedures in the Alberta Capital Health Region (Edmonton). Can J Surg. 2001;44(1):51-8.
[59] Halm EA, Lee C, Chassin MR. Is volume related to outcome in health care? A systematic review and methodologic critique of the literature. Ann Intern Med. 2002;137(6):511-20.
[60] Luft HS. The relation between surgical volume and mortality: an exploration of causal factors and alternative models. Med Care. 1980;18(9):940-59.
[61] Hannan EL, Stone CC, Biddle TL, DeBuono BA. Public release of cardiac surgery outcomes data in New York: what do New York state cardiologists think of it? Am Heart J. 1997;134(6):1120-8.
[62] Schneider EC, Epstein AM. Influence of cardiac-surgery performance reports on referral practices and access to care. A survey of cardiovascular specialists. N Engl J Med. 1996;335(4):251-6.
[63] Chassin MR, Hannan EL, DeBuono BA. Benefits and hazards of reporting medical outcomes publicly. N Engl J Med. 1996;334(6):394-8.
[64] Chen J, Radford MJ, Wang Y, Marciniak TA, Krumholz HM. Do "America's Best Hospitals" perform better for acute myocardial infarction? N Engl J Med. 1999;340(4):286-92.
[65] Canto JG, Every NR, Magid DJ, Rogers WJ, Malmgren JA, Frederick PD, et al. The volume of primary angioplasty procedures and survival after acute myocardial

infarction. National Registry of Myocardial Infarction 2 Investigators. N Engl J Med. 2000;342(21):1573-80.
[66] Hannan EL, Popp AJ, Feustel P, Halm E, Bernardini G, Waldman J, et al. Association of surgical specialty and processes of care with patient outcomes for carotid endarterectomy. Stroke. 2001;32(12):2890-7.
[67] Donabedian A. Evaluating the quality of medical care. Milbank Mem Fund Q. 1966;44(3):166-206.
[68] The U.S. Organ Procurement and Transplantation Network and the Scientific Registry of Transplant Recipients. The 2010 OPTN / SRTR Annual Report: Transplant Data 2000-2009. Available from http://www.srtr.org/annual_reports/2010/
[69] Tsao SY, Lee WC, Loong CC, Chen TJ, Chiu JH, Tai LC. High-surgical-volume hospitals associated with better quality and lower cost of kidney transplantation in Taiwan. Journal of the Chinese Medical Association : JCMA. 2011;74(1):22-7. Epub 2011/02/05.
[70] Epstein AM. Volume and outcome--it is time to move ahead. N Engl J Med. 2002;346(15):1161-4.
[71] Nallamothu BK, Saint S, Eagle KA. Volume and outcome. N Engl J Med. 2002;347(9):693-6.
[72] Urschel JD, Urschel DM. The hospital volume-outcome relationship in general thoracic surgery. Is the surgeon the critical determinant? J Cardiovasc Surg (Torino). 2000;41(1):153-5.
[73] Birkmeyer JD, Finlayson EV, Birkmeyer CM. Volume standards for high-risk surgical procedures: potential benefits of the Leapfrog initiative. Surgery. 2001;130(3):415-22.
[74] Birkmeyer JD, Skinner JS, Wennberg DE. Will volume-based referral strategies reduce costs orjust save lives? Health Aff (Millwood). 2002;21(5):234-41.
[75] Chassin MR. Assessing strategies for quality improvement. Health Aff (Millwood). 1997;16(3):151-61.
[76] Krakauer H, Shekar SS, Kaye MP. The relationship of clinical outcomes to status as a Medicare-approved heart transplant center. Transplantation. 1995;59(6):840-6.
[77] Gordon TA, Bowman HM, Tielsch JM, Bass EB, Burleyson GP, Cameron JL. Statewide regionalization of pancreaticoduodenectomy and its effect on in-hospital mortality. Ann Surg. 1998;228(1):71-8.
[78] Robinson JL, Nash DB, Moxey E, O'Connor JP. Certificate of need and the quality of cardiac surgery. Am J Med Qual. 2001;16(5):155-60.
[79] Dudley RA, Johansen KL. Invited commentary: Physician responses to purchaser quality initiatives for surgical procedures. Surgery. 2001;130(3):425-8.
[80] Milstein A, Galvin RS, Delbanco SF, Salber P, Buck CR, Jr. Improving the safety of health care: the leapfrog initiative. Eff Clin Pract. 2000;3(6):313-6.
[81] Gjertson DW, Terasaki PI. The large center variation in half-lives of kidney transplants. Transplantation. 1992;53(2):357-62. Epub 1992/02/01.
[82] Gjertson DW, Terasaki PI, Cecka JM, Takemoto S. Reduction of the center effect by HLA matching. Transplantation proceedings. 1993;25(1 Pt 1):215-6. Epub 1993/02/01.
[83] Cho YW, Cecka JM. Center effect in the UNOS Renal Transplant Registry. Clinical transplants. 1992:333-46. Epub 1992/01/01.

[84] Cho YW, Cecka JM. Organ Procurement Organization and transplant center effects on cadaver renal transplant outcomes. Clinical transplants. 1996:427-41. Epub 1996/01/01.
[85] Benlahrache C, Cecka M, Mickey MR, Cicciarelli J. The center effect. Clinical transplants. 1987:325-37. Epub 1987/01/01.
[86] Porte RJ, Ploeg RJ, Hansen B, van Bockel JH, Thorogood J, Persijn GG, et al. Long-term graft survival after liver transplantation in the UW era: late effects of cold ischemia and primary dysfunction. European Multicentre Study Group. Transplant international : official journal of the European Society for Organ Transplantation. 1998;11 Suppl 1:S164-7. Epub 1998/07/17.
[87] Evans RW, Manninen DL, Dong F. The center effect in kidney transplantation. Transplantation proceedings. 1991;23(1 Pt 2):1315-7.
[88] Morris PJ, Johnson RJ, Fuggle SV, Belger MA, Briggs JD. Analysis of factors that affect outcome of primary cadaveric renal transplantation in the UK. HLA Task Force of the Kidney Advisory Group of the United Kingdom Transplant Support Service Authority (UKTSSA). Lancet. 1999;354(9185):1147-52. Epub 1999/10/08.
[89] Schaubel DE, Jeffery JR, Mao Y, Semenciw R, Yeates K, Fenton SS. Trends in mortality and graft failure for renal transplant patients. Cmaj. 2002;167(2):137-42. Epub 2002/08/06.
[90] Hariharan S, Johnson CP, Bresnahan BA, Taranto SE, McIntosh MJ, Stablein D. Improved graft survival after renal transplantation in the United States, 1988 to 1996. N Engl J Med. 2000;342(9):605-12. Epub 2000/03/04.
[91] Rosemurgy AS, Bloomston M, Serafini FM, Coon B, Murr MM, Carey LC. Frequency with which surgeons undertake pancreaticoduodenectomy determines length of stay, hospital charges, and in-hospital mortality. J Gastrointest Surg. 2001;5(1):21-6.
[92] Nallamothu BK, Saint S, Ramsey SD, Hofer TP, Vijan S, Eagle KA. The role of hospital volume in coronary artery bypass grafting: is more always better? J Am Coll Cardiol. 2001;38(7):1923-30.
[93] Siegel E, Gillings D, Campbell S, Guild P. A controlled evaluation of rural regional perinatal care: impact on mortality and morbidity. Am J Public Health. 1985;75(3):246-53.
[94] Finlayson SR, Birkmeyer JD, Tosteson AN, Nease RF, Jr. Patient preferences for location of care: implications for regionalization. Med Care. 1999;37(2):204-9.
[95] Nathens AB, Jurkovich GJ, Maier RV, Grossman DC, MacKenzie EJ, Moore M, et al. Relationship between trauma center volume and outcomes. JAMA. 2001;285(9):1164-71.
[96] Nathens AB, Maier RV. The relationship between trauma center volume and outcome. Adv Surg. 2001;35:61-75.
[97] Birkmeyer JD. Should we regionalize major surgery? Potential benefits and policy considerations. J Am Coll Surg. 2000;190(3):341-9.
[98] Chassin MR, Kosecoff J, Park RE, Winslow CM, Kahn KL, Merrick NJ, et al. Does inappropriate use explain geographic variations in the use of health care services? A study of three procedures. JAMA. 1987;258(18):2533-7.

[99] Leape LL, Park RE, Solomon DH, Chassin MR, Kosecoff J, Brook RH. Does inappropriate use explain small-area variations in the use of health care services? JAMA. 1990;263(5):669-72.

Chapter 15

Expanding Opportunities for Kidney Transplantation

Cheguevara Afaneh, Meredith J. Aull, Anthony Watkins, Jim Kim and Sandip Kapur

Additional information is available at the end of the chapter

http://dx.doi.org/10.5772/54219

1. Introduction

Despite the increased use of living donors and marginal donor kidneys, there still exists a significant discrepancy between the organ supply and demand in renal transplantation [1]. This has led to excessive waiting times affecting patient survival. More than half of all patients with end-stage renal disease (ESRD) over the age of 60 die before receiving a kidney transplant [2]. These patients face a mortality rate of 6% per year while awaiting an acceptable donor. Thus, transplant surgeons and physicians have turned to other potential sources of allografts to meet the ever growing demand. Potential resources include maximizing the utilization of pediatric donors, increasing use of marginal donors, and transplanting hepatitis C (HCV) positive donor kidneys into HCV positive recipients. Finally, the advent of kidney paired donation has significantly improved and maximized the use of living donor renal transplants.

The following chapter will discuss these sources of allografts and their associated outcomes. The goal of these donors is to maximize the potential opportunities for any patient on the deceased donor waiting list. Ultimately, these modalities will lead to improved patient survival and slightly offset the burden of the deceased donor waitlist.

2. Pediatric donor

2.1. Introduction

The first attempt at using pediatric donors was in 1972 when en bloc kidneys were successfully transplanted in adult recipients [3]. By the late 1990's, single pediatric donors were being successfully transplanted into adult recipients [4, 5]. This use of pediatric donors in adults has not disadvantaged the pediatric recipient population. In 2005, the United

Network for Organ Sharing (UNOS) mandated that pediatric recipients will be prioritized young adult deceased donor kidneys known as the Share-35 policy [6].

Pediatric kidneys can be transplanted as individual organs or en-bloc as dual kidneys. Some strongly advocated the use of single kidneys from pediatric donors, as opposed to en-bloc transplantation, to avoid the potential for technical complications [7]. Additionally, opponents of single pediatric donor kidney argue that the hyperfiltration syndrome associated with single kidneys leads to early graft failure in adult recipients [8, 9]. Pediatric donor size has been implicated as one of the important risks for graft failure. Initial studies demonstrated that technical complications, most notably graft thrombosis, was significantly higher in small pediatric donors (<10 kg) [9]. Moreover, as a result, pediatric donors represent the highest discard group with rates approaching 40% in donors less than 10 kg.

In the following sections, we will discuss the advantages and disadvantages of the various types of pediatric donors. Short and long-term outcomes will be discussed with attention to perioperative outcomes associated with each.

2.2. Small pediatric donor

Several groups, including our own, have demonstrated the safety and feasibility of using young and small pediatric donors. Initial concerns regarding the use of these donors were related to both technical complications and allograft function. Given the high discard rate in this group, a discussion of their proper utilization and outcomes is important.

Small pediatric donors, defined as weighing <10 kg and ages 5 years or younger, have been successfully transplanted into adult recipients. Balachandran et al. described a successful series of 27 small pediatric donors transplanted into adult recipients weighing >60 kg [10]. All kidneys were transplanted as single kidneys both with and without aortic cuffs (Carrel patch, Figure 1), with an end-to-side anastomosis to the recipient external iliac vessels. The majority of patients underwent rabbit antithymocyte globulin (r-ATG) induction therapy. In this series, no patient experienced a vascular complication and only 2 kidneys had primary non-function (both from the same donor). Patient and graft survival in this cohort at 2 years were 100% and 92.5%, respectively, which was not significantly different to their comparison group of standard adult kidney recipients of adult deceased donor kidneys. Borboroglu et al. also described a successful series of 15 single pediatric donors less than 2 years of age transplanted into adult recipients [11]. The 2 years graft survival rate was 93% with a vascular thrombosis rate of 6.7%.

In a review of over 12,000 pediatric donors, Bresnahan et al. demonstrate inferior graft survival in recipients of these kidneys compared to standard adult donors [8]. Pediatric donors 5 years of age or younger had the worst 1 year graft survival (76.3% in en-bloc kidney recipients and 72.2% in single kidney recipient). In this series, pediatric donors had a graft thrombosis rate of 10% in donors 5 years of age or less, 6% in donors aged 6 to 11 years, and 5% in donors aged 12-17 years. The rate of primary non-function was 5%. Others have also described the increased incidence of vascular complications in these young and small pediatric donors [12].

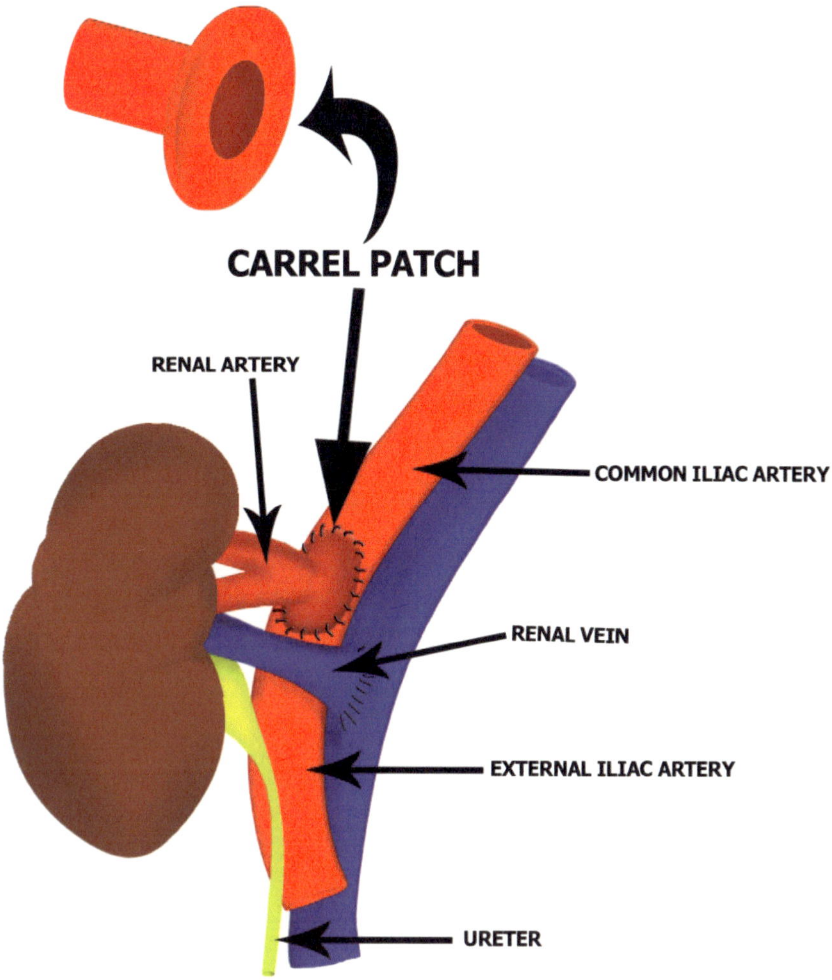

Figure 1. A pediatric kidney is implanted into the external iliac artery with the use of a Carrel patch.

The inferior outcome of small pediatric donors was partly explained in the past by hyperfiltration injury. Hyperfiltration injury describes the compensatory mechanisms in the pediatric kidney that increase the glomerular capillary pressure in response to the inadequate filtration ability of the small graft. This concept was used to explain why transplanting en-bloc pediatric donors lead to improved outcomes as more "renal mass" was transplanted [8, 9]. However, opponents of this approach cite that en-bloc transplantation is a technically more challenging procedure with a relatively high surgical complication rate as well as a graft thrombosis rate of >10% [10, 13].

2.3. En-bloc vs. single kidney transplantation

Initial transplants from pediatric donors consisted of en-bloc transplantation in the recipient (Figure 2). As previously stated, this was described in 1972, and was the primary method used for several years [3]. Solitary pediatric renal allografts were then later performed in the 1990's. The initial concerns regarding the use of single pediatric donors were two-fold: technical complications and poor graft survival.

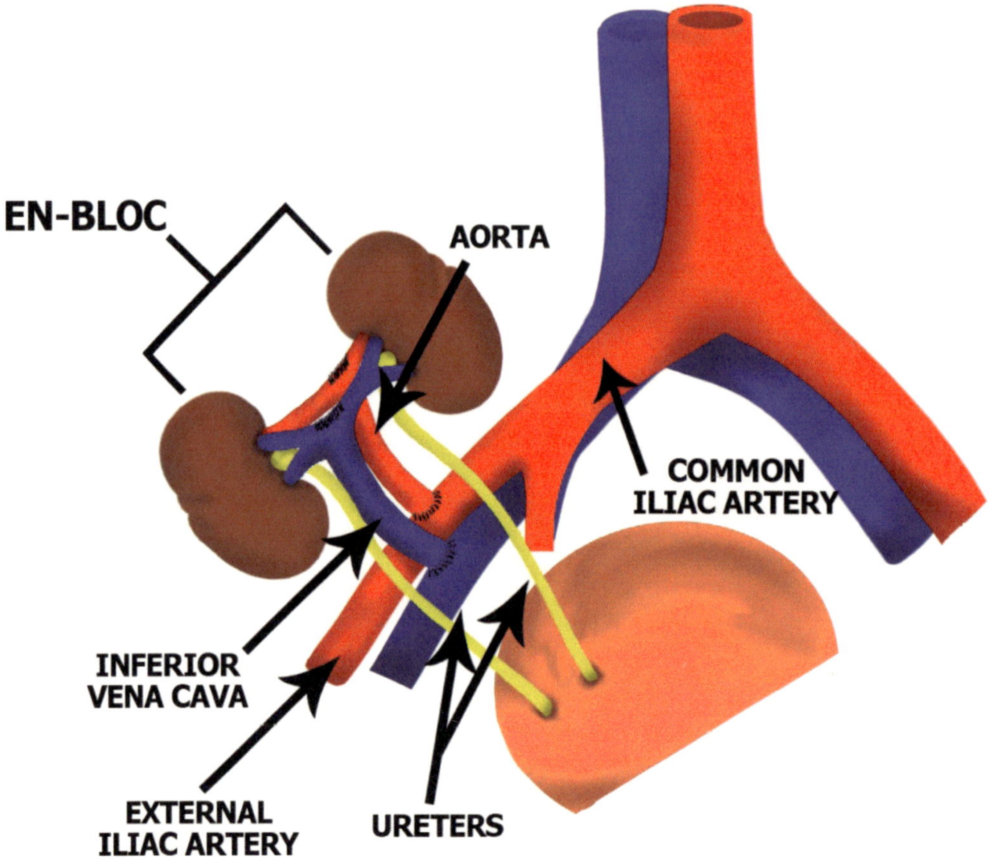

Figure 2. En-bloc pediatric kidney transplant. The following figure depicts en-bloc transplantation of pediatric kidneys into an adult recipient. The anastomosis is performed to the external iliac artery. The donor aorta and inferior vena cava are anastomosed to the recipient vessels as shown.

Technical concerns regarding the use of single pediatric donors were the major concerns initially. Bresnahan and colleagues found that recipients of en-bloc pediatric donor allografts were less likely to develop graft thrombosis compared to single pediatric donor allografts (OR 0.688, $P<0.01$) [8]. A series of 20 en-bloc pediatric donor allografts demonstrated no vascular complications [14]. Borboroglu et al. compared 15 single pediatric donors to 33 en-bloc pediatric donors [11]. Four recipients of en-bloc pediatric donors experienced arterial thrombosis, whereas only one recipient of a single pediatric donor developed arterial thrombosis. Moreover, three recipients of en-bloc pediatric donors experienced ureteral complications, whereas none occurred in the single pediatric donor group. In a series of 27 single pediatric donor allografts, no recipient developed vascular thrombosis postoperatively [10].

Inferior graft survival has also been implicated as a reason to avoid using single pediatric donors. The initial studies by Bresnahan et al. demonstrated poorer graft survival in recipients of single versus en-bloc pediatric donor allografts at 1 year (72.2% versus 76.3%, respectively [8]. Additionally, a study utilizing the Scientific Registry of Transplant Recipients (SRTR) data demonstrated that recipients of single pediatric donors had a 78% increased risk of graft loss compared to en-bloc donors [9]. Graft survival of en-bloc pediatric donor allografts was similar to standard deceased donors. However, a more recent analysis of the SRTR database demonstrated that single pediatric donors >35 kg had similar graft survival to SCD [15]. Moreover, graft survival of single pediatric donors 10-35 kg was similar to SCDs. A later study by Balachandran et al. demonstrated better outcomes than their initial studies. The 2 years graft survival rate in single pediatric donor recipients had improved to 92.5% [10]. Similarly, Borboroglu et al. demonstrated similar graft survival between single versus en-bloc pediatric donor allografts [11]. Effectively, the use of single pediatric donors compared to en-bloc pediatric donors has resulted in more cumulative graft years in recipients.

3. Marginal donor kidneys

3.1. Overview

The lack of available kidneys for transplantation in ESRD has lead to an increase use of suboptimal donors. As a result, more institutions are using expanded criteria donors (ECD) and deceased after cardiac death donors (DCD), sometimes referred to as marginal donors, to lessen the shortage [16-19]. The increased utilization of these organs has expanded the donor pool by 30% [19]. Nevertheless, there has been a concomitant increase in the rate of delayed graft function (DGF) and even primary non-function in DCD grafts [16-18]. Utilization of these kidneys may contribute to the donor pool, although it is important to maximize the outcomes of these allografts.

3.2. Hypothermic machine perfusion

Towards the end of the twentieth century, static cold storage was introduced to preserve kidneys procured from deceased donors, which lead to a decreased incidence of DGF and improvements in survival of DCD allografts [20]. Hypothermic machine perfusion (HMP) is an alternative to static cold storage (Figure 3). Several reports have demonstrated improvements in immediate graft function with the use of HMP compared to static cold storage [21-24]. Additionally, HMP permits longer preservation times without significant consequences to the allograft. Current notions suggest that HMP prevents and/or ameliorates injury to the kidney suffered as a result of preagonal hemodynamic and metabolic perturbations to the donor [25, 26].

Various studies have demonstrated that vascular flow and resistance data of hypothermic machine perfused organs had a decrease in ischemic injury to the allograft prior to implantation compared to static cold storage [27-29]. Additionally, biochemical markers of ischemic injury can be measured and used to assess and evaluate pretransplant ischemic organ damage. In a study by Moers et al, 306 deceased donor kidneys, including DCD donors, undergoing HMP were evaluated for relative concentrations of biomarkers associated with renal and tubular injury [30]. In this study, elevated levels of total glutathione-S-transferase (GST), N-acetyl-β-D-glucosaminidase (NAG), and heart-type fatty acid bind protein (H-FABP) were independent predictors of DGF. Thus, perhaps the phenomenon observed is an increase in ischemic injury to the kidney. The benefits of HMP may be somewhat negated if the allograft is removed prematurely and placed in static cold storage.

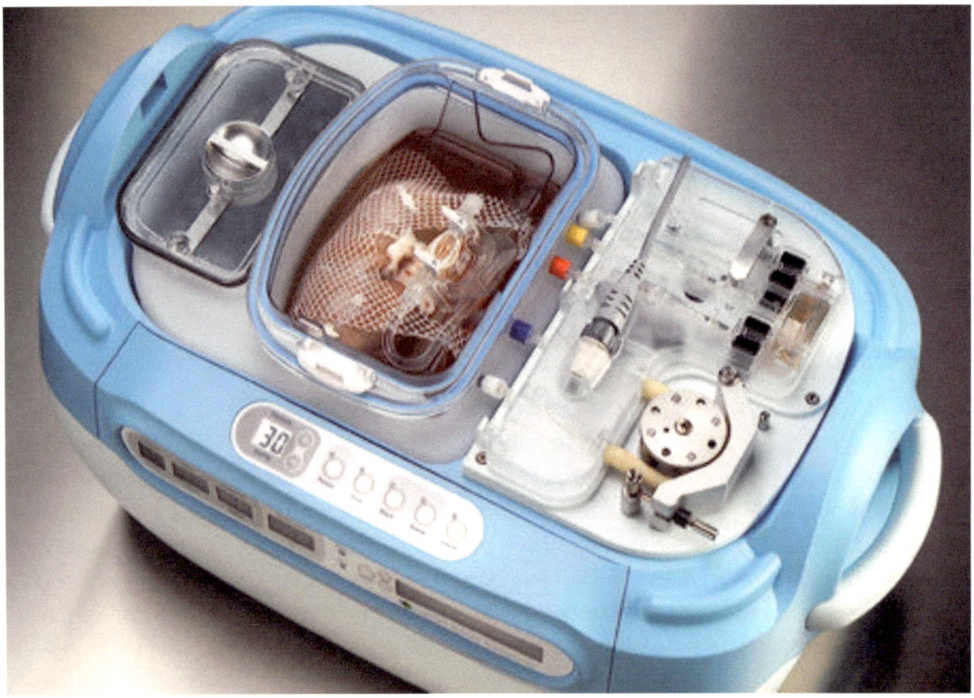

Figure 3. LifePort® Kidney Transporter. The figure depicts the LifePort ® Kidney Transporter that gently pumps the kidney with cold storage solution which can increase the cold ischemia duration compared to static cold storage and potentially improve allograft outcomes in marginal donor kidneys.

3.3. Allograft outcomes

ECD allografts have decreased graft survival rates in comparison to SCD. In general, these kidneys have a life expectancy of 6 to 8 years, whereas standard or ideal kidneys last about 10 to 12 years [31]. Prolonging allograft survival by preventing or minimizing mitigating factors for the development of DGF is imperative since DGF is a known risk factor for decreased allograft survival. Marginal donors are known to have a higher incidence of DGF, which could affect survival.

Several studies have examined the incidence and effects of DGF in marginal donor kidneys. A study by Serur et al evaluated deceased donors over more than a 40 years period and demonstrated that the most significant risk factors for short-term graft survival were DGF and acute rejection, not just the mere utilization of ECD allografts [32]. A large prospective, international, randomized controlled trial examined the efficacy of rATG versus basiliximab in patients at high risk of DGF [33]. Patients were maintained on a cyclosporine-based triple drug immunosuppression regimen and eligibility criteria included ECD or DCD allografts, SCD allografts with greater than 24 hours of cold ischemia time (CIT), repeat transplants, panel-reactive antibody value exceeding 20% before transplantation, donors with acute tubular necrosis (ATN), recipient black race, or one or more HLA mismatches. The incidence of DGF was not significantly different between patients receiving rATG and basiliximab. However, the incidence of biopsy-proven acute rejection was significantly lower in patients receiving rATG. Additionally, severe rejection episodes requiring antibody therapy were less frequent in the rATG group.

Marginal donors were initially shown to have worse outcomes than SCD. Several earlier studies demonstrated worse graft survival in kidneys from ECDs [34, 35]. More recent data, however, suggests that ECD kidneys have similar short and intermediate survival as SCD kidneys; instead, allograft function is slightly worse in the ECD group [31]. This finding is not the general consensus as the more recent trend is to match the donor age to the recipient age to optimize outcomes. For example, Chavalitdhamrong et al. demonstrated that recipients over the age of 60 years receiving ECDs from donors over the age of 70 had better survival than recipients aged 41 to 60 years [36].

Numerous studies have also demonstrated an advantage and decreased risk of DGF in marginal donors preserved by HMP compared to static cold storage [37, 38]. However, other factors, such as race, have also been implicated as risk factors for DGF. Several studies have demonstrated that African-American recipients were more likely to develop DGF [39, 40]. Hariharan and colleagues observed lower rates of graft failure in Hispanic recipients and higher graft failure rates in kidneys from Hispanic donors (compared to white) [41].

4. Hepatitis C virus & transplantation

4.1. Introduction

Hepatitis C Virus (HCV) infection is a common condition among ESRD patients and kidney transplant recipients with infection rates between 11% and 49% [42-46]. The best screening test for HCV is nucleic acid testing, or NAT. Because organ transplantation can transmit the hepatitis C virus, the consensus remains that HCV positive donors should only be transplanted into HCV positive recipients [47, 48]. Initial studies suggested that patients with HCV infection have an increased risk of death following kidney transplantation [42, 44, 45]. More recent studies have demonstrated that HCV positive patients who receive a kidney transplant have superior survival than their counterparts who remain on hemodialysis [49, 50]. Thus, kidney transplantation remains the treatment of choice for HCV positive patients with ESRD and preserved liver function without any evidence of cirrhosis.

4.2. Benefits of transplantation

The use of HCV positive donors may have potential benefits to the respective HCV positive recipients. First, HCV positive recipients transplanted with a HCV positive donor have waiting times that are almost 1 year less than their counterparts who wait for a HCV negative donor [51]. Nevertheless, HCV positive donor kidneys were about 2.6 times more likely to be discarded than HCV negative donors. HCV positive donors could receive high quality organs, especially when the donor is young. As previously discussed, there is a clear survival benefit to transplanting HCV positive recipients with HCV positive donors compared to remaining on the deceased donor waiting list. The use of hypothermic machine perfusion has been shown to decrease the viral load of the allograft prior to implantation [52]. The reported reduction in viral load in the kidney is anywhere from 75% up to 99% if the allograft was perfused for 20 hours and additional flushes were used. Finally, there may be a cost-benefit analysis to using HCV positive donors [53].

4.3. Special transplant considerations

The use of HCV positive donors is not without potential risks. First and foremost, superinfection with a different genotype of HCV could occur with transplantation [54]. This coupled with immunosuppression can lead to a more aggressive HCV infection and increased risk of developing active liver disease [55, 56]. Secondly, recent data suggests that the HCV positive recipient transplanted with an HCV positive donor generally experiences an increase in infectious complications [57]. Moreover, Rao and Ma demonstrated that the HCV positive recipient experienced not only more infectious complications, but also more serious life-threatening infections [56]. The use of induction therapy does not correlate with the level of viremia and has been shown to be safe and efficacious without increasing the risk of infections complications [58, 59]. Finally, HCV positive recipients with ESRD have a higher cardiovascular mortality [60].

4.4. Outcomes following transplantation

The short-term outcomes following transplantation of HCV positive donors into HCV positive recipients have generally been acceptable. Short-term patient survival rates at 1 and 3 years have been reported to be as high as 93% and 83%, respectively, while graft survival rates were 91% and 77%, respectively [51]. The longest study of this cohort of patients comes from Spain with a 10 years total follow-up [61]. Patients had 5- and 10-year survival rates of about 85% and 73%, respectively. The death-censored 5- and 10-year graft survival rates were 69% and 47%, respectively. Graft survival, however, was significantly lower in HCV positive recipients receiving HCV positive donors. The use of a HCV positive donor was not a risk factor for mortality, graft loss or advanced liver disease in this study. Mahmoud and colleagues demonstrated an increased incidence of transplant glomerulopathy among HCV positive renal transplant recipients [62].

5. Kidney paired donation

5.1. Introduction

Up to one-third of all kidney transplant candidates presenting for living donor renal transplantation with a potential living donor will have a blood type or cytotoxic-dependent cytotoxicity (CDC) crossmatch incompatibility [63]. In the past, these patients would be deemed unsuitable pairs and transplantation would not proceed. Some transplant centers may attempt to use desensitization protocols to overcome the immunologic incompatibility; however, these protocols carry the risk of additional immunosuppression. This added risk does not guarantee successful transplantation and, if successfully transplanted, places the recipient at an increased risk of an acute rejection episode [64, 65].

Kidney paired donation (KPD) was introduced as an effective tool to overcome immunologic barriers, such as blood type or CDC crossmatch incompatibility among donor/recipient pairs [66-68]. This initially began as a concept of swapping living donors in individual transplant centers with two or three paired donor exchanges to permit transplantation [69]. This has expanded to various nationwide registries of incompatible donor/recipient pairs of major transplant centers, including our own in the National Kidney Registry [66].

5.2. Living donor chains

An important element of maximizing the benefits of KPD is the addition of an altruistic, or non-directed, donor. These donors wish to donate their kidney, however they do not have an intended recipient. Utilizing these altruistic donors in KPD registries permits the creation of transplant chains with an extra donor to spare. This extra donor is called a bridge donor and is able to donate at a later time (Figure 4). This potentially can create non-simultaneous extended altruistic donor (NEAD), or in other cases the bridge donor can even donate to the deceased donor waitlist [70].

Many different registries exist in the United States and these registries have facilitated the majority of KPD transplants performed to date. One of the important practical lessons learned over time is that it may be more beneficial to have bridge donors donate to a candidate on the deceased donor waiting list [66]. Sometimes it may take longer than expected to find a suitable recipient entered into a registry to match with a bridge donor. The bridge donor's circumstances could change while awaiting donation, such as work or professional changes, economic inability to donate or the donor might renege on their decision to donate. Ultimately this would result in loss of the bridge donor and any future transplant generated by the bridge donor. The exception to this rule is blood type 'O' bridge donors who may be kept within the registry due to their ability to generate future transplant chains [71].

In order for chains to be successful, many logistical aspects need to be addressed. For example, only major transplant centers with operating room availability 24 hours a day should participate, as acute changes can occur regarding scheduling and require flexibility on the donor and recipient hospitals parts. Transplant coordinators with sound understanding of the KPD process are necessary to manage the complex logistical problems that may arise, and to manage entry of donors and recipients into the registry, obtain match offers, and participate in conference calls to coordinate and facilitate continuation of chains[66]. Transplant coordinators need to have GPS access to track organs shipped from other transplant centers.

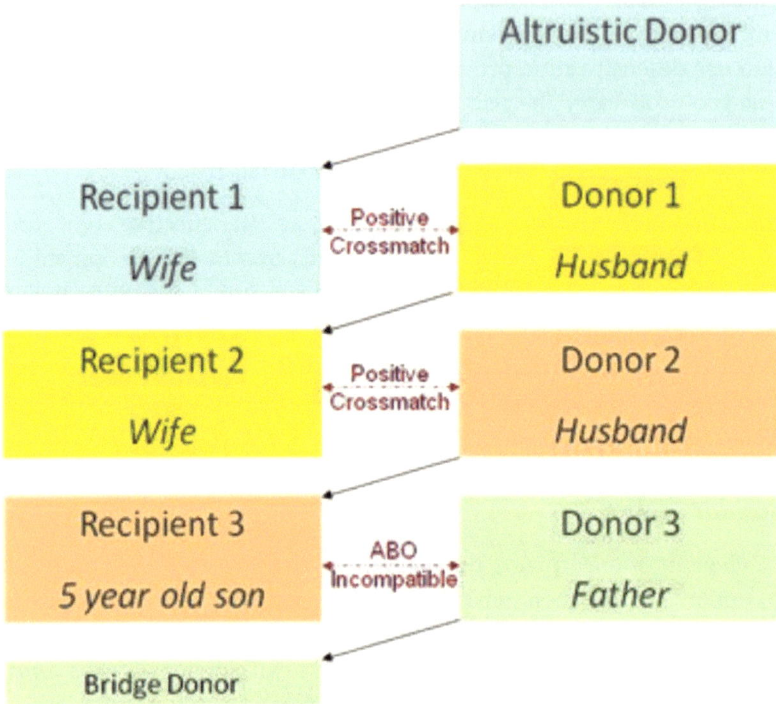

Figure 4. Bridge Donor. The following figure depicts a chain of incompatible donor/recipients who are a part of a chain, beginning with an altruistic donor and ending with a bridge donor who may facilitate another chain.

5.3. Benefits of kidney paired donation

Kidney paired donation offers multiple benefits. First, transplant candidates are removed from the UNOS waiting list. These patients avoid the morbidity and mortality of initiating or remaining on hemodialysis as well as enjoying a survival benefit (U.S. Renal Data System, USRDS 2010 Annual Data Report: Atlas of Chronic Kidney Disease and End-Stage Renal Disease in the United States, National Institutes of Health, National Institute of Diabetes and Digestive and Kidney Diseases, Bethesda, MD, 2010). These patients benefit from receiving a living donor renal transplant, which has better graft survival than a deceased donor allograft. Moreover, these patients, who may undergo various desensitization protocols, avoid the added immunosuppression and risks involved in blood group incompatible transplants. These highly sensitized patients benefit from receiving a living unrelated transplant via a bridge donor. Furthermore, those candidates without a living donor would benefit from having additional patients removed from the deceased donor waiting list.

In general, allografts from living donors have better outcomes than allografts from deceased donors. First, graft half-life is significantly longer in living donor allografts than deceased donors [72]. Second, the incidence of DGF is significantly lower in living donors, thus recipients are receiving a better quality allograft. Even if allografts are shipped across the country with cold ischemia times that may exceed 12 hours, outcomes remain superior to deceased donors [68]. The benefits of higher quality organs could translate into improvements in quality of life for the recipient [73]. KPD maximizes opportunities for transplantation for all transplant candidates.

6. Summary

The supply of available allografts for kidney transplantation does not meet the demands of the growing number of patients listed for transplantation. Thus, other sources of available allograft must be sought to alleviate the burden of the deceased donor waiting list. The use of pediatric donors, en-bloc, or even better as single organs that can be split for two recipients represents a potential source of allografts. Marginal donors are also being increasingly used with respectable graft survival rates. The use of HCV positive donors for HCV positive recipients leads to the transplantation of HCV positive patients significantly faster than waiting for an HCV negative donor, which lessens the burden of those awaiting HCV negative organs. Finally, successful implementation of KPD transplant registries has lead to the transplantation of high quality organs with considerable graft life into patients with blood type incompatible or crossmatch positive donors. Finding a solution to the shortage of suitable organs remains a challenge that must continue to be addressed in the field of transplantation.

Author details

Cheguevara Afaneh, Meredith J. Aull, Anthony Watkins, Jim Kim and Sandip Kapur
Department of Surgery, Division of Transplant Surgery, New York-Presbyterian Hospital- Weill Cornell Medical College, New York, NY, USA

Acknowledgement

The authors gratefully acknowledge the expert assistance of Ms. Johanna Martin in creating figures 1 & 2 depicted in the chapter.

7. References

[1] Leichtman, A.B., et al., Kidney and pancreas transplantation in the United States, 1997-2006: the HRSA Breakthrough Collaboratives and the 58 DSA Challenge. Am J Transplant, 2008. 8(4 Pt 2): p. 946-57.

[2] Danovitch, G.M., et al., Current status of kidney and pancreas transplantation in the United States, 1994-2003. Am J Transplant, 2005. 5(4 Pt 2): p. 904-15.

[3] Meakins, J.L., E.J. Smith, and J.W. Alexander, En bloc transplantation of both kidneys from pediatric donors into adult patients. Surgery, 1972. 71(1): p. 72-5.

[4] Banowsky, L.H., et al., Results of single kidneys from donors aged 9 to 60 months: results in 144 adult recipients. Transplant Proc, 1997. 29(8): p. 3271-3.

[5] Lackner, J.E., F.H. Wright, and L.H. Banowsky, Long-term function of single pediatric kidneys less than 48 months of age transplanted into adult recipients compared with adult cadaveric and living-related transplants. Transplant Proc, 1997. 29(8): p. 3283-7.

[6] Cecka, J.M., Kidney transplantation in the United States. Clin Transpl, 2008: p. 1-18.

[7] El-Sabrout, R. and K. Buch, Outcome of renal transplants from pediatric donors <5 yr of age. Clin Transplant, 2005. 19(3): p. 316-20.

[8] Bresnahan, B.A., et al., Risk factors for renal allograft survival from pediatric cadaver donors: an analysis of united network for organ sharing data. Transplantation, 2001. 72(2): p. 256-61.

[9] Pelletier, S.J., et al., Recovery and utilization of deceased donor kidneys from small pediatric donors. Am J Transplant, 2006. 6(7): p. 1646-52.

[10] Balachandran, V.P., et al., Successful transplantation of single kidneys from pediatric donors weighing less than or equal to 10 kg into standard weight adult recipients. Transplantation, 2010. 90(5): p. 518-22.

[11] Borboroglu, P.G., et al., Solitary renal allografts from pediatric cadaver donors less than 2 years of age transplanted into adult recipients. Transplantation, 2004. 77(5): p. 698-702.

[12] Gourlay, W., et al., Transplantation of pediatric cadaver kidneys into adult recipients. J Urol, 1995. 153(2): p. 322-5 6.

[13] Sureshkumar, K.K., et al., Superiority of pediatric en bloc renal allografts over living donor kidneys: a long-term functional study. Transplantation, 2006. 82(3): p. 348-53.

[14] Sharma, A., et al., En bloc kidney transplantation from pediatric donors: comparable outcomes with living donor kidney transplantation. Transplantation, 2011. 92(5): p. 564-9.

[15] Kayler, L.K., et al., Single kidney transplantation from young pediatric donors in the United States. Am J Transplant, 2009. 9(12): p. 2745-51.

[16] Deroure, B., et al., Expanding the criteria of renal kidneys for transplantation: use of donors with acute renal failure. Nephrol Dial Transplant, 2010. 25(6): p. 1980-6.

[17] Matsuoka, L., et al., Pulsatile perfusion reduces the incidence of delayed graft function in expanded criteria donor kidney transplantation. Am J Transplant, 2006. 6(6): p. 1473-8.

[18] Rudich, S.M., et al., Renal transplantations performed using non-heart-beating organ donors: going back to the future? Transplantation, 2002. 74(12): p. 1715-20.

[19] Vaziri, N., et al., Analysis of machine perfusion benefits in kidney grafts: a preclinical study. J Transl Med, 2011. 9: p. 15.

[20] Maathuis, M.H., H.G. Leuvenink, and R.J. Ploeg, Perspectives in organ preservation. Transplantation, 2007. 83(10): p. 1289-98.

[21] Kwiatkowski, A., et al., The early and long term function and survival of kidney allografts stored before transplantation by hypothermic pulsatile perfusion. A prospective randomized study. Ann Transplant, 2009. 14(1): p. 14-7.

[22] Kwiatkowski, A., et al., Machine perfusion preservation improves renal allograft survival. Am J Transplant, 2007. 7(8): p. 1942-7.

[23] Moustafellos, P., et al., The influence of pulsatile preservation in kidney transplantation from non-heart-beating donors. Transplant Proc, 2007. 39(5): p. 1323-5.

[24] Wight, J.P., et al., Pulsatile machine perfusion vs. cold storage of kidneys for transplantation: a rapid and systematic review. Clin Transplant, 2003. 17(4): p. 293-307.

[25] Brook, N.R., et al., Non-heart beating donor kidneys with delayed graft function have superior graft survival compared with conventional heart-beating donor kidneys that develop delayed graft function. Am J Transplant, 2003. 3(5): p. 614-8.

[26] Nicholson, M.L., et al., A comparison of renal preservation by cold storage and machine perfusion using a porcine autotransplant model. Transplantation, 2004. 78(3): p. 333-7.

[27] Danielewicz, R., et al., An assessment of ischemic injury of the kidney for transplantation during machine pulsatile preservation. Transplant Proc, 1997. 29(8): p. 3580-1.

[28] Stubenitsky, B.M., et al., Pretransplantation prognostic testing on damaged kidneys during ex vivo warm perfusion. Transplantation, 2001. 71(6): p. 716-20.

[29] Tesi, R.J., et al., Pulsatile kidney perfusion for preservation and evaluation: use of high-risk kidney donors to expand the donor pool. Transplant Proc, 1993. 25(6): p. 3099-100.

[30] Moers, C., et al., The value of machine perfusion perfusate biomarkers for predicting kidney transplant outcome. Transplantation, 2010. 90(9): p. 966-73.

[31] Stratta, R.J., et al., Intermediate-term outcomes with expanded criteria deceased donors in kidney transplantation: a spectrum or specter of quality? Ann Surg, 2006. 243(5): p. 594-601; discussion 601-3.

[32] Serur, D., et al., Deceased-donor kidney transplantation: improvement in long-term survival. Nephrol Dial Transplant, 2011. 26(1): p. 317-24.

[33] Brennan, D.C., et al., Rabbit antithymocyte globulin versus basiliximab in renal transplantation. N Engl J Med, 2006. 355(19): p. 1967-77.

[34] Ojo, A.O., et al., Survival in recipients of marginal cadaveric donor kidneys compared with other recipients and wait-listed transplant candidates. J Am Soc Nephrol, 2001. 12(3): p. 589-97.

[35] Port, F.K., et al., Donor characteristics associated with reduced graft survival: an approach to expanding the pool of kidney donors. Transplantation, 2002. 74(9): p. 1281-6.

[36] Chavalitdhamrong, D., et al., Patient and graft outcomes from deceased kidney donors age 70 years and older: an analysis of the Organ Procurement Transplant Network/United Network of Organ Sharing database. Transplantation, 2008. 85(11): p. 1573-9.

[37] Asher, J., et al., Factors predicting duration of delayed graft function in non-heart-beating donor kidney transplantation. Transplant Proc, 2005. 37(1): p. 348-9.
[38] Matsuno, N., et al., Early graft function in kidney transplantation from non-heart-beating donors. Ann Transplant, 2004. 9(2): p. 21-2.
[39] Irish, W.D., et al., Nomogram for predicting the likelihood of delayed graft function in adult cadaveric renal transplant recipients. J Am Soc Nephrol, 2003. 14(11): p. 2967-74.
[40] Ojo, A.O., et al., Delayed graft function: risk factors and implications for renal allograft survival. Transplantation, 1997. 63(7): p. 968-74.
[41] Hariharan, S., T.J. Schroeder, and M.R. First, Effect of race on renal transplant outcome. Clin Transplant, 1993. 7(3): p. 235-9.
[42] Fritsche, C., et al., Hepatitis C is a poor prognostic indicator in black kidney transplant recipients. Transplantation, 1993. 55(6): p. 1283-7.
[43] Ponz, E., et al., Hepatitis C virus infection among kidney transplant recipients. Kidney Int, 1991. 40(4): p. 748-51.
[44] Stempel, C.A., et al., Hepatitis C--its prevalence in end-stage renal failure patients and clinical course after kidney transplantation. Transplantation, 1993. 55(2): p. 273-6.
[45] Ynares, C., et al., Impact of pretransplant hepatitis C antibody status upon long-term patient and renal allograft survival--a 5- and 10-year follow-up. Transplant Proc, 1993. 25(1 Pt 2): p. 1466-8.
[46] Pereira, B.J. and A.S. Levey, Hepatitis C virus infection in dialysis and renal transplantation. Kidney Int, 1997. 51(4): p. 981-99.
[47] Kidney Disease: Improving Global, O., KDIGO clinical practice guidelines for the prevention, diagnosis, evaluation, and treatment of hepatitis C in chronic kidney disease. Kidney Int Suppl, 2008(109): p. S1-99.
[48] Pereira, B.J., et al., Transmission of hepatitis C virus by organ transplantation. N Engl J Med, 1991. 325(7): p. 454-60.
[49] Knoll, G.A., et al., The impact of renal transplantation on survival in hepatitis C-positive end-stage renal disease patients. Am J Kidney Dis, 1997. 29(4): p. 608-14.
[50] Maluf, D.G., et al., Hepatitis C virus infection and kidney transplantation: predictors of patient and graft survival. Transplantation, 2007. 83(7): p. 853-7.
[51] Kucirka, L.M., et al., Underutilization of hepatitis C-positive kidneys for hepatitis C-positive recipients. Am J Transplant, 2010. 10(5): p. 1238-46.
[52] Roth, D., et al., Transmission of hepatitis C virus by kidney transplantation: impact of perfusion techniques and course of viremia post transplant. Pediatr Nephrol, 1995. 9 Suppl: p. S29-34.
[53] Kiberd, B.A., Should hepatitis C-infected kidneys be transplanted in the United States? Transplantation, 1994. 57(7): p. 1068-72.
[54] Widell, A., et al., Hepatitis C superinfection in hepatitis C virus (HCV)-infected patients transplanted with an HCV-infected kidney. Transplantation, 1995. 60(7): p. 642-7.

[55] Legendre, C., et al., Harmful long-term impact of hepatitis C virus infection in kidney transplant recipients. Transplantation, 1998. 65(5): p. 667-70.
[56] Rao, K.V. and J. Ma, Chronic viral hepatitis enhances the risk of infection but not acute rejection in renal transplant recipients. Transplantation, 1996. 62(12): p. 1765-9.
[57] Lopez-Medrano, F., et al., Impact of hepatitis C virus infection on the risk of infectious complications after kidney transplantation: data from the RESITRA/REIPI cohort. Transplantation, 2011. 92(5): p. 543-9.
[58] Luan, F.L., et al., Impact of immunosuppressive regimen on survival of kidney transplant recipients with hepatitis C. Transplantation, 2008. 85(11): p. 1601-6.
[59] Rodrigues, A., et al., Hepatitis C virus genotypes and the influence of the induction of immunosuppression with anti-thymocyte globulin (ATG) on chronic hepatitis in renal graft recipients. Transpl Int, 1998. 11 Suppl 1: p. S115-8.
[60] Kalantar-Zadeh, K., C.J. McAllister, and L.G. Miller, Clinical characteristics and mortality in hepatitis C-positive haemodialysis patients: a population based study. Nephrol Dial Transplant, 2005. 20(8): p. 1662-9.
[61] Morales, J.M., et al., Long-term experience with kidney transplantation from hepatitis C-positive donors into hepatitis C-positive recipients. Am J Transplant, 2010. 10(11): p. 2453-62.
[62] Mahmoud, I.M., et al., The impact of hepatitis C virus viremia on renal graft and patient survival: a 9-year prospective study. Am J Kidney Dis, 2004. 43(1): p. 131-9.
[63] Segev, D.L., et al., Kidney paired donation and optimizing the use of live donor organs. JAMA, 2005. 293(15): p. 1883-90.
[64] Gloor, J. and M.D. Stegall, Sensitized renal transplant recipients: current protocols and future directions. Nat Rev Nephrol, 2010. 6(5): p. 297-306.
[65] Jordan, S.C., et al., Intravenous gammaglobulin (IVIG): a novel approach to improve transplant rates and outcomes in highly HLA-sensitized patients. Am J Transplant, 2006. 6(3): p. 459-66.
[66] Leeser, D.B., et al., Living donor kidney paired donation transplantation: experience as a founding member center of the National Kidney Registry. Clin Transplant, 2012. 26(3): p. E213-22.
[67] Roth, A.E., et al., Utilizing list exchange and nondirected donation through 'chain' paired kidney donations. Am J Transplant, 2006. 6(11): p. 2694-705.
[68] Segev, D.L., et al., Transporting live donor kidneys for kidney paired donation: initial national results. Am J Transplant, 2011. 11(2): p. 356-60.
[69] Kwak, J.Y., et al., Exchange-donor program in renal transplantation: a single-center experience. Transplant Proc, 1999. 31(1-2): p. 344-5.
[70] Roodnat, J.I., et al., Altruistic donor triggered domino-paired kidney donation for unsuccessful couples from the kidney-exchange program. Am J Transplant, 2010. 10(4): p. 821-7.
[71] Veale, J. and G. Hil, National Kidney Registry: 213 transplants in three years. Clin Transpl, 2010: p. 333-44.

[72] Lamb, K.E., S. Lodhi, and H.U. Meier-Kriesche, Long-term renal allograft survival in the United States: a critical reappraisal. Am J Transplant, 2011. 11(3): p. 450-62.

[73] Neri, L., et al., Impaired renal function is associated with worse self-reported outcomes after kidney transplantation. Qual Life Res, 2011. 20(10): p. 1689-98.